EVIDENCE-BASED EDUCATION IN THE CLASSROOM

Examples From Clinical Disciplines

EVIDENCE-BASED EDUCATION IN THE CLASSROOM

Examples From Clinical Disciplines

Editors

Jennifer C. Friberg, EdD, CCC-SLP, F-ASHA

Cross Endowed Chair, Scholarship of Teaching and Learning
Professor, Department of Communication Sciences and Disorders
Illinois State University
Normal, Illinois

Colleen F. Visconti, PhD, CCC-SLP

Program Director, Speech-Language Pathology Program
Professor, Communication Sciences and Disorders Department
Baldwin Wallace University
Berea, Ohio

Sarah M. Ginsberg, EdD, CCC-SLP, F-ASHA

Professor, Communication Sciences and Disorders Program
Eastern Michigan University
Ypsilanti, Michigan

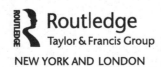

Routledge
Taylor & Francis Group

NEW YORK AND LONDON

First published in 2021 by SLACK Incorporated

Published in 2024 by Routledge
605 Third Avenue, New York, NY 10158

and by Routledge
4 Park Square, Milton Park, Abingdon, Oxon, OX14 4RN

Routledge is an imprint of the Taylor & Francis Group, an informa business

Cover Artist: Justin Dalton

Cover illustration by Molly Friberg.

Library of Congress Cataloging-in-Publication Data

Names: Friberg, Jennifer C., 1974- editor. | Visconti, Colleen F., 1963-
  editor. | Ginsberg, Sarah M., 1966- editor.
Title: Evidence-based education in the classroom : examples from clinical
  disciplines / editors, Jennifer C. Friberg, Colleen F. Visconti, Sarah
  M. Ginsberg.
Description: Thorofare, NJ : SLACK Incorporated, [2021] | Includes
  bibliographical references and index.
Identifiers: LCCN 2021011358 (print) | ISBN 9781630917142 (paperback)
Subjects: MESH: Education, Medical | Evidence-Based Medicine
Classification: LCC R737 (print) | NLM W 18 | DDC
  610.71/1--dc23
LC record available at https://lccn.loc.gov/2021011358

ISBN: 9781630917142 (pbk)
ISBN: 9781003524083 (ebk)

DOI: 10.4324/9781003524083

DEDICATION

We dedicate this book to those who continue to inspire our passion for nurturing evidence-based educational practices in the college classroom: our students and our collaborators. On all days and in different ways, you challenge us to be the best educators we can be.

CONTENTS

ACKNOWLEDGMENTS

An edited volume such as this results from the efforts of many and, to that end, represents a true collaborative effort across the board. We are thankful to all who helped us bring this project to fruition, but we wish to specifically acknowledge those who were particularly instrumental in helping design and execute this project:

- To each of our almost 70 chapter contributors, thank you for generously sharing your time and talents. We appreciate your dedication to using evidence to inform your teaching. Your cases have inspired us to consider new pedagogies in our own course design and implementation.

- To our past, current, and future students, know that you are the true inspiration for this work. Our shared passion for evidence-based education was borne through our sincere desire to help each of you learn deeply and well.

- To Melissa Jenkins, who assisted in the editing and formatting of this volume, thank you for making our loads lighter and using your eagle eye to reference check and prepare this book for publication.

- To Brien Cummings and the good folks at SLACK Incorporated, we are tremendously appreciative of your enthusiasm for this project and your advocacy for evidence-based teaching and learning in clinically based disciplines.

ABOUT THE EDITORS

Jennifer C. Friberg, EdD, CCC-SLP, F-ASHA is the Cross Endowed Chair in the Scholarship of Teaching and Learning and a Professor of Communication Sciences and Disorders at Illinois State University in Normal, Illinois. A speech-language pathologist by discipline, Friberg primarily serves as an educational developer at her institution, with a focus on the scholarship of teaching and learning (SoTL). She maintains an active research agenda, with current projects focused on the application of SoTL, mentoring in SoTL, and the sharing of SoTL beyond individual classroom settings. Along with her coeditors for this project, Friberg is a coauthor of *Scholarship of Teaching and Learning in Speech-Language Pathology and Audiology: Evidence-Based Education*. Additionally, she is the coeditor of the recently published text *Applying the Scholarship of Teaching and Learning Beyond the Individual Classroom* and is the founding associate editor for the journal *Teaching and Learning in Communication Sciences & Disorders*.

Colleen F. Visconti, PhD, CCC-SLP is a Professor and Program Director of the Speech-Language Pathology program in the Communication Sciences and Disorders Department at Baldwin Wallace University in Berea, Ohio. She led the undergraduate program in Communication Sciences and Disorders prior to recently developing an innovative graduate program in speech-language pathology. Her SoTL research has focused on developing culturally responsive practitioners through a service-oriented study abroad program, clinical decision making, and the use of problem-based learning within the classroom. Her work has been shared through webinars, presentations, and various publications. She is a coauthor of *Scholarship of Teaching and Learning in Speech-Language Pathology and Audiology: Evidence-Based Education* and is a founding editorial board member of *Teaching and Learning in Communication Sciences & Disorders*.

Sarah M. Ginsberg, EdD, CCC-SLP, F-ASHA is a Professor of Communication Sciences and Disorders at Eastern Michigan University in Ypsilanti, Michigan. Her SoTL work has appeared in *To Improve the Academy*, the *Journal of the Scholarship of Teaching and Learning*, and *Contemporary Issues in Communication Science and Disorders*. She is a coauthor of *Scholarship of Teaching and Learning in Speech-Language Pathology and Audiology: Evidence-Based Education* and is the founding editor of *Teaching and Learning in Communication Sciences & Disorders*.

CONTRIBUTING AUTHORS

Hilary Applequist, DNP, APRN-NP, ACHPN
(Chapter 20)
Assistant Professor
BSN-DNP Program
Nebraska Methodist College
Omaha, Nebraska

Cassandra Barragan, PhD, MSW (Chapter 9)
Assistant Professor
School of Social Work
Eastern Michigan University
Ypsilanti, Michigan

Dana Battaglia, PhD, CCC-SLP (Chapter 1)
Associate Professor
Department of Communication Sciences
and Disorders
Adelphi University
Garden City, New York

Ann R. Beck, PhD (Chapter 25)
Professor and Chair
Department of Communication Sciences
and Disorders
Illinois State University
Normal, Illinois

Carole Bennett, PhD, PMHCS-BC (Chapter 21)
Associate Professor
School of Nursing
Georgia Southern University
Statesboro, Georgia

Sarah Bolander, DMSc, PA-C, DFAAPA
(Chapter 24)
Associate Professor
Physician Assistant Program
Midwestern University
Downers Grove, Illinois

Chelsey M. Bahlmann Bollinger, PhD
(Chapter 16)
Assistant Professor
Department of Early, Elementary and
Reading Education
James Madison University
Harrisonburg, Virginia

Elizabeth Bourne, PhD, BAppSc(SpPath), CPSP
(Chapter 32)
Associate Lecturer
Work Integrated Learning
Faculty of Medicine and Health
University of Sydney
Sydney, Australia

Tim Brackenbury, PhD, CCC-SLP (Chapter 26)
Professor
Department of Communication Sciences
and Disorders
Bowling Green State University
Bowling Green, Ohio

Judi Brooks, PhD, RD (Chapter 10)
Professor
School of Health Sciences
Eastern Michigan University
Ypsilanti, Michigan

Melissa A. Carroll, PhD, MS (Chapter 33)
Associate Professor
Doctor of Physical Therapy Program
DeSales University
Center Valley, Pennsylvania

Susan L. Caulfield, PhD (Chapter 11)
Professor
School of Interdisciplinary Health Programs
Western Michigan University
Kalamazoo, Michigan

Darlene Chalmers, PhD, RSW (Chapter 31)
Associate Professor
Faculty of Social Work
University of Regina
Regina, Saskatchewan, Canada

Andrea Coppola, OTD, OTR/L (Chapter 23)
Assistant Professor
Department of Occupational Therapy
Springfield College
Springfield, Massachusetts

Julie L. Cox, PhD, CCC-SLP/L (Chapter 2)
Assistant Professor
Speech Pathology and Audiology
Western Illinois University
Macomb, Illinois

Mary Culshaw, PhD, OTR/L (Chapter 7)
Assistant Professor
Master's in Occupational Therapy Program
Moravian College
Bethlehem, Pennsylvania

Kathy Doody, PhD (Chapter 13)
Associate Professor
Exceptional Education Department
State University of New York College at Buffalo
Buffalo, New York

Amy Egli, MHA, LDH, CDA, EFDA
(Chapter 12)
Clinical Assistant Professor
Dental Hygiene Program
University of Southern Indiana
Evansville, Indiana

Krystina Eymann, MSN, RN (Chapter 20)
Assistant Professor
Undergraduate Nursing Department
Nebraska Methodist College
Omaha, Nebraska

Karen A. Fallon, PhD, CCC-SLP (Chapter 3)
Professor
Department of Speech-Language Pathology
and Audiology
Towson University
Towson, Maryland

Diane Fenske, LMSW (Chapter 10)
Part-Time Lecturer
School of Social Work
Eastern Michigan University
Ypsilanti, Michigan

Katrina Fulcher-Rood, PhD, CCC-SLP
(Chapter 13)
Associate Professor
Speech-Language Pathology Department
State University of New York College at Buffalo
Buffalo, New York

April Garrity, PhD, CCC-SLP
(Chapters 14 and 28)
Associate Professor
Department of Rehabilitation Sciences
Georgia Southern University–
Armstrong Campus
Savannah, Georgia

Jennine M. Harvey-Northrop, PhD, CCC-SLP
(Chapter 19)
Associate Professor
Department of Communication Sciences
and Disorders
Illinois State University
Normal, Illinois

Amber Herrick, MS, PA-C (Chapter 24)
Director of Didactic Education
Physician Assistant Program
Midwestern University
Downers Grove, Illinois

Leslie A. Hoffman, PhD (Chapter 29)
Assistant Professor
Department of Anatomy, Cell Biology
and Physiology
Indiana University School of Medicine
Bloomington, Indiana

Polly R. Husmann, PhD (Chapter 30)
Assistant Professor
Department of Anatomy, Cell Biology
and Physiology
Indiana University School of Medicine
Bloomington, Indiana

Keiko Ishikawa, PhD, CCC-SLP
(Chapters 14 and 28)
Assistant Professor
Department of Speech and Hearing Science
University of Illinois at Urbana–Champaign
Champaign County, Illinois

Casey Keck, PhD, CCC-SLP (Chapters 14 and 28)
Assistant Professor
Department of Rehabilitation Sciences
Georgia Southern University–
Armstrong Campus
Savannah, Georgia

Louise C. Keegan, PhD, CCC-SLP, BC-ANCDS
(Chapter 7)
Program Director
Master of Science in Speech-Language Pathology
Moravian College
Bethlehem, Pennsylvania

Marla Kniewel, EdD, MSN, RN (Chapter 20)
Professor, Director
MSN Program
Nebraska Methodist College
Omaha, Nebraska

Nancy E. Krusen, PhD, OTR/L (Chapter 34)
Program Director and Associate Professor
Division of Occupational Therapy Education
University of Nebraska Medical Center
Omaha, Nebraska

Eric Kyle, PhD (Chapter 20)
Associate Professor, Director
Contextual Education
Lutheran School of Theology at Chicago
Chicago, Illinois

Carey Leckie, OT, OTD, OTR, CHT (Chapter 23)
Assistant Professor
Department of Occupational Therapy
Springfield College
Springfield, Massachusetts

Mary-Jon Ludy, PhD, RDN, FAND (Chapter 26)
Chair and Associate Professor
Department of Public and Allied Health
Bowling Green State University
Bowling Green, Ohio

M. Nicole Martino, MS, OTR/L (Chapter 34)
Adjunct Faculty
Department of Clinical Research & Leadership
School of Medicine and Health Sciences
The George Washington University
Washington, DC

Lydia McBurrows, DNP, RN, CPNP-PC
(Chapter 10)
Associate Professor
School of Nursing
Eastern Michigan University
Ypsilanti, Michigan

Jean McCaffery, OT, EdD, OTR (Chapter 23)
Associate Professor
Department of Occupational Therapy
Springfield College
Springfield, Massachusetts

Lauren H. Mead, MA, CCC-SLP (Chapter 5)
Speech and Language Pathologist
Ridge Zeller Therapy
Chandler, Arizona

Andi Beth Mincer, PT, EdD (Chapter 15)
Physical Therapy Program
Department of Rehabilitation Sciences
Georgia Southern University
Statesboro, Georgia

Irene Mok, MRC, BA (Chapter 32)
Conjoint Associate Lecturer
Sydney Medical School
Faculty of Medicine and Health
University of Sydney
Sydney, Australia

Joy Myers, PhD (Chapter 16)
Assistant Professor
Department of Early, Elementary and
Reading Education
James Madison University
Harrisonburg, Virginia

Margaret Nicholson, MEd, BSc, Dip Nut Diet,
Dip Ed (Health), AdvAPD (Chapter 32)
Senior Lecturer/Clinical Placement Lead
School of Life and Environmental Sciences
Faculty of Science
University of Sydney
Sydney, Australia

Gillian Nisbet, PhD, MMEd, DipNutr, BSc(Hons)
(Chapter 32)
Senior Lecturer
Work Integrated Learning
Faculty of Medicine and Health
University of Sydney
Sydney, Australia

Brent Oliver, PhD, RSW (Chapter 31)
Associate Professor
Department of Child Studies and Social Work
Mount Royal University
Calgary, Alberta, Canada

Christina Y. Pelatti, PhD, CCC-SLP (Chapter 8)
Associate Professor
Department of Speech-Language Pathology
and Audiology
Towson University
Towson, Maryland

D. Mark Ragg, PhD, LMSW, BSW (Chapter 6)
Professor
School of Social Work
Eastern Michigan University
Ypsilanti, Michigan

Amanda Reddington, LDH, MHA, CDA, EFDA
(Chapter 12)
Clinical Assistant Professor
Dental Hygiene Program
University of Southern Indiana
Evansville, Indiana

Haleigh M. Ruebush, MS, CCC-SLP/L
(Chapter 2)
Instructor
Speech Pathology and Audiology
Western Illinois University
Macomb, Illinois

Ken Saldanha, PhD, MSW, BEd (Chapter 6)
Associate Professor
School of Social Work
Eastern Michigan University
Ypsilanti, Michigan

Eric J. Sanders, PhD, CCC-SLP (Chapter 7)
Assistant Professor
Department of Rehabilitation Sciences
Moravian College
Bethlehem, Pennsylvania

Allison Sauerwein, PhD, CCC-SLP (Chapter 17)
Assistant Professor
Applied Health Department
Southern Illinois University Edwardsville
Edwardsville, Illinois

Amanda G. Sawyer, PhD (Chapter 16)
Associate Professor
Middle, Secondary and Mathematics
Education Department
James Madison University
Harrisonburg, Virginia

Jean Sawyer, PhD, CCC-SLP (Chapter 18)
Professor
Department of Communication Sciences
and Disorders
Illinois State University
Normal, Illinois

Audra F. Schaefer, PhD (Chapters 29 and 30)
Assistant Professor
Department of Neurobiology and
Anatomical Sciences
University of Mississippi Medical Center
Jackson, Mississippi

Heather Schmuck, MS, RT(R) (Chapter 12)
Clinical Associate Professor
Radiologic and Imaging Sciences Program
University of Southern Indiana
Evansville, Indiana

Pamela Schuetze, PhD (Chapter 13)
Professor
Department of Psychology
State University of New York College at Buffalo
Buffalo, New York

Scott Seeman, PhD (Chapter 25)
Associate Professor
Department of Communication Sciences
and Disorders
Illinois State University
Normal, Illinois

K. Chisomo Selemani, MA, CCC-SLP
(Chapter 35)
Associate Professor and Coordinator of the
BW-Zambia Program
Communication Sciences and
Disorders Department
Baldwin Wallace University
Berea, Ohio

Maryam S. Sharifian, PhD (Chapter 16)
Assistant Professor
Department of Early, Elementary and
Reading Education
James Madison University
Harrisonburg, Virginia

Amanda B. Silberer, PhD, CCC-A (Chapter 2)
Associate Professor
Speech Pathology and Audiology
Western Illinois University
Macomb, Illinois

Lisa R. Singleterry, PhD, RN, CNE (Chapter 11)
Assistant Professor
Bronson School of Nursing
Western Michigan University
Kalamazoo, Michigan

Heidi Verticchio, MS (Chapter 25)
Clinic Director
Department of Communication Sciences
and Disorders
Illinois State University
Normal, Illinois

Lisa A. Vinney, PhD, CCC-SLP
(Chapters 4, 19, and 22)
Associate Professor
Department of Communication Sciences
and Disorders
Illinois State University
Normal, Illinois

Kaitlyn P. Wilson, PhD, CCC-SLP (Chapter 8)
Assistant Professor
Department of Speech-Language Pathology
and Audiology
Townson University
Towson, Maryland

Stephanie P. Wladkowski, PhD, LMSW,
APHSW-C (Chapter 9)
Associate Professor
School of Social Work
Eastern Michigan University
Ypsilanti, Michigan

Andrea Gossett Zakrajsek, OTD, OTRL, FNAP
(Chapter 10)
Professor
School of Health Sciences
Eastern Michigan University
Ypsilanti, Michigan

INTRODUCTION

This is not a book *about* case studies. Rather, it is a book *of* case studies that depicts ways in which innovative course instructors across a variety of clinical disciplines have used or collected data to inform their own course design, development, or implementation. What each of the chapters in this text have in common is a tie to research-informed ways of teaching in clinical disciplines. This evidence, whether collected or applied by chapter authors as a result of a SoTL investigation, informed changes in pedagogy (the practice of teaching). We consider the cases featured in this text as examples of evidence-based education (EBE), a concept we first introduced almost a decade ago as part of our first scholarly collaboration (Ginsberg et al., 2012). We defined this idea as follows (Ginsberg et al., 2012, p. 29):

> EBE is an educational approach in which current, high-quality scholarship of teaching and learning is integrated with pedagogical content knowledge and teaching-learner interaction to make educational decisions in order to maximize student learning outcomes.

We envisioned EBE as parallel in concept to evidence-based practice (EBP), a cornerstone of professional practice embraced by many (if not all) clinical disciplines. EBP holds that practitioners should consider three things when planning for any work with a client: patient/family needs, clinical expertise, and scientific evidence (American Speech-Language-Hearing Association, n.d.). We saw immediate and important commonalities between clinical practice guided by EBP and course design/implementation that we felt necessitated a similarly oriented approach. For, if we planned our clinical encounters with a systematic trifecta of considerations, why would we not approach our academic encounters in a similar manner? With this in mind, our model for EBE was born (Figure I-1).

Before EBE was even a spark of an idea in our minds, McKinney (2007) explored ideas about professional roles in academia, represented across a teaching continuum. Essentially, McKinney (2007) shared that while *good teachers* are individuals who have the best of intentions about course design and delivery, they are guided by their own instincts and perceptions, rather than by available research on teaching and learning. She defined *scholarly teachers* as those who seek out evidence-informed ways in which a course might be designed or presented. Finally, she posited that *scholars of teaching and learning* produce the research used by scholarly teachers. One instructor might be a good teacher at one point in a semester and a scholarly teacher at another. We agree that the identities identified by McKinney each speak to the makeup of most instructors' academic persona; however, we posit that our EBE model subsumes all aspects of McKinney's continuum into one purposeful practice: good teaching (through a focus on teacher/learning interactions), scholarly teaching (borne from specific pedagogical content knowledge; Shulman, 1986), and the scholarship of teaching and learning (creation or application of evidence from scholarly endeavors).

We contend that it is not enough to solely read or produce research focused on teaching and learning. It must be applied to have an effect on our students and their acquisition of knowledge and skills in the individual classroom context to improve learning (McKinney et al., 2019). Thus, application of SoTL is at the heart of our efforts in compiling the cases featured in this text. Through our work with each other and our contributors, we aimed to highlight innovative approaches to clinical teaching and learning aligned with our vision for EBE. Understanding that there are more similarities than differences across clinical disciplines in terms of evidence-informed teaching practices, we sought to represent a variety of perspectives and practices for our readers' consideration and, potentially, application to their own teaching and/or learning contexts. Through a competitive call for contributors, we reached out to representatives of clinically based disciplines far and wide, using disciplinary email listservs, social media, word of mouth, and various other venues to reach as many clinical instructors as possible. While dozens of proposals were submitted for review, we ultimately selected 35 chapters for inclusion in this volume. Seventy professionals representing 24 institutions, 14 disciplines, and 3 countries authored these chapters. We celebrate the diversity represented in this project and hope that our readers will as well.

Figure I-1. Interactive cycle of evidence-based education.

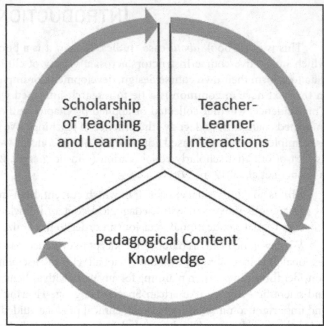

Organizing the chapters in this book was not an easy task, due in large part to a wide array of topics and individual experiences shared by our contributing authors. In the end, we chose to engage in an informal, but systematic, thematic study of each chapter's content to derive categories that allowed for the arrangement of our chapters in a manner that was both cohesive and reflected typical teaching/learning practices in any type of course. Thus, we separated our book's content into five different parts:

1. **Planning for Evidence-Based Teaching and Learning:** This section of the text contains eight chapters focused on the course planning process. Topics such as co-teaching, collaborative course design, flipped classroom models, and print versus digital text are explored in this first part of the book.

2. **Teaching and Learning Together:** The 11 chapters in this section share contributors' experiences with evidence-informed approaches to group learning, interprofessional education/practice, team-based learning, peer review, and curricular integration. Each chapter features a description of collaborations across a variety of stakeholders to support instruction and student learning.

3. **Learning From Models, Cases, and Simulations:** Across the five chapters featured in this section of our text, contributors share ways in which they have harnessed case-based learning to introduce real-world experiences for their students in contexts that include a client-based approach to experiential learning.

4. **Learning to Think Critically and Reflectively:** Contributors in this fourth section of the text report the use of evidence to inform deep learning through reflection and critical thinking, using mindfulness training, visual thinking strategies, and a variety of reflective pedagogies.

5. **Learning to Apply Beyond the Classroom:** The final four chapters of this text explore ways in which learning can be encouraged outside of the traditional classroom environment, with a focus on topics such as assessment and study abroad.

Each chapter in this volume presents a case study of how literature and/or data were applied to solve a teaching or learning problem. Readers should note that each chapter is arranged in a standardized format, telling a story of each case's EBE adventures across the following topics: a description of the learning context, a review of literature tied to the pedagogy described, original data (if collected), an overview of how the original data or literature reviewed was applied to the learning context, considerations for other educators in clinical settings who might seek to use similar pedagogies, and resources for readers to extend their learning on the pedagogy described in each chapter. This similar organization for each chapter was important to us as editors of this text for a few simple reasons. First, with a volume as diverse as this, having standard headings and format allows for cohesion across topics and contributors. Additionally, we wanted our readers to have a predictable framework for each chapter that was both organized and easily searchable.

As we edited this text, each of us found ourselves inspired to try new and different approaches—grounded in evidence—in the courses that we teach. We hope a similar interest and excitement is sparked in our readers!

—Jennifer C. Friberg, EdD, CCC-SLP, F-ASHA
—Colleen F. Visconti, PhD, CCC-SLP
—Sarah M. Ginsberg, EdD, CCC-SLP, F-ASHA

REFERENCES

American Speech-Language-Hearing Association. (n.d.). *Evidence-based practice (EBP)*. https://www.asha.org/research/ebp/evidence-based-practice/

Ginsberg, S. M., Friberg, J. C., & Visconti, C. F. (2012). *Scholarship of teaching and learning in speech-language pathology and audiology: Evidence-based education*. Plural Publishing.

McKinney, K. (2007). *Enhancing learning through the scholarship of teaching and learning: The challenges and joys of juggling*. Anker Publishing, Inc.

McKinney, K., Friberg, J. C., & Moore, M. (2019). Introduction to applying SoTL beyond the individual classroom: Overview, framework, and two examples. In J. C. Friberg & K. McKinney (Eds.), *Applying the scholarship of teaching and learning beyond the individual classroom*. Indiana University Press.

Shulman, L. S. (1986). Those who understand: Knowledge growth in teaching. *Educational Researcher, 15*(2), 4-14.

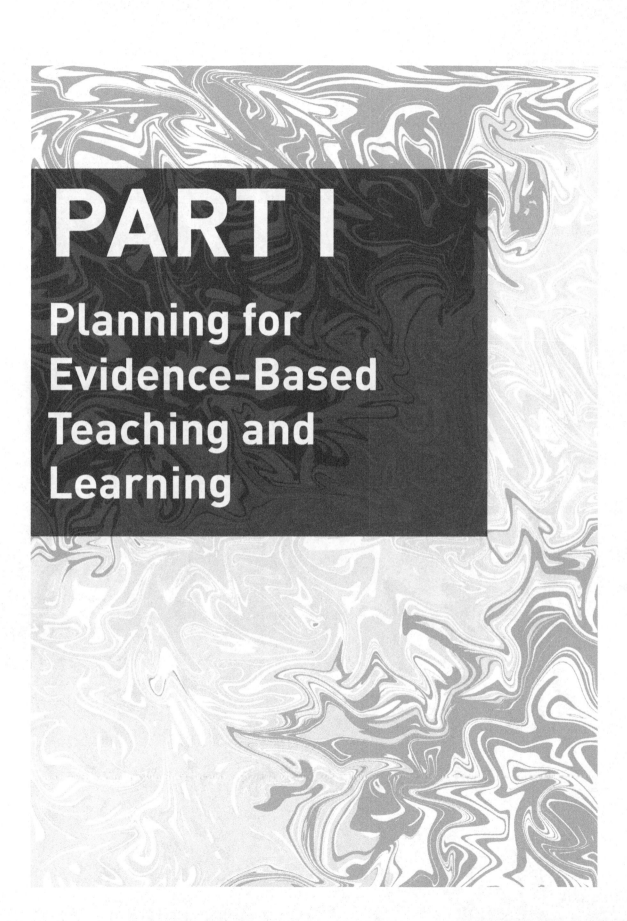

PART I

Planning for Evidence-Based Teaching and Learning

1

UNIVERSAL DESIGN FOR LEARNING AND TECHNOLOGY
Using Data to Inform Pedagogy

Dana Battaglia, PhD, CCC-SLP

DESCRIPTION OF TEACHING/LEARNING CONTEXT

When I began my journey on the tenure track almost a decade ago, I taught courses based on my own classroom experiences; I would lecture and then allow time for questions and answers. I quickly fell flat using this approach. Simply lecturing did not offer students the learning experience they deserved. Additionally, I was bored and questioning whether higher education was the direction I should pursue in my career. Being open to trying new approaches, monitoring student success, reflecting on how students can best engage, and using their own abilities and interaction styles, I sought guidance from the available literature.

While reviewing the evidence on pedagogy in higher education, I familiarized myself with different, yet overlapping, approaches, such as reflective practice (Clegg, 2000) and problem-based learning (Savin-Baden, 2000). In an attempt to synthesize this information, while finding my own academic voice, I learned that there are many ways of knowing content, and subsequently, demonstrating knowledge of said content (Laurillard, 2002). Hence, my affinity for universal design for learning (UDL; McGuire et al., 2006) was born. Expanding my knowledge in pedagogy in higher education fueled my need to ask more questions. I began to ask students how they feel about their own progress in the class, ask how I am doing to meet their needs, and then adjust accordingly.

At the end of every semester, I provide students with a course-specific evaluation. Within the course evaluation, I ask questions about content, specific assignments, and pedagogical approaches. In addition, blind to these evaluations, I generate my own teaching reflection, thinking of which strategies and topics worked and those that did not. Then, I review both my reflection as well as student feedback, triangulating these and prioritizing changes.

Friberg, J. C., Visconti, C. F., & Ginsberg, S. M. (Eds.). *Evidence-Based Education in the Classroom: Examples From Clinical Disciplines* (pp. 3-12).

This chapter describes how data collected in the form of task-specific, self-generated course reviews has informed and evolved my pedagogical practices. This investigation is a mixed research design, collecting qualitative and quantitative data on development and modification of pedagogical practices to teach graduate level students in the Communication Sciences and Disorders department. The specific course in question is at the graduate level, entitled Autism Spectrum Disorders for Speech-Language Pathologists. This is a required course in an accredited program. Students who complete this program will eventually become licensed and certified speech-language pathologists.

I will describe modifications to course design in an effort to increase student engagement, following up with reflection. How these initiatives connect to the scholarship of teaching and learning will be discussed throughout. Thus, this chapter serves as an example of application of both reflection and review in the spirit of extending UDL practices and maximizing student outcomes.

REVIEW OF LITERATURE

Originally conceptualized in the area of architecture to bring accessibility to the forefront of the construction industry (Mace et al., 1991), UDL is defined as offering all individuals multiple means of representation (e.g., signage appearing both in the [English] alphabet and Braille), engagement (e.g., being able to choose to mobilize from floor to floor by stairs, elevator, escalator, or ramp), and expression (e.g., using either push buttons or eye scanners to gain access to areas of a building or provide feedback on an experience). By planning building construction using these principles, retrofitting for additional forms of access is essentially unnecessary.

The translational use of UDL in pedagogy has been supported in the literature, primarily in the last decade (King-Sears, 2009; Rao & Meo, 2016; Spooner et al., 2007). Application of principles of UDL guides educators to provide all students with access to content, engagement, and learning throughout a course. In doing so, course materials are readily accessible to all students regardless of interest, abilities, or other factors that may potentially affect learning (Hall et al., 2012, 2014; McGuire et al., 2006; Meyer et al., 2014; Rose et al., 2005). Using this framework, use of UDL principles in higher education and pedagogy may be as follows:

- Course content/materials are offered to all individuals across multiple means of representation (e.g., displaying information visually and auditorily).
- Course concepts are illustrated across modalities (e.g., face to face, online, and using practice activities) to engage students.
- Expression of ideas by instructor and students occurs across a variety of formats (e.g., class participation, different evaluation structures, discussion boards).

While grounded in the spirit of serving individuals with disabilities, subscribing to UDL philosophy and implementation offers an enhanced learning experience for all students (Al-Azawei et al., 2016). Al-Azawei and colleagues (2016) conducted a literature review and shared the positive effects of using UDL in both K–12 and university environments. Additionally, there is a small and emerging body of literature exploring the intersection of UDL and differentiated instruction in the K–12 domain (Hall et al., 2014). Furthermore, studies in this area have examined academic outcomes and engagement with UDL-based digital learning environments (Hall et al., 2014; Rappolt-Schlichtmann et al., 2013), with positive outcomes for all learners.

Prensky (2001, 2011) refers to students in the 21st century as *digital natives*. Digital citizenship is defined as behavior of confident and competent individuals who are engaged in a broader online context (e.g., a community), both socially and professionally. Well-developed digital citizens are able to construct and engage in virtual identities, navigating the complex journey toward becoming a well-rounded digital citizen (Mattson, 2017). As our students are now digital natives and developing digital citizenship, there is a need for thoughtful planning of activities and creativity (Walser, 2008) that incorporates technology. When accomplished effectively, an instructor will have a highly efficient and engaging classroom without walls, using traditional methods of student interaction combined with technology. Engaging in the process of teaching using technology is integral (Carr et al., 1998; Mishra & Koehler, 2003) while offering students multiple means of representation, engagement, and expression. Hence, the intersection between use of technology and UDL naturally emerges when reflecting upon one's teaching practices. Evidence of the value of joining both technology and UDL has recently been shared with the scientific community (Hall et al., 2015; Rappolt-Schlichtmann et al., 2013), particularly in the areas of science and reading comprehension.

Active science learning requires that students build skills and create connections while engaging the process of exploration. Consider an assignment where a journal documenting phases of the scientific process is maintained by a student. For students with different abilities, the simple act of maintaining a notebook, rather than the inquiry or exploration, may be a roadblock to learning. Rappolt-Schlichtmann and colleagues (2013) explored the use of a web-based science notebook to support elementary school students, utilizing principles of UDL. The online science notebook offered students a space to: (1) collect, organize, and display data and observations; (2) reflect upon said observations; and (3) both demonstrate understanding and receive formative feedback from the teacher. Results indicated that the online science notebooks framed according to UDL principles improved outcomes in science knowledge, as compared with traditional paper-and-pencil science notebooks. The authors further conducted a qualitative analysis exploring student and teacher interest and excitement using these notebooks. Collectively, both students and teachers described high levels of excitement and/or interest in using this instructional method (Rappolt-Schlichtmann et al., 2013).

Subsequently, Hall and colleagues (2014) reviewed the efficacy of Strategic Reader, which is a web-based program created by the Center for Applied Special Technology (CAST). Targeting reading comprehension, this technology blends a digital reading environment with UDL principles. Hall and colleagues (2014) found robust evidence of increased growth in comprehension using this program in online versus offline conditions for students with learning disabilities. Results suggest that designing curriculum using both an online component and UDL can substantially facilitate acquisition of curricular concepts.

In summary, the relationship between UDL practices and use of technology appears to be both intuitive and synergistic. Using technology with UDL in mind in higher education can help students overcome barriers to accessing curriculum. These barriers are no longer simply obtaining new information. Rather, potential barriers can be those precluding the ability to focus or access content due to personal circumstances. The next section discusses both quantitative and qualitative data collected on both technology and UDL, which I have attempted to implement in my classroom.

ORIGINAL DATA

Given this review of the interface between UDL and technology use in pedagogy in higher education, merging these two domains seemed a natural fit for students as digital natives who are continually learning digital citizenship. Online platforms, such as Blackboard and Moodle, are readily available on most college campuses. Hence, using technology as a facilitator of active engagement seems not only innovative but rather logical. The question here is, how can UDL, supported through technology, be applied to pedagogical practices to maximize student outcomes, per (student) self-report?

I have 10 topics (formal lectures) that are explicitly taught over the 15-week semester related to the role of the speech-language pathologist and autism spectrum disorders. Each of these 10 topics has a corresponding technology used with the intent of acting as a springboard for discussion. See Table 1-1 for a summary of technologies used over the course of the semester.

TABLE 1-1

Technology Used in All Ten Formal Topics to Facilitate Universal Design for Learning

TECHNOLOGY	DESCRIPTION	USE IN COURSE
PowerPoints	Each topic has a corresponding PowerPoint sharing vital content.	Offers foundational concepts and spurs discussion during face-to-face meetings.
Podcasts	I audio-record lectures using a high-quality digital recorder. I then podcast these out to the class immediately following the class meeting.	This support assists students who would like to review the class lecture while mobile. Podcasting further supports students who have been absent, without isolating them.
Panopto	A lecture recording software solution that allows instructors to record their presentations, screens, and themselves all at once. This media content is then sequentially linked together into one cohesive video.	There are occasions when the class does not meet face to face. Further, this platform supports teaching using a flipped classroom in which the formal lecture is delivered in advance of the face-to-face class meeting, allowing in-seat time to be utilized for active learning exercises.
Video demonstrations	I share intervention videos of myself early on in clinical practice, demonstrating flaws in my methods. I also use YouTube videos during the goal-writing unit.	This evokes discussion on how the clinical session could have been improved, facilitating critical thinking and clinical application. Together, we review a session, and then reverse engineer the activity, asking students to write a goal based on the session they just observed.
Anonymous surveys*	At the end of each class, I send out an anonymous Google Form, asking students what they learned that was truly new for them and what they still have questions about.	I spend time between class meetings preparing responses or follow-up questions to expand particular thoughts and concepts. I begin the next class by addressing those specific questions before moving on to the next topic.
Self-studies*	At the beginning of each new topic, I disseminate a self-study guide with specifically designed, open-ended questions.	Students are asked to complete these forms at their own pace and in their own way. The self-studies were also posted to the online course site immediately following each unit. These forms are not collected or graded. Rather, similar questions in style and content appear on the cumulative final exam.

Note: Items that have (*) indicate new approaches applied in Spring 2019 semester.

Measuring Universal Design for Learning and Technology Use

In the spring of 2019, students were surveyed to determine their perceptions of UDL and technology use. Table 1-2 presents the data collected from that survey. Additionally, upon completion of the course, students were surveyed again to ascertain their perceptions related to the design of the course. Table 1-3 presents this data. Data suggests that UDL was implemented effectively in class, and that the two newest initiatives (anonymous surveys and self-studies) warrant further development. A third piece of evidence regarding monitoring change is my own teaching reflection. Summaries of my reflections of each technology used in my course are presented in Table 1-4.

In addition to these findings, students provided narrative feedback on their end-of-semester course evaluation forms specific to the topics of UDL and technology. Overwhelmingly, students reported their experiences in the class to be engaging, helping to support learning and further their understanding of dense, complex, and synergistic content. Excerpts of student feedback on technology use are reported below:

- "Very helpful to have Panopto [recordings] and recorded lectures during class."
- "I liked the online option! Was very clear and Dr. Battaglia kept us informed and gave great reminders!"
- "I like the online delivery because it gives us the opportunity to review the material multiple times."
- "Just as informative as in-person classes."

Excerpts of student feedback on UDL use are reported below:
- "I loved how we had lecture and hands on assignments in class."
- "Loved all the activities. Facilitated my understanding better."
- "The activities helped me bridge the gap between textbook knowledge and clinical impressions."

APPLICATION OF LITERATURE/DATA

Initially blind to student reviews, I triangulate my reflection with student feedback (both quantitative and qualitative) to inform decisions moving forward. Data suggests that students responded positively to the use of PowerPoints, podcasts, video demonstrations, and Panopto to support their learning. As a result, those aspects of this course will be retained and/or expanded. Data also suggest that my two newest initiatives (i.e., anonymous surveys and self-studies) were not overwhelmingly well-received. Hence, I plan to make changes on these. In the qualitative analyses, students did not make specific requests or suggestions for future modification. Therefore, intended changes will be based on literature reviewed in pedagogy (Ginsberg et al., 2012; Lang, 2016) and will be continually monitored.

In addition to maintaining anonymous surveys in their current form, I will also add an anonymous survey halfway through the course (around midterm season) asking the following three questions (Ginsberg et al., 2012):
1. What happens in this class that supports my learning?
2. What happens in this class that hinders my learning?
3. What would I like to see more of in this class?

The hope here is that roadblocks to learning particular content can be determined by way of weekly surveys, intersected with questions on delivery style. I can therefore make pedagogical changes in the second half of the class to enhance the student experience. Collecting data, in a systematic and evidence-based manner, will allow further reflection on my teaching and the learning of my students.

TABLE 1-2

Student Responses to Questions About Technology Implementation (*n* = 20)

STATEMENT	STRONGLY AGREE	AGREE	NEUTRAL	DISAGREE	STRONGLY DISAGREE
The PowerPoints were a useful aid to learning in this course.	14	6	0	0	0
Podcasts via Google Drive were a useful tool for review and study purposes.	14	6	0	0	0
Panopto, used for delivering online lectures and video streaming, was effectively used to provide additional content to our face-to-face meetings.	14	6	0	0	0
Video demonstrations were a useful aid to learning in this course.	15	4	0	0	0
Anonymous surveys were helpful in communicating my understanding of each topic.	8	5	6	1	0
Self-studies, handed out at the beginning of each class, were helpful in guiding my learning.	8	3	6	2	1

TABLE 1-3

Student Responses to Questions About Universal Design for Learning (*n* = 20)

STATEMENT	STRONGLY AGREE	AGREE	NEUTRAL	DISAGREE	STRONGLY DISAGREE
Provides students with course content using multiple means of representation (e.g., visual, auditory)	18	2	0	0	0
Engages students using multiple means (e.g., illustrating concepts face to face, online and using practice activities)	17	3	0	0	0
Affords students with multiple opportunities for expression (e.g., in-class discussion, group-based case studies, one-on-one meetings)	18	2	0	0	0

Self-studies will also be modified in an effort to support student learning. It is unclear to me at present if students are utilizing the self-studies as they were intended. This tool was never meant to add hours of additional work on student workload or to incite panic in the student. I will now add a statement at the bottom of this form, stating that "If completing this form takes more than 10 minutes of your time, please either review the podcast and lecture once more or schedule an appointment to meet with me so we can discuss further." It is my hope that increased frequency of engagement with the content will help students review and retain information in a way that works for them.

APPLICATION TO CROSS-DISCIPLINARY CONTEXTS

UDL was originally proposed as a proactive solution to accommodating differently abled individuals when building structures from an architectural perspective. Hence, utilizing UDL principles in speech-language pathology and pedagogy is inherently translational. Principles of universal design can easily be applied to other clinical disciplines. When thinking about clinical populations and habilitation (or rehabilitation), the idea of using an alternative method to achieve the same

TABLE 1-4

My Own Reflections on Each of the Six Technology Domains

ACTIVITY	REFLECTION
PowerPoints	PowerPoints were generally helpful. I would like to restructure some of the slide sequences and condense two social skills lectures into one. This will allow me to add more counseling to my family involvement unit. I would like to add a unit explicitly dedicated to cultural and linguistic diversity, rather than infusing these notions throughout the course.
Podcasts	I believe podcasts were useful for those students who accessed them. I am not convinced that all students did so. However, I feel it was a good way to offer students equal access to the content, whether they were physically present or had to miss a class for sick or personal reasons.
Panopto	I think Panopto has greatly enhanced the student learning experience. This technology far exceeds use of a narrated PowerPoint, in that students can see *you* while engaging in each slide. I think this helps make teaching more human while using a mode of teaching that may be perceived as sterile (i.e., technology).
Video demonstrations	Video demonstrations of my own clinical practice were helpful for students to see my human failures and successes. Considering they were dated, the quality of the videos was sometimes compromised. However, they were important pieces of information to supplement traditional lectures. Links to YouTube videos enhanced the teaching and learning experience through small group discussions and guided activities in class.
Anonymous surveys	I am not sure if students were forthcoming with anonymous surveys. While it did help with some points I apparently missed, I am not sure that all students trusted that the surveys were anonymous, and therefore did not respond. In addition, I have noticed that for some units there are several responses and others there are none.
Self-studies	The intention is for this to be self-guided. I mirror questions on the final to be similar to questions on the self-studies. I am not sure that students complete them or if this is a helpful practice (yet).

outcome is, indeed, the underlying concept of UDL. Extending this notion to the higher education teaching and learning experience, multiple means of representation, expression, and engagement stand to have great impact. Essentially, in thinking of scholarship on teaching and learning, any pedagogical scenario that attempts UDL and monitors outcomes is most efficacious.

For instance, students in an occupational therapy anatomy and movement course are provided with lectures in advance using PowerPoint, handouts, and video components. The students are allowed to use their laptops in class or print the presentations ahead of time for either computer entry or hand recording. During the lecture, the students are provided with models to understand the underlying anatomy and then are asked to work with each other to identify the structures on their partners. Once the structures are identified, these structures are connected to functional tasks in the classroom. The instructor can break down students into groups where one or two students demonstrate the activity, while the remaining student in the group identifies how anatomy creates motion and affects participation in occupation. By providing the students with PowerPoint lectures in advance, the students can choose which way is best for them to interact with the lecture material. Some students will take notes on their computers, others will print and write on the sheet, or some students will opt for listening to the lecturer and use the PowerPoint as a guide. For some students, having the ability to use a computer interface improves their ability to enter notes or attend to the lecture. For students with special needs, such as students with low vision who need larger print, having the lecture in advance provides options for accessing the material (i.e., increasing the screen size or print size when printing).

Videos embedded in the lecture also provide increased access to the material for those who learn better through listening and observing than reading and writing. Providing students with the opportunity to move in the classroom and experience how structures cause movement allows for kinesthetic learning as well. For example, a lecture on upper extremity musculature might include someone putting dishes in a cabinet or taking cooking trays out of the oven. By providing this kinesthetic motion, the person performing the task can feel the action of the muscles they are learning about. Furthermore, it provides the opportunity for observers to interact with the lecture material in real life scenarios that make the material more accessible. In all, the lecture described provides demonstration, as well as visual, auditory, and kinesthetic methods of instruction to improve access to the material across all learning styles and educational requirements. It also provides the occupational therapy instructor the ability to embed occupation into foundational material.

ADDITIONAL RESOURCES

- CAST provides a wealth of information regarding UDL. Several technology initiatives are created and managed through CAST, as well as helpful resources to self-study UDL, and bring these principles to the forefront in your own place of work:
  - http://www.cast.org/
- The TEDx "Why We Need Universal Design" is eye opening as a first-person narrative regarding different abilities we all share, and the possibilities that the UDL framework can offer:
  - https://www.youtube.com/watch?v=bVdPNWMGyZY
- The following desk reference is helpful to understand the wide-reaching application of UDL in higher education:
  - Tobin, T. J., & Behling, K. T. (2018). *Reach everyone, teach everyone.* West Virginia University Press.

REFERENCES

Al-Azawei, A., Serenelli, F., & Lundqvist, K. (2016). Universal design for learning (UDL): A content analysis of peer reviewed journals from 2012 to 2015. *Journal of the Scholarship of Teaching and Learning, 16*(3), 39-56. https://doi.org/10.14434/josotl.v16i3.19295

Carr, A. A., Jonassen, D. H., Litzinger, M. E., & Marra, R. M. (1998). Good ideas to foment educational revolution: The role of systemic change in advancing situated learning, constructivism, and feminist pedagogy. *Educational Technology, 38*(1), 5-15.

Clegg, S. (2000). Knowing through reflective practice in higher education. *Educational Action Research, 8*(3), 451-469. doi:10.1080/09650790000200128

Ginsberg, S. M., Friberg, J. C., & Visconti, C. F. (2012). *Scholarship of teaching and learning in speech-language pathology and audiology: Evidence-based education.* Plural Publishing.

Hall, T. E., Cohen, N., Vue, G., & Ganley, P. (2015). Addressing learning disabilities with UDL and technology: Strategic reader. *Learning Disability Quarterly, 38*(2), 72-83. https://doi.org/10.1177/0731948714544375

Hall, T. E., Meyer, A., & Rose, D. H. (2012). *Universal design for learning in the classroom: Practical applications.* Guilford Press.

Hall, T. E., Vue, G., Strangman, N., & Meyer, A. (2014). Differentiated instruction and implications for UDL implementation. *National Center on Accessing the General Curriculum.* https://www.cast.org/products-services/resources/2014/ncac-differentiated-instruction-udl

King-Sears, M. (2009). Universal design for learning: Technology and pedagogy. *Learning Disability Quarterly, 32*(4), 199-201.

Lang, J. M. (2016). *Small teaching: Everyday lessons from the science of learning.* Jossey-Bass Inc.

Laurillard, D. (2002). *Rethinking university teaching. A framework for the effective use of learning technologies* (2nd ed.). Routledge Falmer.

Mace, R., Hardie, G., & Place, J. (1991). Accessible environments: Toward universal design. In W. E. Preiser, J. C. Vischer, & E. T. White (Eds.), *Design intervention: Toward a more humane architecture.* Van Nostrand Reinhold.

Mattson, K. (2017). *Digital citizenship in action: Empowering students to engage in online communities.* International Society for Technology in Education.

McGuire, J. M., Scott, S. S., & Shaw, S. F. (2006). Universal design and its applications in educational environments. *Remedial and Special Education, 27*(3), 166-175.

Mishra, P., & Koehler, M. J. (2003). Not "what" but "how:" Becoming design-wise about educational technology. In Y. Zhao (Ed.), *What teachers should know about technology: Perspectives and practices* (pp. 99-122). Information Age Publishing.

Meyer, A., Rose, D. H., & Gordon, D. (2014). *Universal design for learning: Theory and practice.* CAST Professional Publishing.

Prensky, M. (2001). Digital natives, digital immigrants. *On the Horizon, 9*(5), 1-6. https://doi.org/10.1108/107481 20110424816

Prensky, M. (2011). Digital natives and homo sapiens digital. In M. Thomas (Ed.), *Deconstructing digital natives: Young people, technologies, and the new digital literacies* (pp. 15-29). Routledge.

Rao, K., & Meo, G. (2016). Using universal design for learning to design standards-based lessons. *Sage Open, 6*(4), 1-12. https://doi.org/10.1177/2158244016680688

Rappolt-Schlichtmann, G., Daley, S. G., Lim, S., Lapinski, S., Robinson, K. H., & Johnson, M. (2013). Universal design for learning and elementary school science: Exploring the efficacy, use, and perceptions of a web-based science notebook. *Journal of Education Psychology, 105*(4), 1210-1225. https://doi.org/10.1037/a0033217

Rose, D. H., Meyer, A., & Hitchcock, C. (Eds.). (2005). *The universally designed classroom: Accessible curriculum and digital technologies.* Harvard Education Press.

Savin-Baden, M. (2000). *Problem-based learning in higher education: Untold stories.* Society for Research in Higher Education & Open University Press.

Spooner, F., Baker, J. N., Harris, A. A., Ahlgrim-Delzell, L., & Browder, D. M., (2007). Effects of training in universal design for learning on lesson plan development. *Remedial Special Education, 28*(2), 108-116.

Walser, N. (2008). Teaching 21st century skills: What does it look like in practice? *Harvard Education Letter, 24*(5), 1-3.

2

BREAKING OUT OF THE SILOS
A Case Study in Co-Teaching in Speech-Language Pathology

*Julie L. Cox, PhD, CCC-SLP/L; Amanda B. Silberer, PhD, CCC-A;
and Haleigh M. Ruebush, MS, CCC-SLP/L*

DESCRIPTION OF TEACHING/LEARNING CONTEXT

The challenge to develop critical thinking skills in graduate student clinicians has become increasingly difficult. Our faculty have been focused on this issue for years, but more recently, it has been openly discussed in professional meetings and national conferences (American Speech-Language-Hearing Association [ASHA], Council of Academic Programs in Communication Sciences and Disorders). Despite the size or research level of the university that is offering the clinical program, the trend remains that students are often missing the big picture. Student clinicians appear to be having more trouble than ever taking coursework and applying it in the clinical setting. One trend that has been identified by our faculty is that students are addressing patients based solely on a simplified definition of their primary communication diagnosis instead of fully considering the range of abilities and deficits. Even more alarming is that some students are also struggling to carry over learned clinical skills from one patient to another. In our department, we have tried implementing changes to our curriculum and to our clinical assignments that focus on teaching students to see communication abilities not as isolated silos for each of the Big 9 disorders (ASHA, n.d.-a), but as layers of information. To accomplish this, we have assigned simulated diagnostics for complex disorders, provided more hands-on opportunities in the classroom, increased article reviews, and incorporated group clinician meetings to initiate peer discussions and learning from one another. Some of these changes have yielded positive changes, but overall, the impact has not been as global as we had hoped.

Friberg, J. C., Visconti, C. F., & Ginsberg, S. M. (Eds.). *Evidence-Based
Education in the Classroom: Examples From Clinical Disciplines* (pp. 13-20).
© 2021 Taylor & Francis Group.

Students continued to struggle with making important connections between the layers of information required for identification and holistic treatment of speech and language disorders. The instructors of two of our first-year graduate courses, Motor Speech Disorders and Aphasia, requested to have their courses be scheduled back-to-back so they could co-teach periodically throughout the semester. It was hypothesized that co-teaching courses across disorders would lead to more connections and carryover from course material to clinical practice. The courses were scheduled as individual 50-minute courses 3 days per week, but they were scheduled back-to-back so there could be a co-teaching component when appropriate. This chapter aims to show the effect co-teaching could have on strengthening the connection between courses and clinic by teaching students how to think more holistically. Overall, we planned on providing hands-on experiences that would allow the students to integrate and synthesize content across two graduate courses into a more blended and realistic schema.

REVIEW OF LITERATURE

Co-teaching has varied definitions in the literature with just as varied implementation methods. Wenzlaff and colleagues (2002, p. 14; as cited in Ferguson & Wilson, 2011) stated that co-teaching is "two or more individuals who come together in a collaborative relationship for the purpose of shared work" resulting in an outcome that could not be achieved alone. It has also been defined as sharing the responsibility for instruction of the content (Roth et al., 2005). Regardless of the definition, co-teaching has been found to be a successful instructional technique in special education and K–12 education (Bacharach et al., 2008; Bouck, 2007; Ferguson & Wilson, 2011; Graziano & Navarrete, 2012); however, there is less evidence for higher education (Chanmugam & Gerlach, 2013; Gillespie & Israetel, 2008).

Over the past 3 decades of educational research, seven unique co-teaching strategies have been identified, including one teach, one observe; one teach, one drift; station teaching; parallel teaching; supplemental teaching; alternative (differentiated) teaching; and team teaching (Table 2-1; Bacharach et al., 2008; Graziano & Navarrete, 2012; Lock et al., 2016). The co-teaching model best fitting our needs within our higher education environment was to implement a modified version of team teaching. The foundation of this model was well-constructed and well-planned team teaching that provided students with opportunities to integrate information. Although teaching philosophies and clinical approaches do not have to be a match between the instructors, differences should be discussed prior to co-teaching to present information to the students in a clear and meaningful way.

Much of the literature on co-teaching discusses not only the logistics of lesson planning and leading the class sessions, but also on the relationship between the co-teachers (Bacharach et al., 2008; Chanmugam & Gerlach, 2013; Ferguson & Wilson, 2011; Lock et al., 2016). Sharing the balance of power is the foundation of successful team-teaching. Neither instructor is in charge, nor is there a mentor-mentee relationship between the instructors. Rather, they are a team. Students tend to buy in more readily when they experience the enthusiasm, passion, and respect of the instructors without the added challenge of trying to determine a singular authority figure (Bacharach et al., 2008). With blended content, we also wanted to be sure that students were not confused about the importance of the material and its clinical application (e.g., speech is more important than language or vice versa depending on the primary instructor).

Simply deciding to co-teach two courses, though, is still not adequate for a well-integrated learning experience. The curricular decisions must also be based on the level of similarity or overlap of course content. One reason these particular two courses were so easily blended is the foundational neurological etiology of both disorders that are typically taught in their silos. Vinney and Harvey (2017) reported a collaborative effort between courses on aphasia and motor speech disorders at their university. Their experiment was quite different in that they provided structured and co-created pre-course learning modules to integrate the neuroanatomy and neurophysiology of

Table 2-1

Summary of Seven Co-Teaching Strategies

STRATEGY	DESCRIPTION
1. One teach, one observe	One instructor has the primary responsibility for leading the class session, while the other instructor observes the students for specific behaviors that may indicate learning or confusion.
2. One teach, one drift	This is an extension of one teach, one observe, where one instructor still has the primary teaching responsibility, but in this model, the instructor who drifts will assist students with their work or help to answer questions, etc.
3. Station teaching	Each instructor is responsible for a portion of the content. Students are divided into groups and will rotate to each instructor.
4. Parallel teaching	Each instructor teaches half the class but is addressing the same content for the purpose of lowering the student-to-instructor ratio.
5. Supplemental teaching	One instructor teaches the class at a typical pace, while the other instructor works with students who need extra support.
6. Alternative (differentiated) teaching	Instructors each provide their own, unique approach to teaching the content with the same learning outcome for all students.
7. Team teaching	Well-planned lessons with an invisible flow of instruction and no division of authority. Both instructors are actively involved in the class and are able to share in the teaching, interject information, and answer questions.

Adapted from Bacharach, N., Heck, T. W., & Dahlberg, K. (2008). Co-teaching in higher education. *Journal of College Teaching & Learning, 5*(3), 9-16; Graziano, K. J., & Navarrete, L. A. (2012). Co-teaching in a teacher education classroom: Collaboration, compromise, and creativity. *Issues in Teacher Education, 21*(1), 109-126; Lock, J., Clancy, T., Lisella, R., Rosenau, P., Ferreria, C., & Rainsbury, J. (2016). The lived experiences of instructors co-teaching in higher education. *Brock Education Journal, 26*(1), 22-35.

the two disorders; however, they established a strong link between the two courses. The connection they demonstrated spurred us to think of how we could implement more crossover in the content, especially between the same two disorders. Furthermore, this type of curriculum could potentially be developed across disorders of similar etiologies or disorders that often co-occur within or between professions.

Course content is obviously very important, but the real missing piece, as we were seeing students navigate their graduate program, was just as often in their ability to think critically about communication disorders, not just repeat memorized information. There are specific standards that applicants must meet to be eligible for the Certificate of Clinical Competence in speech-language pathology (ASHA, n.d.-a). Many of these standards are met during their graduate program and are typically evaluated through both academics and clinical requirements. Currently, the Standards for the Certificate of Clinical Competence indicate that "experiences should allow students to: interpret, integrate, and synthesize core concepts and knowledge; demonstrate appropriate professional and clinical skills; and incorporate critical thinking and decision-making [emphasis added] skills while engaged in identification, evaluation, diagnosis, planning, implementation, and/or intervention" (ASHA, n.d.-b). Our purpose was to provide deliberate training opportunities for students in hopes that the explicit overlap between acquired disorders of speech and language would be readily recognized, retained, and implemented using enhanced critical thinking skills.

Our concern lies in the fact that critical thinking across the scope of practice is difficult to assess in courses taught in silos. Students often become so focused on their grades in each course (silo) that they seem to have trouble connecting the information across disorders with actual patients in the clinical setting. In fact, our highest achieving academic students may be our lowest performing clinicians. This factor, amongst others, plays a part in how we organize our curriculum, specifically aimed at improving critical thinking. Often, in an effort to follow the standards, course design is structured around what to think and not necessarily how to think. Critical thinking, however, is complex and encompasses many thought processes including, but not limited to, planning, monitoring, evaluating, and reflecting (Behar-Horenstein & Niu, 2011). These processes can be incorporated into any well-designed course, whether taught individually or co-taught. It was our hope, though, that we could bring critical thinking even more to the forefront by modeling our own discussions and highlighting the need for the complex level of thought when delivering high-quality patient care. Furthermore, previous authors have found that when they consciously worked to improve their teaching practices through co-teaching, their own knowledge base broadened, and the students often noticed and displayed higher levels of engagement with the course material (Ferguson & Wilson, 2011).

Application of Literature/Data

Our program is designed for students to take four consecutive semesters of courses and clinic before being assigned for full-time, off-campus internships. Length of time, lack of resources, limited faculty, and minimal client diversity all contribute to the importance of capitalizing on each opportunity we have to facilitate students making connections across courses and clinic. Adding more courses to the curriculum was not an option, so in an effort to help develop clinical/critical thinking, the instructors for Motor Speech Disorders and Aphasia collaborated to foster the overlap between disorders. Each course was developed independent of the other—syllabi, exams, and projects; however, each major unit (e.g., neurology, assessment, treatment) offered an opportunity for team teaching.

Weekly preparation meetings were scheduled and used to discuss team teaching sessions, as well as the individual courses and ways we could build in more opportunities to collaborate (Chanmugam & Gerlach, 2013). The focus of the meetings was most often preparation for the upcoming co-taught session. In order to do so, we also discussed progress in our individual courses to ensure that students were prepared for the information that would be presented in the co-teaching section. It was important to us that students were grasping individual course concepts of neurology, assessment, and treatment so that both speech and language disorders could be discussed as they related to one another. The planning process was quite detailed, and it became apparent that collaborating in this way made us better teachers in terms of structure, delivery, and learning activities in both our individual and team teaching sessions.

We anticipated students would initially feel overwhelmed and/or anxious about this design because it was different than anything we had done before in our program. The first class period of the semester was dedicated to answering questions and offering explanations about the logistics of co-teaching and how it would blend with individual courses. Students were concerned about how the courses would be graded. At least for the first time, we had predicted this may be an issue, so we had already decided to keep the course grades separate. It was, however, important to collect data for the purposes of our research so we assessed the learning activities completed during the co-teaching sections using a rating scale. The ratings assigned to student work were not included in their overall course grades. There were no additional questions or concerns other than questions specific to grading.

For this first collaboration, we planned four team teaching sessions over the semester. A session was scheduled for each major unit: neurology, assessment, and treatment. In addition to these three units, there was a final case study session where both instructors participated with students during an in-class case study. The instructors were present to answer questions and provide clarifications, if needed. On team teaching days, both instructors were present and actively engaged in the learning activities throughout the entire 100 minutes. Content-based lectures and discussions were often the focus of individual class times, but this type of delivery was purposely limited during team teaching sessions. Class periods were planned around one or two learning activities that encouraged critical thinking and active participation.

The planned activity for the neurology unit was reflective of what we envisioned for the team teaching sessions. First, students were divided into small groups and charged with outlining the neurological process/pathway used for expressive language with conversion to speech output. Next, the names of all of the cortical and subcortical structures were listed on individual cards and were placed in a bucket for each student to randomly select. Based upon the structure that each student selected, they were asked to physically form a line representing the correct order for the expressive language and speech output process. Once the students physically lined up, one by one they described their structure and its function as it related to the process (e.g., "I am Broca's area; I sequence motor movements for speech"). Finally, the level of difficulty increased when students were asked to discuss potential deficits of a specific lesion at the site of a stroke. These activities facilitated discussion, engagement, and active participation for the students. Additionally, it pushed them to apply knowledge they had learned recently, or even not so recently, but from undergraduate courses and clinical experiences. Obviously, this type of activity would be successful in any course, but implementing it as we did for this session provided the opportunity for students to truly connect the related processes of message formulation and the motoric output component.

Then, at the end of the semester, we provided a case study that would include important data for our research. The case study was designed to assess knowledge and skills that were gained as a function of individual courses and the co-teaching portion. Students received the following case:

> Pearl is a 72-year-old female. Eight weeks ago, she experienced a left cerebrovascular accident, which resulted in right hemiparesis and difficulty with her expressive language. She spent the first 2 weeks in a community hospital and then an additional 6 weeks in a rehabilitation hospital. She has now been discharged to go home but will continue with outpatient speech/language services. The speech therapy discharge summary revealed Pearl followed 1-step commands 9/10 trials independently, completed basic naming tasks 8/10 trials independently, formulated grammatically correct sentences of 3 to 4 words in 6/10 trials with extended time, presented a S/Z ratio of 2.3, produced a maximum phonation duration of 10 seconds, and had an overall speech intelligibility of 76%.
>
> Pearl is retired from her career as a legal assistant and lives on her own in a studio apartment near her two sons. Pearl is now embarrassed about her speech and language characterized by phonological and semantic substitutions, soft and slurred speech, as well as a lack of error awareness. While her family is supportive, they do not understand her speech and sometimes tease Pearl about the "funny" things she says. Her family frequently states "Mom, think about what you are saying." She has been declining visits and phone calls from her friends and family. Another fear that she has is that she will not be able to live alone and will end up in a nursing home.

After reading about Pearl, students, who were acting as the outpatient speech-language pathologist, were asked to hypothesize what communication diagnoses she had and then provide details on what formal and informal assessments they would use. Students developed three short-term goals using realistic expectations that were based on the results of the assessments. They were to provide detailed therapy activities that would address each goal with emphasis on the cueing hierarchies. In addition, though, students were also expected to understand the differences in the levels of care where we work with our patients, and incorporate patient/family needs into their treatments as that is an often overlooked component to evidence-based practice. We felt a case study, such as the one provided, would require students to take a holistic view of the patient when considering her communication status blended with professional issues for the speech-language pathologist and quality-of-life issues for the patient. This is an example of the critical thinking we hope to promote in discussions with our student clinicians; thus, it seemed to be a great way to prepare them for that in an academic setting.

It was important to get the students' feedback about this model, so they were given an opportunity to answer questions using a semi-structured survey. The aim of the survey was to give the students an opportunity to provide information as to what was and was not beneficial as it related to the co-teaching component. Most of the feedback was positive with students commenting that they did feel they were able to connect the material between the two courses when given the explicit opportunity to do so. There were some suggestions for improvement in terms of logistics, but the most encouraging suggestion was that students wanted more co-teaching across these two courses. As planning is currently underway for the upcoming semester, we do hope to foster more meaningful connections between the courses and implement information from other courses when relevant.

The students who were in the inaugural cohort to receive our co-taught format for Motor Speech Disorders and Aphasia are currently in their final semester of coursework and clinic on-campus, and will begin full-time internships in a few months. Coincidentally, at the same time these students were being assigned more clients as progressing through the program, our local hospital lost their speech-language pathology coverage and our clinic experienced a greater volume of referrals for patients with more complex medical and communication diagnoses. It was observed by our faculty supervisors that the students were largely ready for this new challenge and were prepared to think critically about their patients for the purposes of assessment and treatment of co-occurring communication disorders. It is nearly impossible to determine whether the co-teaching component we added to our curriculum was the singular reason for the subjectively improved performance from our student clinicians when we have implemented several new experiences for them. However, we believe the explicit, hands-on practice with these two commonly co-occurring disorders in the classroom setting could have only been a supportive factor.

Co-teaching, with all of its advantages, is not without its disadvantages. The most significant consideration when adopting a teaching and learning model such as this one is that there will be an increased time commitment for both instructors. There is the obvious increased time commitment spent in the classroom on the blended days. Additionally, 30 to 60 minutes a week were carved out into our already busy schedules to meet specifically about this collaboration. Over the length of a semester, that added up rather quickly. Another consideration that may come more from administrators is the division of labor. In our case, we each taught an individual course worth 3 semester hours. Our workloads were based on those hours, and there was really no confusion to speak of. Of greater concern could be if two or more instructors were to co-teach just one course. Just like with billable time in the clinical setting, administrators are not likely to count the full course for each member of the faculty member involved in the co-teaching. However, for the most effective and best practice of a co-teaching model, each instructor should commit the full course time each day for the greatest learning outcomes of the students (Bacharach et al., 2008; Chanmugam & Gerlach, 2013; Ferguson & Wilson, 2011; Lock et al., 2016). Finally, it should be recognized that co-teaching is not for everyone. Fortunately, the two of us (Cox and Ruebush) work very well together, but we discussed the difficulties this type of collaboration could create if this was attempted with someone with whom the working relationship was not as compatible. Much like the dreaded group projects in courses, this model could easily lead to undue stress and an imbalance of work and power. Both instructors should be fully committed to the model and understand one another's teaching philosophies and learning objectives.

At the time this chapter was written, the instructors were well underway for planning the second semester of co-teaching the same two courses. As we prepare, we spent some time exploring our own teaching styles using the work of Anthony Grasha (1994). Surprisingly, we found that we had similar scores across all five teaching styles: expert, formal authority, personal model, facilitator, and delegator. It should be noted that there is no one style better than the others, and that each comes with its own set of strengths and weaknesses. In fact, all instructors display each style at different times, and the overall blend is what makes a teacher unique (Grasha, 1994). That said, the lowest style displayed by each of us was that of facilitator. Our discussion led us to a thought that perhaps this is perceived as the most challenging because of the known ASHA standards that must be met in the courses. It is also known that the work of a facilitator is more time-intensive than other styles of teaching (Grasha, 1994). Although neither of us were greatly surprised by our scores, our plan to continue co-teaching was further reinforced. By engaging in our blended class sessions, we are able to actively put forth the effort to engage in a more facilitative role rather than that of an expert or formal authority that is likely more often observed in a traditional day of lecture on some individually taught days. Now as we plan to blend the two courses a few more times within the upcoming term, we are able to readily focus on the facilitator piece of our teaching styles, which may allow the students even more opportunities for critical thinking and application of material.

APPLICATION TO CROSS-DISCIPLINARY CONTEXTS

Based on the positive feedback we gained from the students following their semester of two strategically and periodically co-taught courses, we see the applications that could be possible in any clinical discipline. In any case where multiple deficits can arise from a single etiology, co-teaching across the deficit areas may be beneficial, although it is acknowledged that there are other ways to manage this within curricular design. Due to the acquired neurological cause, Dysphagia and Cognition Caused by Brain Injury or Progressive Decline are two additional courses that could be together or with Motor Speech Disorders and/or Aphasia. There are so many across course connections that could be developed if faculty are on board to adopt this model and develop them. For example, on the pediatric side of our field, courses related to child language, articulation and phonology, and application in the public schools could complement each other extremely well and help students make those important connections of how communication disorders are evaluated and treated in a very common work setting for a speech-language pathologist. Not only could blended courses within the field of speech-language pathology help show overlapping etiologies, but it can also demonstrate the similarities in a holistic communication assessment and the development of treatment plans. In addition to the blended content, we felt we were also able to highlight the importance of intraprofessional (within our profession) collaboration with two speech-language pathologists teaching the students simultaneously. Students were able to observe us sharing ideas; challenging one another to think differently; and accepting alternative ideas, opinions, and teaching practices based on discussion.

Based on that unexpected benefit that we experienced, we foresee there could be incredible opportunities for interprofessional (outside our profession) collaboration within and across courses and even clinical programs. For example, at a university where there are graduate programs of both speech-language pathology and occupational therapy, courses could be co-taught where discussions of patient cases could be facilitated from both professional perspectives. The same could be said for occupational therapy and physical therapy or speech-language pathology and dietetics. Nearly any clinical field could also have overlap with counseling as that should be a part of the provision of all patient education. Dealing with individual patient needs, as well as their families and caregivers can be the most rewarding or the most challenging aspects of the job. These pieces of clinical work cross over into many other disciplines or professions, which is one way that interprofessional education could benefit from blended content and co-taught models.

Another broad contextual area where we could develop interprofessional curricular changes is professional ethics. All clinical professions, not just speech-language pathology, have a code of ethics or a similar document to guide the respective fields, including physical and occupational therapies (American Occupational Therapy Association, 2015; American Physical Therapy Association, 2020). As such, a blended or co-taught ethics course across disciplines could bring in many viewpoints about ethical patient scenarios from a variety of professional lenses. Certainly there would be curricular and administrative challenges with such a model, but with the increased push across most, if not all, clinical disciplines for more interprofessional collaboration, it only seems logical to begin the process during the training programs at universities with a variety of such clinical opportunities.

ADDITIONAL RESOURCES

- The work of Grasha provides information on five different teaching styles that can apply to educators at any level:
  - Grasha, A. F. (1994). A matter of style: The teacher as expert, formal authority, personal model, facilitator, and delegator. *College Teaching, 42*(4), 142-149. http://www.montana.edu/gradschool/documents/A-Matter-of-STyle-Grashab.pdf
- The ASHA website contains all of the necessary information for certification of new members, including the requirements for all education programs for speech-language pathology and audiology:
  - http://www.asha.org
- This article found in *Teaching and Learning in Communication Sciences & Disorders* was what pushed the authors into new ways to present the content of specific communication disorders:
  - Harvey-Northtop, J. M., & Vinney, L. A. (2019). Bridging the gap: An integrated approach to facilitating foundational learning of neuroanatomy and neurophysiology in graduate-level speech-language pathology coursework. *Teaching and Learning in Communication Sciences & Disorders, 1*(2).

REFERENCES

American Occupational Therapy Association. (2015). Occupational therapy code of ethics. *American Journal of Occupational Therapy, 69*(3). https://doi.org/10.5014/ajot.2015.696S03

American Physical Therapy Association. (2020, August 12). Code of ethics for the physical therapist. https://www.apta.org/uploadedFiles/APTAorg/About_Us/Policies/Ethics/CodeofEthics.pdf

American Speech-Language Hearing Association. (n.d.-a). Certification standards for speech-language pathology frequently asked questions: Forms and documentation. https://www.asha.org/certification/2020-slp-certification-standards/

American Speech-Language Hearing Association. (n.d.-b). Professional development requirements for the 2020 audiology and speech-language pathology certification standards. https://www.asha.org/Certification/Prof-Dev-for-2020-Certification-Standards/

Bacharach, N., Heck, T. W., & Dahlberg, K. (2008). Co-teaching in higher education. *Journal of College Teaching & Learning, 5*(3), 9-16.

Behar-Horenstein, L. S., & Niu, L. (2011). Teaching critical thinking skills in higher education: A review of the literature. *Journal of College Teaching & Learning, 8*(2), 25-42.

Bouck, E. C. (2007). Co-teaching...not just a textbook term: Implications for practice. *Preventing School Failure, 51*(2), 46-51.

Chanmugam, A., & Gerlach, B. (2013). A co-teaching model for developing future educators' teaching effectiveness. *International Journal of Teaching and Learning in Higher Education, 25*(1), 110-117.

Ferguson, J., & Wilson, J. C. (2011). The co-teaching professorship: Power and expertise in the co-taught higher education classroom. *Scholar-Practitioner Quarterly, 5*(1), 52-68.

Grasha, A. F. (1994). A matter of style: The teacher as expert, formal authority, personal model, facilitator, and delegator. *College Teaching, 42*(4), 142-149.

Gillespie, D., & Israetel, A. (2008, August). *Benefits of co-teaching in relation to student learning* [paper presentation]. 116th Meeting of the American Psychological Association, Boston, MA.

Graziano, K. J., & Navarrete, L. A. (2012). Co-teaching in a teacher education classroom: Collaboration, compromise, and creativity. *Issues in Teacher Education, 21*(1), 109-126.

Lock, J., Clancy, T., Lisella, R., Rosenau, P., Ferreria, C., & Rainsbury, J. (2016). The lived experiences of instructors co-teaching in higher education. *Brock Education Journal, 26*(1), 22-35.

Roth, W-M., Tobin, K., Carambo, C., & Dalland, C. (2005). Coordination in co-teaching: Producing alignment in real time. *Science Education, 89*(4), 675-702.

Vinney, L. A., & Harvey, J. M. T. (2017). Bridging the gap: An integrated approach to facilitating foundational learning of neuroanatomy and neurophysiology in graduate-level speech-language pathology coursework. *Teaching and Learning in Communication Sciences & Disorders, 1*(2), 1-24.

3

PRINT VERSUS DIGITAL TEXT
Considerations for Classroom and Clinical Teaching

Karen A. Fallon, PhD, CCC-SLP

DESCRIPTION OF TEACHING/LEARNING CONTEXT

The transition to a digital age has brought many changes to the academic landscape. Among these is an increased emphasis on the use of ebooks for academic reading. The availability of digital media for purchase, rental, and loan has increased substantially in recent years, offering benefits such as lower costs and increased convenience (e.g., accessibility, portability; Dalton, 2014; Daniel & Woody, 2013). At the postsecondary level, electronic/digital textbooks are an increasingly available alternative to traditional print textbooks. Electronic textbooks are often encouraged as a means to battle the growing costs of traditional textbooks and occasionally even required by some universities (Hamer & McGrath, 2011; Young, 2010). As with any transition, the growing push to incorporate digital media into our reading practices leads to important questions concerning the prudence of using electronic media platforms, particularly in educational contexts.

The current chapter examines the issue of reading in a university setting. Historically, university students have been asked to read and retain extensive amounts of written material presented at an advanced reading level (Hamer & McGrath, 2011). University instructors face important pedagogical decisions when designing didactic and clinical courses. Critical considerations include choosing the most effective platforms upon which to deliver academic information (e.g., ebooks versus print books), student reading practices, and student reading preferences. Evidence from the current literature base along with data from the present study will be used to discuss instructional implications for the university classroom and clinical teaching settings.

Friberg, J. C., Visconti, C. F., & Ginsberg, S. M. (Eds.). *Evidence-Based Education in the Classroom: Examples From Clinical Disciplines* (pp. 21-27).

REVIEW OF LITERATURE

With the advent of the digital age and the infusion of digital materials in academic settings, research on this topic has grown steadily in the last decade. One area of focus in this relatively new body of literature addresses the issue of text format (digital versus print). Research has focused on several questions including those of student preferences, effects of format on comprehension, and self-perceptions of ability with different text formats.

Text Format Preferences of University Students

It has long been anticipated that ebooks would replace traditional paper textbooks in university settings. However, the expected shift has yet to emerge (Cumaoglu et al., 2013; Dalton, 2014; Daniel & Woody, 2013). Although ebooks have recently commanded an increasing share of the general marketplace, their use has yet to grow substantially in university settings (National Association of College Bookstores, 2011). Existing research consistently suggests that electronic textbooks remain unpopular with undergraduate and graduate students and that overwhelmingly, college students prefer to read print over digital text for academic reading (Daniel & Woody, 2013; Kong et al., 2018; Mizrachi et al., 2018; Woody et al., 2010). A preference for print seems to increase when required to read longer text passages, such as in academic textbook reading (Kong et al., 2018; Mizrachi et al., 2018) A survey by the National Association of College Bookstores (2011) reports that university students prefer paper texts to electronic textbooks for textbook reading. Several reported reasons for students' reluctance to adopt digital textbooks include eye strain, a tendency to become distracted with other web activities (e.g., email, surfing the internet), and insufficient cost savings (Dalton, 2014; Myrberg & Wiberg, 2015; Young, 2010).

Reading Comprehension

Studies present a mixed picture of the effect of text format on reading comprehension and retention of material. Some studies suggest that students comprehend more from paper-based reading material (Akbar et al., 2015; Delgado et al., 2018; Kong et al., 2018; Myrberg & Wiberg, 2015; Rasmusson, 2015). This research suggests that experiences and performance tend to be task specific, reporting that performance can be affected by several moderators including the length of the reading passage, time constraints, and the text genre (e.g., expository versus narrative). Specifically, studies suggest a print advantage for longer text passages, time-constrained tasks (as opposed to self-paced), and expository/informational texts (Delgado et al., 2018; Kong et al., 2018).

One hypothesis to explain a potential advantage for better comprehension from printed text is that people tend to use a more shallow processing style when reading digital text. This "shallowing hypothesis" (Annisette & Lafreniere, 2017) suggests that people's typical interaction with digital text involves quick interactions with immediate rewards (e.g., Google search, number of hits on social media) rather than deep processing that requires sustained attention. Because of this, people tend to interact more "shallowly" with digital material (Annisette & Lafreniere, 2017) and are therefore less likely to use digital text for more challenging, in-depth reading tasks.

Although several recent studies suggest a print advantage for reading comprehension, there is also a significant database that indicates there is no difference between the two platforms (Hamer & McGrath, 2011; Kretzschmar et al., 2013; Margolin, 2013; McVicker, 2019; Taylor, 2011; Yi-Chin et al., 2014). These studies support the assertion that text format does not affect comprehension ability in secondary and postsecondary students. Margolin (2013) compared reading comprehension ability across three mediums (computer screen, e-reader, and paper text) and found similar text comprehension among the three formats. With no clear superior platform for comprehension and the potential for moderating factors to affect performance, the research on student perceptions and preferences for text format warrants consideration.

Self-Perceptions of Reading Ability in University Students

Although general comprehension ability (i.e., the ability to score satisfactorily on a quiz that measures understanding of reading material) does not appear to be affected by text format, research suggests other factors that may potentially affect the reading process. Studies that have investigated student perceptions of their reading ability relative to text format have found a perceived difference in text format, with university students feeling that they perform better when reading paper-based text (Daniel & Woody, 2013; Hamer & McGrath, 2011).

In explanation of these perceptions, university students consistently cite distractibility as a primary impeding factor of digital text. Study participants frequently report that they have difficulty concentrating and controlling their urge to engage in other web-based activities, such as checking email or other social media when it is all a "click away" (Hamer & McGrath, 2011). Participants also report a memory advantage with printed text (Myrberg & Wiberg, 2015) suggesting that handling the paper reading materials, taking handwritten notes, and marking the text (e.g., underlining, circling) aids the learning process. Perceived health and physical issues including eye strain, light sensitivity, and headaches are also cited in the literature as factors leading to perceptions of paper text as a superior format (Daniel & Woody, 2013; Margolin, 2013).

ORIGINAL DATA

With a continuously growing digital culture, it is important that the research literature provides evidence to guide practitioners and educators in the most effective implementation of various text formats. The present study sought to add to the relatively small text format database and address current questions of an evolving digital age as they relate to university student learning.

Research Questions

The current study used a survey design to investigate the following research questions:
- Which text format (print or digital) do university students use most frequently for academic reading?
- Which text format (print or digital) do university students prefer for academic reading?
- What are the reasons for the text format practices and preferences of university students?

Method

Participants in the study included 262 college students ranging in age from 18 to 30 years. The participants all attended a mid-sized state university in central Maryland. Participants were recruited via email, social media, and face-to-face requests. The survey consisted of a 30-item online questionnaire developed using the Anthology web-based platform. Participants of the study were asked to complete a 3- to 5-minute web-based survey with questions focused on their reading format preferences and practices. Questions also gathered data concerning the reasons for students' preferences and practices. The Anthology survey system was used to distribute and collate survey results.

Results

A total of 234 completed surveys were collected and analyzed using descriptive statistics. Overwhelmingly, students preferred paper-based formats to digital text formats with 83% of participants (n = 202) reporting that they prefer print to digital text for academic reading. With respect to text practices, university students reported that they use paper-based text with greater frequency than electronic textbooks with 98% (n = 230) of participants reporting regular use of paper textbooks and only 56% (n = 132) of students indicating that they had used an electronic textbook for one or more classes.

The most common reasons students preferred paper-based print included: (1) less eye strain when reading print than when reading digital text, (2) better comprehension of the material when reading print, (3) greater ability to attend to the reading task without the distractions of the internet, and (4) fewer headaches when reading print. When students reported a preference for digital text ($n = 31$), they cited convenience/portability, accessibility, and lower cost as the top reasons for preferring electronic text.

Data further showed that the frequency of the textbook use or necessity for success in a given class was a factor in student preferences. Specifically, participants indicated that when a book was used frequently for exams and assignments, students preferred to have a paper copy of the textbook. If the book was not utilized frequently, students would rather have the convenience and cost savings of an electronic textbook. In other words, if students were actually going to need the book to be successful in a class, they preferred a paper copy.

Application of Literature/Data

Although the majority of the participant sample consists of "digital natives" (i.e., a generation of individuals who have grown up in a digital era surrounded by digital technology such as computers and the internet; Prensky, 2001), respondents strongly preferred and more frequently used print over digital text formats for academic reading. These results are consistent with the current literature base and further offer important implications for higher education and classroom pedagogy.

Print Still Has Its Place

The first and most apparent implication is the importance of offering university students a print option for all academic reading materials. Results from the current study show a continued trend of university students to prefer printed text despite predictions that university students would eventually become acclimated to digital formats. Students prefer paper and perceive this as a format that will more successfully facilitate text comprehension and learning. University students worldwide report that they feel they focus, learn, and retain printed information better than information presented via digital formats. The issue of distractibility was the most frequently cited problem for students in the current study who reported that access to the web and other digital functions presented too great a temptation and impeded the reading and retention process. Health considerations including eye strain and headaches add further data to suggest the need to hit pause on the growing push to move academic texts to a digital format.

Consider Moderating Factors When Implementing Digital Text

Although students prefer a paper format, it has become nearly impossible to ignore digital technologies in contemporary educational settings. Further, some researchers suggest that student preferences may not be the best criteria upon which to make pedagogical decisions (Daniel & Woody, 2013) because students often make learning decisions based on efficiency rather than effectiveness (Gurung et al., 2010; Wesp & Miele, 2008). Additionally, performance on reading comprehension tasks may not necessarily align with self-perceptions of learning (Mizrachi et al., 2018). So, although student preferences should be taken into consideration, it is also important to consider learning effectiveness when selecting text formats.

With no clear picture offered by the current literature regarding the most effective text format, the data from the current study and existing literature base suggest the need for educators to use a variety of text formats to support the needs of diverse learners. In addition, it is important for educators to understand the moderating factors that can affect learning and retention and design classroom and clinical instruction accordingly. Specifically, instructors designing university courses should take the following into consideration:

- Length of text passages: Research suggests that university students prefer print and comprehend and retain information presented in print better when the text passages are longer (Kong et al., 2018). Therefore, when reading textbook assignments, research articles, etc., it is important that students be afforded a print option. Conversely, when shorter amounts of text are called for, digital formats may be more acceptable.
- Text genre: The potential print advantage for informational texts should also be considered. More complex, information-rich text may be better suited to print formats, whereas less complex more straightforward classroom activities (e.g., lab exercises, Kahoot! quizzes) may be more suited to convenient digital formats (e.g., phones, tablets, laptops).
- Time constraints: Research suggests that students struggle more with digital-based tasks when under a timed condition but perform better if the task is untimed (Sidi et al., 2017). Studies also suggest that students are often overconfident with digital-based reading, which leads to poorer learning outcomes (Ackerman & Lauterman, 2012; Sidi et al., 2017). Educators should consider making digital tasks (e.g., quizzes and exams) untimed.

Teach Students to Be Metacognitive Learners

Although the majority of today's university students are digital natives, research consistently suggests that they may struggle with the challenge of effectively using digital texts for learning. It is important for students to understand the pros and cons of both print and digital text formats and how to apply each format effectively. This requires that students have the metacognitive knowledge to be aware of which type of print format works best for them and the metacognitive regulation to use strategies that best support effective learning. Although university professors often take for granted that their students are independent, self-regulated learners, empirical evidence indicates that this is not always the case and that metacognitive strategies can and should be taught to university students (Isakson & Isakson, 2017; Jairam & Kiewra, 2009)

Research consistently suggests that learners can be taught metacognitive strategies and that, in doing so, learning can be improved (Biemiller & Meichenbaum,1992; Nietfeld & Shraw, 2002; Thiede et al., 2003). Readers will need to implement metacognitive strategies to maximize their comprehension and retention of text using a variety of text formats. University instructors can assist in this process by designing university courses to include some guidance on strategies to optimize learning by providing strategies for successful print reading versus screen reading. Some specific strategies for both print and electronic format (Hamer & McGrath, 2011) may include:

- Read chapter headings and subheadings
- Clarify purpose
- Access background knowledge
- Look at/review graphics
- Read end-of-chapter summaries and questions
- Take and reread notes
- Reread portions of text
- Define words
- Review graphics

When considering which strategies to choose for each format, research suggests that some strategies may be more effective for electronic screen reading and others for reading print. Instructors can provide instruction and modeling of strategies that support both comprehension as well as concentration (Hamer & McGrath, 2011). It is also important that instructors remain flexible in their promotion of strategy use and encourage students to use the strategies that work best for them relative to the print format. For this application, it is critically important that students possess well-developed metacognitive awareness so that they can most effectively select and apply strategies that will be most effective for their learning.

ADDITIONAL RESOURCES

- American Institutes for Research, & Literacy Information and Communication System. (2015, August). *Promoting teacher effectiveness: Evidence-based instruction and teacher induction.* https://lincs.ed.gov/publications/te/ebi.pdf
- Jabr, F. (2013, April 11). The reading brain in the digital age: The science of paper versus screens. *Scientific American.* https://www.scientificamerican.com/article/reading-paper-screens/
- Mangen, A., Walgermo, B. R., & Brønnick, K. (2013). Reading linear texts on paper versus computer screen: Effects on reading comprehension, *International Journal of Educational Research, 58,* 61-68.
- Mohktari, K. (2017). *Improving reading comprehension through metacognitive reading strategies instruction.* Rowman & Littlefield.
- Pressley, M., & Afflerbach, P. (1995). *Verbal protocols of reading: The nature of constructively responsive reading.* Lawrence Erlbaum.
- Singer, L., & Alexander, P. (2017). Reading across mediums: Effects of reading digital and print texts on comprehension and calibration. *Journal of Experimental Education, 85*(1), 155-172.

ACKNOWLEDGMENTS

The author gratefully acknowledges Morgan Schmincke, McKenzie Sesterhenn Ochoa, Katrina Vain, and Amanda Keister for their contributions to the project.

REFERENCES

Ackerman, R., & Lauterman, T. (2012). Taking reading comprehension exams on screen or on paper? A metacognitive analysis of learning texts under time pressure. *Computers in Human Behavior, 28,* 1816-1828.

Akbar, R., Taqi, H., Dashti, A., & Sadeq, T. (2015). Does e-reading enhance reading fluency? *English Language Teaching, 8*(5), 195-207.

Annisette, L., & Lafreniere, K. (2017). Social media, texting, and personality: A test of the shallowing hypothesis. *Personality and Individual Differences, 115,* 154-158.

Biemiller, A., & Meichenbaum, D. (1992). The nature and nurture of the self-directed learner. *Educational Leadership, 50,* 75-80.

Cumaoglu, G., Sacici, E., & Torun, K. (2013). E-book vs. printed materials: The preferences of university students. *Contemporary Educational Technology, 4*(2), 121-135.

Dalton, B. (2014). E-text and e-books are changing the literacy landscape. *Phi Delta Kappan, 96*(3), 38-43.

Daniel, D., & Woody, W. (2013). E-textbooks at what cost? Performance and use of electronic v. print texts. *Computers and Education, 62,* 18-23.

Delgado, P., Vargas, C., Ackerman, R., & Salmeron, L., (2018). Don't throw away your printed books: A meta-analysis on the effects of reading media on reading comprehension. *Educational Research Review, 25,* 23-38.

Gurung, R., Wiedert, J., & Jeske, A. (2010). Focusing on how students study. *Journal of the Scholarship of Teaching and Learning, 10*(1), 28-35.

Hamer, A., & McGrath, J. (2011). On-screen versus on-paper reading: Students' strategy usage and preferences. *NADE Digest, 5*(3), 25-39.

Isakson, R., & Isakson, M. (2017). Preparing college students to learn more from academic texts through metacognitive awareness of reading strategies. In K. Mokhtari (Ed.), *Improving reading comprehension through metacognitive reading strategies instruction* (pp. 155-176). Rowman & Littlefield.

Jairam, D., & Kiewra, K. A. (2009). An investigation of the SOAR study method. *Journal of Advanced Academics, 20*(4), 602-629.

Kong, Y., Seo, Y., & Zhai, L. (2018). Comparison of reading performance on screen and on paper: A meta-analysis. *Computers & Education, 123,* 138-149

Kretzschmar, F., Pleimling, D., Hosemann, J., Füssel, S., Bornkessel-Schlesewsky, I., & Schlesewsky, M. (2013). Subjective impressions do not mirror online reading effort: Concurrent EEG-eyetracking evidence from the reading of books and digital media. *PLoS ONE, 8*(2), e56178. https://doi.org/10.1371/journal.pone.0056178

Margolin, S. L. (2013). E-readers, computer screens, or paper: Does reading comprehension change across media platforms? *Applied Cognitive Psychology, 27*(4), 512-519.

McVicker, C. J. (2019). Plugged and unplugged readers: Studying the preferences of readers. *The Reading Teacher, 72*(6), 731-740.

Mizrachi, D., Salaz, A., Kurbanoglu, S., & Boustany, J. (2018). Academic reading format preferences and behaviors among university students worldwide: A comparative survey analysis. *PLoS ONE, 13*(5), 1-32.

Myrberg, C., & Wiberg, N. (2015). Screen vs. paper: What is the difference for reading and learning? *Insights: The UKSG Journal, 28*(2), 49-54. http://doi.org/10.1629/uksg.236

National Association of College Bookstores. (2011, March). *UPDATE: Electronic book and eReader device report March 2011.* https://docplayer.net/19120662-Update-electronic-book-and-ereader-device-report-march-2011.html

Nietfeld, J. L., & Shraw, G. (2002). The effect of knowledge and strategy explanation on monitoring accuracy. *Journal of Educational Research, 95,* 131-142.

Prensky, M. (2001). Digital natives, digital immigrants part 1. *On the Horizon, 9*(5), 1-6. https://doi.org/10.1108/10748120110424816

Rasmusson, M. (2015). Reading paper-reading screen: A comparison of reading literacy in two different modes. *Nordic Studies in Education, 34*(1), 3-119.

Sidi, Y., Shpigelman, M., Salmanov, H., & Ackerman, R. (2017). Understanding metacognitive inferiority on screen by exposing cues for depth of processing. *Learning and Instruction, 51,* 61-73.

Taylor, A. K. (2011). Students learn equally well from digital as from paperbound texts. *Teaching of Psychology, 38,* 278-281.

Thiede, K. W., Anderson, M. C., & Therriault, D. (2003). Accuracy of metacognitive monitoring affects learning of texts. *Journal of Educational Psychology, 95,* 66-73.

Wesp, R., & Miele, J. (2008). Student opinion of the quality of teaching activities poorly predicts pedagogical effectiveness. *Teaching of Psychology, 35,* 360-362.

Woody, W., Daniel, D., & Baker, C. (2010). E-books or textbooks? Students prefer textbooks. *Computers and Education, 55,* 945-948.

Yi-Chin, L., Yu-Ling, L., & Ying-Shao, H. (2014). The effects of meta-cognitive instruction on students' reading comprehension in computerized reading contexts: A quantitative meta-analysis. *Educational Technology & Society, 17*(4), 186-202.

Young, J. R. (2010, October 24). The end of the textbook as we know it. *The Chronicle of Higher Education.* https://www.chronicle.com/article/to-save-students-money-colleges-may-force-a-switch-to-e-textbooks/

4

ESTABLISHING SUCCESSFUL CO-TEACHING RELATIONSHIPS

Jennifer C. Friberg, EdD, CCC-SLP, F-ASHA
and Lisa A. Vinney, PhD, CCC-SLP

DESCRIPTION OF TEACHING/LEARNING CONTEXT

Several semesters ago, we developed an independent study experience for undergraduate students in our speech-language pathology program. This independent study was borne through a unique set of circumstances that unfolded in three distinct phases, each described in the following list. These are described in what might seem at first glance to be unnecessarily deep detail; however, the subsequent literature review on the topic of co-teaching later in this chapter will bear out the need for our expertise, perspectives, and collegiality:

1. Supportive colleagues: Our initial collaboration together had nothing to do with teaching, but rather with providing support at a difficult time. One of us (Friberg), sought out support from the other (Vinney) to help with an urgent matter. In the spring of 2014, Friberg's mother was diagnosed with advanced laryngeal cancer, and while treatment for this disease certainly falls into a speech-language pathologist's scope of practice, Friberg's expertise lay elsewhere. Looking for answers to difficult questions about the potential impact and outcome of this disease, she approached her colleague (Vinney) for help, as Vinney's areas of professional, teaching, and research expertise directly related to structures and functions affected by laryngeal cancer. Vinney provided support and consultation for Friberg and her family throughout her mother's illness. Our professional relationship was built from these shared experiences.

2. Scholarly collaborators: Across our conversations, we realized that there was no resource available for practitioners or patients/families that discussed the interdisciplinary management of laryngeal cancer. We decided to embark upon a scholarly collaboration, coediting a text representing ways in which professionals, patients, and families interact together following a

Friberg, J. C., Visconti, C. F., & Ginsberg, S. M. (Eds.). *Evidence-Based Education in the Classroom: Examples From Clinical Disciplines* (pp. 29-37).
© 2021 Taylor & Francis Group.

laryngeal cancer diagnosis (Friberg & Vinney, 2017). Our goal for this project was to create a resource that allowed professionals and patients/families to better understand the management of laryngeal cancer. Thus, while one of us (Vinney) was the content expert on the disease of laryngeal cancer, the other (Friberg) served as an expert on the patient/family experience in the management of this condition. Both perspectives were well represented throughout this project.

3. Pedagogical co-facilitators: Now experienced collaborators, we noted that the topic of laryngeal cancer was not one that most undergraduate students had exposure to or experience with as part of their program's curriculum. Knowing that students in our department were always interested in independent study opportunities focused on varied special topics, we worked to develop an independent study for students interested in focused learning about the interprofessional management of laryngeal cancer.

This chapter describes the development of our co-teaching relationship that evolved over time as a result of a series of professional interactions, with a discussion of how we planned and executed our co-taught independent study course. Suggestions for ways in which high-quality co-teaching experiences may be cultivated across clinical disciplines are presented, with a focus on developing a valid rationale for co-teaching and fostering interpersonal relationships to support such endeavors.

REVIEW OF LITERATURE

Co-teaching is defined as instruction facilitated by two persons forming a collaborative relationship to engage in shared work (preparation for and delivery of instruction) with a resultant product that could not have been reached alone (Wenzlaff et al., 2002). Historically, co-teaching has been underused and understudied at the university level. Much of the research and pedagogy of co-teaching originates from K–12 educational models in an effort to address the needs of students qualifying for special education services alongside peers who do not qualify for these services (Bacharach et al., 2008). There are a variety of K–12 co-teaching models (Bacharach et al., 2008; Lock et al., 2017) that stem from this need, described as:

- One teach, one observe: One teacher takes on the main responsibility for instruction while the second instructor observes students and the primary instructor for specific behaviors
- One teach, one drift: While one teacher takes on the role of instructor, the other circulates around the room to help students with learning activities by providing input, facilitating desired student behavior, or grading assignments
- Station teaching: Stations are set up in which each instructor teaches one section of the content while the students rotate through the stations spending an allotted amount of time at each
- Parallel teaching: The ratio of students to instructor is reduced by having both instructors address the same material but with a different set of students
- Supplemental teaching: The needs of all students are addressed within one classroom by one instructor working with those students on grade-level instruction, while the other instructor works with students requiring extra support
- Differentiated teaching: Each instructor teaches the content using a different pedagogical technique in order to provide students with alternatives for mastering content
- Team teaching: Each teacher provides instruction alongside the other and both are equally available to address students' needs

The models described previously may be hard to conceptualize in a university setting for a number of reasons. University teaching loads are traditionally calculated based on the idea of one instructor for one class, providing challenges to course and other assignments. Adding to this, many of the models listed above require only one primary instructor. Thus, it is difficult to determine how a separate instructor's responsibilities would be treated (or "counted") in a university context. Similarly, faculty members often specialize in content that no other member of their faculty may have expertise in, making differentiated and team teaching difficult. Finally, college instruction has traditionally been designed with the expectation that each student requires less individual attention and should take on more responsibility for their learning. Thus, models in which co-teaching is put into place to decrease class sizes or provide additional forms of support may be considered unnecessary by university administrations.

Morelock and colleagues (2017) describe an alternating model of co-teaching in which course planning and pedagogy, assignment and assessment design, and grading responsibilities are shared, but the instruction of each class session is provided individually by one of the co-teachers. This model may more easily map onto calculating collegiate teaching loads (i.e., each instructor might be given credit for teaching half of a class), allowing co-teachers the opportunity to collaborate in determining how the course will be executed and how content connects while still teaching sessions on topics where they have expertise and interest. The major pitfall of this approach is the potential for faculty members to create two courses in one in an effort to be efficient in course planning and execution. In this scenario, co-teachers create two mini-courses, with one instructor teaching the course for a span of weeks, followed by the other instructor taking over for an equal span of weeks. Attention to the co-teaching relationship, conceptualization of the class, and expectations for co-teaching may never be communicated. Instead, each instructor may develop all or part of their instruction, its methods, assignments, and grading strategies in a vacuum. While this approach may save faculty members time, it does not fit the definition of co-teaching (i.e., the teaching relationship is not collaborative, and preparation and delivery of instruction is not shared). Furthermore, the instructional product is not likely to lead to a project that a faculty member could not achieve on their own, as simply dividing the course into two does not satisfy this requirement. Teaching in this way is a missed opportunity that forgoes the advantages of co-teaching (i.e., strengthening educational opportunities for students and enriching faculty's development as scholars and teachers) and instead leads to many challenges highlighted in the literature (i.e., students' confusion over differing expectations, communication, and teaching styles and power struggles between faculty).

Given the earlier information, it is no surprise that much of the research literature in this area is focused on the importance of a sustained and shared relationship between co-teachers (Bacharach et al., 2008; Ferguson & Wilson, 2011; Hsieh & Nguyen, 2015; Lock et al., 2017; Morelock et al., 2017). Successful co-teaching relationships have been described as:

- Contributing differing expertise, backgrounds, perspectives, and styles to the same course; thus, creating a course that neither co-teacher could have executed in isolation
- Encouraging collaboration and discussion in students as well as the instructors
- Establishing trust, respect, and openness
- Viewing the co-teaching relationship as ever-evolving rather than static
- Respectfully communicating and establishing clear expectations about differences of opinion; the sharing of power; and challenges in course development, delivery, and assessment
- Addressing conflicts and their resolutions in a timely manner
- Debriefing about each class period to discuss those elements that worked and those that did not
- Sharing and executing a unified vision for the course
- Holding similar values about teaching and education and approaches toward students and their learning

APPLICATION OF LITERATURE/DATA

Though we had engaged in and observed co-teaching efforts in the past, many of these were in conflict with evidence-informed practices identified in relevant literature. It was evident that extant research on the topic of co-teaching very clearly pointed toward the need to avoid common pitfalls of co-teaching (e.g., splitting a course into two separate parts, using different assessment schemes, establishing different instructor expectations for students) and work toward an ideal where collaborative planning, effective communication, and a mutual vision of the learning context were shared by both co-teachers. Thus, we focused on three main areas in designing our co-teaching experience, each of which are discussed in the following sections.

Different Areas of Expertise

From the description of our teaching/learning context at the start of this chapter, it is evident that we had different types of expertise to bring to the co-teaching of the independent study experience. One of us (Vinney), as an individual with a specialty (both in clinic and in research) on voice and voice disorders, had robust professional knowledge about laryngeal cancer. She could clearly articulate how the communication, respiration, and nutrition of patients with laryngeal cancer could be compromised and how patients with such effects could best be treated. Conversely, the other of us (Friberg) was also a speech-language pathologist; however, her 20 years of professional practice had focused exclusively on clients from school-based populations. While her content expertise in terms of laryngeal cancer was lacking, as the daughter of a laryngeal cancer patient, she could share valuable expertise: the close and personal effect of the disease in the day-to-day lives of patients and their families. We found these different areas of expertise to be synergistic for two reasons. First, we had no competing priorities for the content of the independent study. We agreed easily on important topics to cover and were confident that our own perspectives, though different, would allow students to understand a complex disease with depth. Second, we were excited that our students would have a patient narrative (Friberg's mother) to help connect the different topics of our independent study and help students better understand how theoretical content was applied in the real world.

Content Planning

We took very seriously the initial design of our independent study, consciously setting aside time to collaboratively organize our efforts. Initially, we brainstormed ideas about content we felt was critical to our independent study and how that content might be best ordered to illustrate the management of laryngeal cancer. In terms of planning content for our independent study, we focused our discussions on the following topics:

- Course learning outcomes: Our first conversations around the topic of developing this independent study focused on what we hoped students would learn through enrollment in this experience. We had more latitude here than many co-teachers do, as our learning context was an independent study rather than a required course in our program's curriculum. Thus, we could develop any sort of learning outcomes we felt were important for students around our selected topic. Across our discussions, we weighed which topics were reasonable for undergraduate students to learn and which ones might be most impactful. In the end, we focused on facilitating students' deepened understanding of the roles/responsibilities of speech-language pathologists working with patients diagnosed with laryngeal cancer and other stakeholders involved in the management of this disease.

- Setting up a structure: Because this was an independent study, we were able to customize specific factors of our co-teaching context. We determined that this would be a 1 (academic) credit offering for students, and that we would organize our independent study into weekly, 1-hour meetings over the course of a semester. We used our coedited textbook as a required reading for the course but did identify supplemental materials that we wanted our students to have access to, as well. In establishing a structure for our independent study, we also determined that we would only offer participation in the independent study to students who had either completed or were concurrently enrolled in our department's undergraduate voice disorders course. This was important to ensure that all students had an underlying understanding of laryngeal anatomy and physiology to truly benefit from their independent study experience.

- Assignment/alignment of content: Once we had our learning outcomes and basic independent study structure developed, we brainstormed a list of topics we felt were critical to include in our independent study. We organized these topics into a timeline that helped us to tell the story of a patient's experience with laryngeal cancer, moving from symptoms to diagnosis to treatment selection, with end-of-life care discussed, as well. We thought carefully about whether both of us needed to be at all independent study meetings, or if we might be able to assign different topics to each of us to manage separately. In the end, we opted to both be present for our first independent study meeting to explain to students our different experiences and expertise with laryngeal cancer. Subsequent independent study meetings were assigned to each of us individually to facilitate, although we relied on one another to help plan cases and discussions for each session so that both our perspectives were represented. We also chose to include a graduate teaching assistant as a co-facilitator for several of our independent study meetings, as well.

- Pedagogical approaches: While there are myriad approaches to evidence-based teaching that might have worked for our independent study students, we prioritized the selection of pedagogical approaches that would allow for deep discussions about the management of laryngeal cancer. It was our goal that students would complete assigned readings in advance of each meeting and that our weekly meetings would be used to explain and expand on that material. We started each meeting with a brief question and answer session (15 minutes) to clear up anything that was "muddy" from assigned readings. Following this, each meeting used a mix of case studies (to give students exposure to an array of patient types, severities, etc.) and perspective-taking, which allowed students to view laryngeal cancer from a variety of different lenses. Thus, the majority of each independent study meeting was spent discussing cases and integrating content into these discussions.

- Assessment schemes: Because the structure of the independent study was driven by discussion and critical thinking about the topic of laryngeal cancer, we wanted our assessment scheme to be similarly oriented. We discussed ways in which we might encourage students to reflect on their learning metacognitively, with a focus on helping students to tie new learning from the independent study to prior knowledge from their courses and experiences in light of our course objectives. To that end, we agreed that assessment through weekly reflection papers was ideal to address each students' questions and thinking about the independent study content. We established a set of five questions that students responded to each week based on their readings and our subsequent group discussions (see Additional Resources section for these questions). We determined that the facilitator each week would take the lead in providing feedback for these reflections. Interestingly, while we were able to keep to this plan most of the time, there were times student reflections would necessitate feedback from both of us in order to access our individual expertise. In those situations, we would collaboratively provide feedback to address students' needs.

Communication Planning

Once we had planned the independent study content, it was important that we navigate communication planning strategically, recognizing a need to clarify expectations for each other and creating understandable processes for our students. We explain both processes separately in the following sections.

Co-Teacher to Co-Teacher Communication

As part of our initial planning process, we set up a series of planning meetings to negotiate content planning. These meetings served to design the structure and timeline for our independent study. While we agreed on general pedagogical approaches, we met frequently throughout the first semester this independent study was offered to develop cases for our independent study meetings and envision how these cases would be used with our students. Email was used, as needed, for smaller clarifications.

Communication With Students

More complicated was determining how we would communicate with students because we sought to eliminate any confusion they might feel about who was "in charge" of any aspect of the independent study. To be consistent, we agreed that only one of us (Vinney) would serve as the instructor of record. At our institution, the instructor of record is the individual who receives credit for teaching a course. We note here that we could have easily split students so that both of us received teaching credit for this independent study experience; however, we determined it was easier for one person to act in this role for our specific needs. Thus, Vinney took the lead on sending periodic organizational emails to students and submitting final grades at the end of each semester.

We also developed a detailed syllabus for the independent study experience. While it featured a section with the course timeline and assigned readings, the majority of the document outlined how the independent study would be managed, expectations for students participating in the independent study, and explanations for completing and submitting weekly reflection papers. This seemed to allay student confusion as to which co-teacher was in charge of various topics or sections of the independent study. The syllabus also included guidance to students, such as, "When in doubt, feel free to email both Dr. Vinney and Dr. Friberg and the appropriate person will answer your question." We felt this invitation was critical, as we wanted students to feel welcome to ask questions, even when they were unsure who to address them to.

APPLICATION TO CROSS-DISCIPLINARY CONTEXTS

In higher education, academic programs for most clinical disciplines employ a mix of academic and clinical educators to scaffold student learning in the classroom and in the clinic. We firmly believe that within these contexts, the notion of shared expertise is fairly universal, in that recognition of others' specialized areas of clinical knowledge/expertise allows for wholesale preparation of future professionals. Co-teaching is simply another opportunity to harness the expertise of two or more individuals to educate students well. We would argue that while the content of co-taught courses is necessarily quite different, the considerations for planning and implementing evidence-informed co-teaching are very similar. The following list presents considerations—from our literature review and from our own experiences co-teaching together—we believe are critical to address as part of planning any co-taught experience:

- Start with your "why." Students need to understand why a course is being co-taught from the very start of the course. They are likely nervous about differing instructor expectations, grading, and processes. Sharing the expected benefits of a co-taught course helps students understand the importance of the course design and its potential positive effects on their own learning. Assuring students that all course instructors communicate frequently and have a process that can be easily articulated for grading and feedback is helpful, as well.

- Co-teaching should not be something imposed upon course instructors if it does not make sense. Literature firmly and strongly supports the need for decisions related to the establishment of a co-teaching relationship to be founded in need and benefit, rather than by any other administrative priority or need.

- Clinical disciplines often seek out (through interest or external need, such as accreditation expectations) interprofessional education (IPE) opportunities for students. IPE is a perfect setup for co-teaching, as professionals from different disciplines certainly bring different forms of expertise to planning such experiences; however, we would urge that co-taught IPE courses should take care to reflect best practices from the literature.

- We would suggest that students be considered as possible co-teachers. Many faculty members utilize students as teaching assistants; however, they often lack ownership of any part of the teaching design process. Rather, teaching assistants are told what they will teach and how they should teach it. We suggest that teaching assistants be made partners in the process of deciding how a course will be designed and implemented in order to maximize benefits for all stakeholders.

- Think about your institution's processes and procedures for assigning and giving credit for teaching loads before embarking on co-teaching. In our case, one of us served as the instructor of record and received credit for leading our independent study experience. This worked for us but might not work for all.

- This last notion may be our most important piece of advice: Choose your co-teaching partner with care. Notice we say "choose," rather than have your co-teacher "chosen" for you! We firmly believe our co-teaching experiences have been positive and impactful for our students because we have been aligned in philosophy and practice, something we knew would be the case from our past professional experiences together. Being assigned to work with a colleague you have little experience with might not result in a similar type of synergy, which might affect you and/or your students negatively.

ADDITIONAL RESOURCES

- Suggested reading:
  ○ Morelock, J. R., Lester, M. M. G., Klopfer, M. D., Jardon, A. M., Mullins, R. D., Nicholas, E. L., & Alfaydi, A. S. (2017). Power, perceptions, and relationships: A model of co-teaching in higher education. *College Teaching, 65*(4), 182-191. https://doi.org/10.1080/87567555.2017.1 336610 (Table 4-1)

- Information on co-teaching from the University of California at Berkeley's teaching and learning center:
  ○ https://teaching.berkeley.edu/resources/engage/co-teaching

- Podcast by chapter authors on topic of co-teaching:
  ○ https://ctlt.illinoisstate.edu/podcast/2019/ep052.shtml

TABLE 4-1

Best Practices for Collegiate Co-Teaching That Serve as a Valuable Reference for Common Co-Teaching Issues/Initial Considerations

EVIDENCE-BASED INSIGHTS	RECOMMENDATIONS FOR PRACTICE
Reduced teaching credit from co-teaching can be problematic for promotion and tenure and may not reflect the actual reduction in workload.	Verify with administration the value placed on the co-teaching experience and any implications for the promotion and/or tenure process. Understand that adding a second teacher to a course will rarely reduce the workload by half.
Establishing compatibility with one's partner is important to maintain a strong, communicative relationship.	Select a co-teaching partner with whom you know you can build or broaden a compatible relationship. A good launching point for a co-teaching partnership might be a different form of collaboration (e.g., research partnership).
Joint planning of all co-taught content is critical to ensure that a course is cohesive and runs smoothly.	Establish a process for how the course will be developed, delivered, and assessed in the planning stages with your co-teaching partner.
Unresolved differences in teaching philosophies can strain the co-teaching relationship.	Develop a joint teaching philosophy for the co-teaching experience to ensure each partner understands the other's perspectives regarding the experience.
Students unfamiliar with co-teaching may be confused about what to expect.	Establish expectations for communicating with students regarding the course's content, activities, grading, and general advice.
Students may not understand why the class is being co-taught or how they can benefit.	Explain the benefits of co-teaching to your students and the reasons you decided to teach the course in this structure. Make sure to explicitly state why co-teaching is the best model and how expertise of all co-teachers contributes value to the course experiences.

Adapted from Morelock, J. R., Lester, M. M., Klopfer, M. D., Jardon, A. M., Mullins, R. D., Nicholas, E. L., & Alfaydi, A. S. (2017). Power, perceptions, and relationships: A model of co-teaching in higher education. *College Teaching, 65*(4), 182-191.

REFERENCES

Bacharach, N., Heck, T. W., & Dahlberg, K. (2008). Co-teaching in higher education. *Journal of College Teaching and Learning, 5*(3), 9-16.

Ferguson, J., & Wilson, J. C. (2011). The co-teaching professorship: Power and expertise in the co-taught higher education classroom. *Scholar-Practitioner Quarterly, 5*(1), 52-68.

Friberg, J. C., & Vinney, L. A. (2017). *Laryngeal cancer: An interdisciplinary resource for practitioners.* SLACK Incorporated.

Hsieh, B., & Nguyen, H. (2015). Co-teaching, co-leading, co-learning: Reflecting on the co-teaching model in practicum. *Teaching and Learning Together in Higher Education, 1*(14), 1-10.

Lock, J., Clancy, T., Lisella, R., Rosenau, P., Ferreira, C., & Rainsbury, J. (2017). The lived experiences of instructors co-teaching in higher education. *Brock Education Journal, 26*(1), 22-35. https://doi.org/10.26522/brocked.v26i1.482

Morelock, J. R., Lester, M. M. G., Klopfer, M. D., Jardon, A. M., Mullins, R. D., Nicholas, E. L., & Alfaydi, A. S. (2017). Power, perceptions, and relationships: A model of co-teaching in higher education. *College Teaching, 65*(4), 182-191. https://doi.org/10.1080/87567555.2017.1336610

Wenzlaff, T., Berak, L., Wieseman, K., Monroe-Baillargeon, A. Bacharach, N., & Bradfield-Kreider, P. (2002). Walking our talk as educators: Teaming as a best practice. In E. Guyton, & J. Rainer (Eds.), *Research on meeting and using standards in the preparation of teachers* (pp. 11-24). Kendall-Hunt Publishing.

5

COLLABORATIVE COURSE (RE)DESIGN

Sarah M. Ginsberg, EdD, CCC-SLP, F-ASHA
and Lauren H. Mead, MA, CCC-SLP

DESCRIPTION OF TEACHING/LEARNING CONTEXT

Collaborative Course Design (CCD) was used to update and revise an existing graduate clinical methods course in a graduate speech-language pathology program. In an example of collaboration, this chapter has been written by the faculty member (Ginsberg) and a former student-collaborator (Mead). The course was a speech-language pathology clinical methodology course that had been taught for several years by the same professor. The purpose of the course was to prepare graduate students for their first clinical experience in the university's in-house clinic. However, for students coming from undergraduate speech-language pathology programs, the material felt redundant as they learned much of it in their undergraduate programs. Further, it was not entirely clear to the instructor that the course was adequately preparing graduate students to engage in the clinical process beyond the rudimentary mechanics of clinical methods, such as writing clinical documentation and structuring therapy sessions. The instructor also felt that the course was unsuccessful in that it lacked energy and enthusiasm on the part of both the teacher and the learners. A revision to the course was contemplated in order to increase the effectiveness and prepare students for their first clinical experience. The method for revising the course that was chosen was the use of CCD, or in this case, collaborative course redesign. This chapter shares information regarding how the literature was applied to the process as well as data that were collected from the collaborators and the students enrolled in the course following the redesign.

Friberg, J. C., Visconti, C. F., & Ginsberg, S. M. (Eds.). *Evidence-Based Education in the Classroom: Examples From Clinical Disciplines* (pp. 39-46).
© 2021 Taylor & Francis Group.

REVIEW OF LITERATURE

Collaboration among faculty and students involves enlisting students as equals in order to refine and advance classroom procedures. CCD represents a model for collaboration between instructors and learners in which they work collaboratively to develop specific aspects of a course, such as classroom procedures, course objectives, instructional design, and/or learning assessments (Bovill et al., 2011; Mead, 2018). Examples in the literature suggest that the collaborative course redesign process has been used to improve flagging student ratings (Mihans et al., 2008), to foster improved faculty insights and reflections on students' learning (Cook-Sather, 2008), and to improve course accessibility for a variety of learners (Aguirre & Duncan, 2013).

Several benefits of CCD have been suggested for both faculty members and for students. In working together collaboratively, faculty and students have an opportunity to develop a deeper appreciation of each other and of the teaching and learning process. Faculty gain insights into students' views of learning and the learning experience (Kane & Chimwayange, 2014). By engaging students in the course design process, faculty can develop insights into students' perspectives, knowledge, and application of the relevant content (Bovill et al., 2011; Mihans et al., 2008). This insight into the student perspective can help faculty members refine their teaching methods as well as their expectations of students. CCD can enhance student engagement and ownership in the teaching and learning process, which in turn deepens students' knowledge about course content and dedication to the teaching and learning process. Students may also feel incentivized to maximize their educational experience, as they feel the potential for ownership (Bovill et al., 2011, 2015; Hutchings, 2005; Mead, 2018).

Faculty and students working together collaboratively requires a significant paradigm shift in the dynamic between the participants. In order to be fully effective, students must be given the power to make changes to the course and must perceive that they have the ability to be effective in designing the targeted aspects of the course (Mead, 2018; Mihans et al., 2008). In essence, in order for the collaboration to be effective, both sides must recognize the value of each other's input and work as reciprocal partners. This process requires not only a shift in power and control, but for many faculty members, it requires what may be an uncomfortable relinquishing of control over the teaching process (Bovill et al., 2011; Hutchings, 2005; Mead, 2018; Mihans et al., 2008). The research offers several suggestions to guide the collaborative process for faculty who are looking to develop collaborations for course design and have not done so previously (Bovill et al., 2011, 2015, 2014; Cook-Sather, 2008). Faculty may find that starting with addressing a small portion of the course (e.g., one assessment) may be helpful. Another suggestion is to approach the process as a strictly voluntary one such that there is no pressure for students relative to grades. It is also important to remember that working together toward a common goal, such as designing a course, requires the development of rapport between all of the participants. Helping students feel like respected partners can be particularly critical to the success of the collaborative process (Mead, 2018). Carlile (2012) argued that "a constructive, dynamic and socially-just education requires the teacher and student to consider and make decisions together about how and where learning and schooling takes place" (p. 398). Student-faculty collaboration is one way that faculty members can incorporate student insight into the students' education.

APPLICATION OF LITERATURE/DATA

Given the suggested benefits of CCD and the potential for students to incorporate their insights into their education, CCD was selected as the method to redesign the clinical methods course. Student volunteers were solicited from students who had taken the clinical methodology course the previous semester. Four students volunteered, including Mead, and participated in a collaborative course redesign process with the faculty member, forming a committee and meeting weekly over the course of approximately 12 weeks. The process began with two key elements: (1) the students were explicitly informed that they were full and equal partners in the redesign process, and (2) they were given a set of materials that included the syllabus from the course and brief readings relevant to teaching and learning, specifically a summary of Wiggins and McTighe's (2005) description of backward design, an article regarding the use of authentic assessment (Wiggins, 1990), and a chapter specifically describing course design and preparation (Ginsberg et al., 2012). The first meeting began with a review and discussion regarding course design. For each of the following weeks, the course was redesigned following the backward design principles, beginning with identifying learning objectives that the students felt were needed in order to be successful in the subsequent clinical practica that they would be enrolled in (see Additional Resources). Learning objectives for the course were determined first, the committee then designed assessments of learning and planned appropriate learning activities once the assessments were completed (see Additional Resources). At no time did the faculty member exercise straight veto power regarding suggestions that the students made. Rather, all course design decisions were discussed and then mutually agreed upon once a consensus was reached.

At the end of the 12 weeks of committee work, the clinical methodology course had been redesigned with updated learning objectives, assessments of learning, and learning activities. The committee members reviewed and reflected on their work before developing a new syllabus. On the first day of the course the following semester, the student members of the committee joined the faculty member in class and discussed with the currently enrolled students how and why the course was designed the way it was. The student committee members shared with the current students the value that they felt the course held in preparing them for their clinical practica. The course was then taught for the rest of the semester by the faculty member.

ORIGINAL DATA

Two sets of qualitative data were collected: one set from the student committee members and one set from the students who had been enrolled in the redesigned course. Both studies were approved by the university institutional review board prior to data collection. The semester following the completion of the committee's work, the four committee members each agreed to an informal, qualitative interview with the faculty member to discuss how being a member of the CCD committee influenced their view of education. Analysis of the results suggested that the committee members perceived a strong benefit to them as students in that they found the insights into the educational process "eye opening" and developed an appreciation for the work that faculty put into course development. Perhaps most critically, they noted that it also increased their metacognitive thinking around education as they began to ask themselves questions about the professors' learning objectives and rationale for certain projects and assessments. The committee members demonstrated the higher-level thinking skills surrounding their educational experiences that are associated with a greater depth of learning as they became more actively engaged in their own education (Bovill et al., 2011, 2015; Hadley & Fulcomer, 2010; Hutchings, 2005; Mead, 2018).

Additionally, students enrolled in the redesigned course were given a brief written questionnaire at the beginning of the term after they heard the introduction from the committee, and then again after the course was completed, with all anonymous, completed questionnaires being withheld from the faculty member until after grading was completed. All students enrolled in the course chose to participate in the study. The questionnaires focused on expectations and satisfaction with the course and included several items asking the students how their views of the course were influenced by knowing that the course had been collaboratively designed with students.

Two key themes emerged from data. First, participants had increased expectations for the value of the content because of the involvement of students in the course development. They attributed the usefulness and applicability of specific learning activities to the byproduct of a faculty-student collaboration process and noted after the course that they were more motivated and engaged know-ing that other students felt the material was important to their future success. While their voices were not directly heard in the development of the course, knowing that other students' voices had been heard on pedagogical development still appeared to affect their attitude toward learning (Bovill et al., 2011, 2015; Hutchings, 2005; Mead, 2018). The second theme that appeared primarily in the pre-course evaluation was the presumption of increased faculty transparency. Teacher transparency is the ability of students to understand information from the instructor that allows them to develop insights into the nature of the instructor and their teaching philosophy and is associated with increased student motivation (Ginsberg, 2007). Students in the class reported that knowing that the faculty member had been willing to collaborate with students to design a course suggested to them that the faculty member was open to feedback, was open to requests for clarification, and valued their opinions. They also indicated that they looked forward to potentially participating in the same type of collaborative process in the future.

APPLICATION TO CROSS-DISCIPLINARY CONTEXTS

Viewing students as potential collaborators has opened many doors for this faculty and former student pair. As faculty, the initial emotional response to the collaborative process, once it was underway, was pure energy. The collaboration gave me insights into my students' thinking, often in shockingly honest, but helpful ways (no, they may not be reading the syllabus you slaved over). It forged connections with them that were more meaningful than had been developed in the classroom setting, as I learned how they thought about learning and what graduate education meant to them. And finally, on a personal level, it reinvigorated my commitment and enthusiasm for teaching in a way that, after about 17 years, I was probably ready for (Mead, 2018). If you are reading this and considering how the use of CCD might affect you, I have to be honest and say it was tremendously energizing and gratifying for me as a long-time faculty member. The positive feedback from the students who had completed the redesigned course was also extremely helpful and encouraging as an indicator of the value of the work that went into redesigning this course with four other people, which may have not required any more time to complete but did require adhering to a schedule and also required that I let go of the notion of unilateral decision making.

For the former student, this collaborative process shaped my views not only of my education, but of my professors. It also completely altered my own aspirations as a speech-language patholo-gist and sparked interest in aspects of our field that I had never considered before. In terms of my education, the collaborative process opened my eyes to the work professors put into their courses and helped me to appreciate the learning objectives that were being targeted. After taking part in this process, I stopped complaining about projects and tests and how much work they were, and I started critically thinking about why the professor had chosen these projects and how they were going to make me a better clinician. It also humanized my professors and helped me feel comfort-able with those in positions of authority (e.g., telling your professor that you rarely, if ever, read the whole course syllabus that they put so much time and effort into). This shift in my view of those in positions of authority not only helped me to form a collaborative partnership with the faculty member in this study (we continue to collaborate on articles and chapters), but it also helped me to be more confident in the workforce when collaborating with individuals in positions of authority. Lastly, engaging in this process is what ignited my desire to complete a thesis, and without it, I am not sure that I would have discovered my love for research or made a goal to complete my doctorate. This process opened my eyes to the possibilities in our field and helped me to realize that being a clinician is not the only track that interests me.

Moving forward and considering the application of this approach to numerous opportunities, it can certainly be used to design or redesign part or all of any course. The literature suggests that some faculty choose to collaborate with students who have not yet completed the course or with students who have already succeeded in the course. This is a personal, and perhaps philosophical, choice. As noted above, if you are tentative about the process, we would recommend beginning with one element of a course and (re)designing that in collaboration with students. As a faculty member, having gained appreciation for my students' thinking and wonderful insights, I have continued to create collaborative opportunities both in and out of the classroom. As I prepare to teach a new course, I convene a group of student collaborators who have taken the course in order to learn from them what was valuable to their learning and how the course could be made more valuable. Outside of the classroom, I routinely seek out students to collaborate with me on research projects and other scholarly work, such as publications and patient resource development. Thus far, I have not had a single experience in which I created a prospect for collaboration with a student that was not successful in my view. The quality of the work that resulted from the collaboration has been excellent, and the collaboration made the process more pleasurable. I enjoy learning from my students as much as I enjoy teaching them. Collaboration with students gives faculty the chance to "explore ways for students to become full participants in the design of teaching approaches, courses, and curricula" (Bovill et al., 2011, p. 133).

For students, collaborating and providing input regarding their learning not only increases student ownership of learning, but it also enhances student knowledge of learning, including how learning is supported and how it is assessed (Mead, 2018). As a former student, this collaborative process helped me to reflect on my own learning and to take into consideration how others learn in order to develop a course that would benefit a number of learning styles. I found the first few meetings in which we discussed course design and authentic assessment to be a crucial part of this process. This was the first time in all my years of schooling that I had really learned about learning or reflected on my own learning. The articles and worksheets used in the processes helped to give the student participants some background knowledge about the teaching and learning processes. I personally found it easier to provide input on a class that I had already taken, since I had some background knowledge and was in my clinical placement. However, the ultimate goal of CCD is to gain insight into the student perspective, and course content knowledge is not a necessary component. Students are not content experts yet, and while they have much to learn, they have much to teach us and "to deny students their own expert knowledge is to disempower them" (Delpit, 1988, p. 288).

Additional Resources

- Worksheets created for use with the student collaborating committee:
  - Backward Design Learning Priorities to help identify and sort course objectives and to organize committee's thinking and discussions regarding course development.
  - Backward Design Worksheet to track progress across course development for the committee.
- Two articles in the reference list are particularly practical for instructors considering student-instructor collaboration for the first time:
  - Bovill, C., Cook-Sather, A., Felten, P., Millard, L., & Moore-Cherry, N. (2015). Addressing potential challenges in co-creating learning and teaching: Overcoming resistance, navigating institutional norms and ensuring inclusivity in student-staff partnerships. *Higher Education, 71,* 195-208. https://doi.org/10.1007/s10734-015-9896-4
  - Bovill, C., Felten, P., & Cook-Sather, A. (2014). Engaging students as partners in learning and teaching (2): Practical guidance for academic staff and academic developers. Proceedings from *ICED Conference 2014: Educational Development in a Changing World.* Stockholm, Sweden. http://www.iced2014.se/proceedings/1146_BovillFeltenCook-Sather%20.pdf

Backward Design Learning Priorities

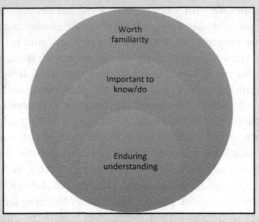

ENDURING UNDERSTANDING	IMPORTANT TO KNOW/DO	WORTH FAMILIARITY

Recommended readings: Fink, L. D. (2003). *Creating significant learning experiences*. Jossey-Bass Inc; Ginsberg, S. M. (2007). Teacher transparency: What students can see from faculty communication. *Journal of Cognitive Affective Learning, 4*(1), 13-24; Wiggins, G., & McTighe, J. (1998). *Understanding by design*. Association for Supervision and Curriculum Development.

Created by Sarah M. Ginsberg, EdD, CCC-SLP, F-ASHA.
© 2021 SLACK Incorporated. Friberg, J. C., Visconti, C. F., & Ginsberg, S. M. (2021). *Evidence-based education in the classroom: Examples from clinical disciplines*. SLACK Incorporated.

Backward Design Worksheet

LEARNING GOALS FOR COURSE	EVALUATION PROCEDURES	LEARNING ACTIVITIES	RESOURCES
1.			
2.			
3.			
4.			

REFERENCES

Aguirre, R. T., & Duncan, C. (2013). Being an elbow: A phenomenological autoethnography of faculty-student collaboration for accommodations. *Journal of Teaching in Social Work, 33,* 531-551. https://doi.org/10.1080/08841233.2013.8 27611

Bovill, C., Cook-Sather, A., & Felten, P. (2011). Students as co-creators of teaching approaches, course design, and curricula: Implications for academic developers. *International Journal for Academic Developers, 16*(2), 133-145. http://dx.doi.org/10.1080/1360144x.2011.568690

Bovill, C., Cook-Sather, A., Felten, P., Millard, L., & Moore-Cherry, N. (2015). Addressing potential challenges in co-creating learning and teaching: Overcoming resistance, navigating institutional norms and ensuring inclusivity in student-staff partnerships. *Higher Education, 71,* 195-208. https://doi.org/10.1007/s10734-015-9896-4

Bovill, C., Felten, P., & Cook-Sather, A. (2014). Engaging students as partners in learning and teaching (2): Practical guidance for academic staff and academic developers. Proceedings from *ICED Conference 2014: Educational Development in a Changing World*. http://www.iced2014.se/proceedings/1146_BovillFeltenCook-Sather%20.pdf

Carlile, A. (2012). "Critical bureaucracy" in action: Embedding student voice into school governance. *Pedagogy, Culture and Society, 20*(3), 393-412. https://doi.org/10.1080/14681366.2012.712053

Cook-Sather, A. (2008). "What you get is looking in a mirror, only better": Inviting students to reflect (on) college teaching. *Reflective Practice, 9*(4), 473-483. http://dx.doi.org/10.1080/14623940802431465

Delpit, L. D. (1988). The silenced dialogue: Power and pedagogy in educating other people's children. *Harvard Educational Review, 58*(3), 280-298. http://lmcreadinglist.pbworks.com/f/Delpit+(1988).pdf

Ginsberg, S. M. (2007). Teacher transparency: What students can see from faculty communication. *Journal of Cognitive Affective Learning, 4*(1), 13-24.

Ginsberg, S. M., Friberg, J., & Visconti, C. (2012). *Scholarship of teaching and learning in speech-language pathology and audiology: Evidence-based education*. Plural Publishing.

Hadley, A. J., & Fulcomer, M. C. (2010). Models of instruction used in speech-language pathology graduate programs. *Communication Disorders Quarterly, 32*(1), 3-12. https://doi.org/10.1177/1525740109332833

Hutchings, P. (2005, January). Building pedagogical intelligence. *Carnegie Perspectives. The Carnegie Foundation for the Advancement of Teaching*. https://cseweb.ucsd.edu/classes/wi05/cse141/pedagogy.pdf

Kane, R. G., & Chimwayange, C. (2014). Teacher action research and student voice: Making sense of learning in secondary school. *Action Research, 12*(1), 52-77. https://doi.org/10.1177/1476750313515282

Mead, L. H. (2018). Faculty perspectives of student-faculty collaborative course design. *Teaching and Learning in Communication Sciences & Disorders, 2*(1), Article 7.

Mihans, R. J., II, Long, D. T., & Felten, P. (2008). Power and expertise: Student-faculty collaboration in course design and the scholarship of teaching and learning. *International Journal for the Scholarship of Teaching and Learning, 2*(2), 1-9. http://digitalcommons.georgiasouthern.edu/ij-sotl/vol2/iss2/16

Wiggins, G. (1990). The case for authentic assessment. *ERIC Digest*, ED328611.

Wiggins, G. & McTighe, J. (2005). *What is backward design? Understanding by Design*. Association for Supervision and Curriculum Development.

6

Using Flipped-Course Pedagogy to Promote Competence in Professional Education

Ken Saldanha, PhD, MSW, BEd
and D. Mark Ragg, PhD, LMSW, BSW

Description of Teaching/Learning Context

In the past 2 decades, major health and human service professional education programs have transitioned from knowledge-based to competence-based outcomes. The shift toward competence-based learning requires programs to retool the curriculum so students can progressively develop and demonstrate complex professional competencies throughout their educational program (Albanese et al., 2010; Bracy, 2018). Competencies include professional roles, ethics, values, knowledge, and interpersonal practice skills (Bogo et al., 2016).

Transitioning into competence-based teaching is difficult. At the instructor level, competence-based teaching and formative assessment is more demanding than knowledge-based instruction given that instructors must observe student performances and then engage them in feedback-based reflection (Fitzgerald et al., 2016). This makes for a difficult transition because ongoing university-related pressures often interfere with a willingness to engage in the change process (Arvandi et al., 2016). For several decades, universities have pressured faculty to prioritize funded projects, diverting energy away from teaching (Elliott, 2016; Robbins et al., 2016). Considering that competing stresses already result in faculty having to use weekend and leisure time to complete course planning and assessment tasks, adopting a more time-intensive instructional model is challenging (Arvandi et al., 2016; Peng, 2017). While the increased burden of competence-based teaching can be partially mitigated by decreasing class sizes, such solutions are unlikely with many university settings pressing for larger classes and increased credit hour production (Schuman, 2014).

Friberg, J. C., Visconti, C. F., & Ginsberg, S. M. (Eds.). *Evidence-Based Education in the Classroom: Examples From Clinical Disciplines* (pp. 47-57).
© 2021 Taylor & Francis Group.

As professional bodies are mandating the adoption of demonstrable outcomes by instructors (although they are already stressed by multiple demands), competency-based professional schools are forced to manage their own adaptations to competence-based outcomes. Consequently, in the spirit of working smarter rather than harder, many instructors and programs are using flipped-class and hybrid learning approaches to restructure teaching and learning (Ayala, 2009). Flipped instruction refers to the delivery of lecture content outside of the classroom so more time can be devoted in class to active learning (Lo et al., 2018).

Review of Literature

In general, the effectiveness research suggests that flipped-course applications are equivocal to traditional face-to-face teaching approaches, with individual studies sometimes finding one approach superior but with small effect sizes (Day, 2018; Hwang & Chen, 2019). While outcomes are comparable, findings indicate that students prefer and retain more when the learning experience is engaging and interactive (Jaggars & Xu, 2016) and there is a high level of instructor interaction with students, not only in the face-to-face elements but also in the online elements of the course (Butz & Stupnisky, 2017; Owston, 2018).

While the earlier discussed findings are helpful in planning course activities, they are largely generic. Beyond providing strong teaching tips for any flipped or online course, they offer no unique insight in planning competence-based professional courses. The goal of competence-based teaching is to achieve specific and applied outcomes and professional competencies that are discipline specific. This requires a synergy among outcome expectations, engagement, learning design, and technology applications (Akçayir & Akçayir, 2018; Brewer & Movahedazarhouligh, 2018). As such, there arises a need for a well-grounded framework that can organize the various course elements comprehensively to achieve the outcomes required in flipped-course teaching (Liang-Yi & Tsai, 2017).

In the literature, there are two correlated pedagogical frameworks guiding professional schools in the transition to competence-based, flipped-course learning: modular design (Botma et al., 2015; Klotz & Wright, 2017) and first principles of instruction (FPI; Merrill, 2002). Modular design provides a framework for organizing the learning sequence around specific outcomes. FPI are learning principles that guide the organization of each module, so the online and face-to-face components progressively build toward achieving the desired competencies.

Modular Design

Modular design was recently introduced as a method for organizing learning (Desiatov, 2014), particularly online learning (Klotz & Wright, 2017). It begins with an analysis of the important outcomes and sub-elements within each competency (Botma et al., 2015). In this analysis, it is important to identify three elements:

1. Specific outcomes that must be achieved and demonstrated for the successful completion of the course
2. Existing knowledge, cognitive, interpersonal, and behavioral elements associated with and foundational or antithetical to the desired outcome
3. Additional knowledge, cognitive, interpersonal, and behavioral components needed to achieve the desired outcome

The above elements become the foundation for learning. Each learning module must activate the pertinent existing material, provide new material, and create opportunities to demonstrate mastery of the new material and its application to real-world situations (Botma et al., 2015). Next, the instructor must sequence the modules and subsumed learning experiences in a manner that ensures that each module progressively certifies mastery of the competency-based outcomes and learning activities within it and in conjunction with other competencies (Botma et al., 2015; Klotz & Wright, 2017). Another requirement of the planning process involves backward design, beginning with the compilation of a list of specific competencies required by the profession (Albanese et al., 2010).

Modularization logically fits with competence-based learning because most professional associations already provide competency frameworks and expected role-behaviors that lend themselves to a modular organization. Given that the competence-based professional literature recommends sequencing the curriculum based on skills and competencies (Albanese et al., 2010; Bracy, 2018), an internal consistency can easily be obtained simply by developing specific learning modules, each with sub-units, that ultimately contribute to the larger competencies.

First Principles of Instruction

Just as modularization provides a structure for the learning sequence, FPI is a meta-design theory providing a structure for facilitating learning within each module (Merrill, 2002). Merrill's framework suggests beginning with an activation of student existing knowledge that is applicable for achieving the module's specific outcomes. New information is then provided and explored in application to the learning goals. The skills required for the learning outcomes must then be demonstrated, prior to engaging students in applied activities and exercises to demonstrate their competence and integrate it into their learning/real world. These principles structure both the online and on-campus segments of each learning module.

The FPI structure in a flipped-learning module suggests online learning followed by on-campus learning. This sequencing promotes the progression from knowledge to applied skills, first within the online learning activities, and then in the on-campus learning. Online learning uses applied learning activities to provide a foundation for on-campus work (Lo et al., 2018). In the on-campus condition, students are engaged in applied learning through demonstrating and receiving feedback on the skill sets of the competence-based outcomes. As feedback on student skill performance is provided, the instructor helps students to integrate the online and face-to-face learning, providing a foundation for the next learning module.

Competence-Based Course Organization

Research indicates that the balance between online and face-to-face learning is important, with 30% to 45% online and 55% to 70% face-to-face to maximize student engagement and performance (Owston, 2018). The face-to-face element remains critical because this is where the learning between the instructor and student is forged (Ding et al., 2012; Reddy et al., 2014; Rousmaniere et al., 2014; Toste et al., 2014). When flipping a course, it is important to plan the use of technology and online activities in a manner that maximizes competency advancement in the face-to-face sessions. In a professional program, consideration must also be given on how to integrate ethical, cognitive, emotional, and interactive material into the online activities (Klotz & Wright, 2017).

Competence-Based Learning

Recent research using the FPI framework identifies how the principles and learning sequences enhance student outcomes (Lo et al., 2018). The framework provides an easy to follow structure that maximizes the strengths of both online and face-to-face pedagogical approaches, with the online work setting the stage for active and applied learning in the on-campus environment (Brewer & Movahedazarhouligh, 2018). The general sequence for competence expansion includes seven elements:

1. Using salient knowledge, values, and ethics associated with the societally entrusted professional role
2. Applying knowledge and professional role functions to assessing client situations
3. Mastering the interpersonal skills required for effective assessment and intervention
4. Building the skills required to engage clients in an effective working alliance

5. Managing socialized habits interfering with effective intervention
6. Integrating knowledge of evidence-supported interventions to adjust understanding, strategy, and skills when approaching client situations
7. Monitoring and evaluating the effect of intervention and professional services

These seven elements are the focus of the learning modules. In teaching and learning, it is important to visualize how the different course elements fit together and complement each other to achieve the required skills and competency outcomes (Toetenel & Rienties, 2016). In competence-based, flipped pedagogy courses, active and applied learning activities are sequenced to progressively build learning outcomes.

APPLICATION OF LITERATURE/DATA

The principles discussed earlier were applied in a series of three foundation practice classes in a school of social work including individual, family, and group counseling. All of the courses were organized identically with an on-campus introduction followed by a series of six 2-week modules. Each module began with online learning prior to an on-campus series of activities.

Online Learning Activities

Consistent with FPI and modularization principles, the first task of each online module focuses on activating, expanding, and directing existing knowledge to respond to professional practice situations. Currently the most promising strategy for delivering information is video-based online presentations, which are found to be effective in building student understanding of the concepts and context for learning (Awidi & Paynter, 2019). Engagement is further enhanced by using media-rich videos containing relevant images and animations (Hua, 2013; Nwosu et al., 2018). The use of integrated audio and visual media allows for greater engagement of learners. Equally important is a deliberate use of scaffolding.

Knowledge Application Scaffolds

Many knowledge-based, flipped courses enhance online content with supplemental resources providing access to online expert information, such as videos, discussion boards, blogs, and websites (Butz & Stupnisky, 2017; Nami et al., 2018). In the application highlighted in this chapter, there was a conscious decision to avoid using links to expert-based discussions and examples. While these can be useful, experts subscribe to a specific model and frequently delve into a conceptual discussion that exceeds the target competencies of a foundation practice course (Greener, 2009).

Demonstration Scaffolds

To prepare students for on-campus applied learning activities, every online module provided additional access to focused and demonstrable examples (through selected video clips and content available at the digital common holdings of the library) to expand and demonstrate the application of knowledge with minimal divergence from the learning goals (Trief & Rosenblum, 2016; Windale, 2010). Based on the goal outcomes, such activities illustrate and challenge students, rather than engage them in alternative and highly specific models of practice required for postgraduate training and certification. It should be noted that such embedded content requires adherence to the fair use statutes in the copyright laws. Over the years, the authors of this chapter have invested significant time and resources to gather and compile an entire repertoire of video examples demonstrating specific professional skills.

Providing video examples of module-related skills is the most prevalent online instructional approach (Hoogerheide et al., 2014). For these courses, examples were created through videotaping simulations using student actors or volunteers. The use of student actors and volunteers allowed the demonstrations to reflect the same situations used in the on-campus role plays and simulations.

Performance Scaffolds

The biggest challenge in the online modules is having students demonstrate a higher skill level, in keeping with the professional requirement called for. In fully online courses, it is becoming common to engage students in role play and simulation exercises using Zoom (Zoom Video Communications, Inc) or other conferencing platforms (Fitch et al., 2016). In this flipped-learning application, simulations and observations (for discussion and feedback) were reserved for the on-campus component. Consequently, the competence performance used applied online exercises to apply module concepts.

In applied exercises, it is important that after skill demonstration, feedback is offered to students so they can begin adjusting their skills (Carless, 2019). It is helpful to offer multiple opportunities for students to engage in skill performances and receive feedback during online learning (Petrovic et al., 2017). As such, applied exercises were developed to focus the feedback using one of two formats. The first, and most complex exercise format, is branched simulation exercises (Wilkening et al., 2017). Branching works well within most quiz development or even presentation application systems. It allows for developing content on a timeline and also includes a system that permits layers (e.g., Articulate Storyline 2 and Articulate 360 [Articulate Global, Inc]). This enables students to make choices that lead to diverse outcomes, each with embedded feedback.

The second exercise format was applied video-enhanced quizzes. Research has found that videos followed by quizzes help students apply their learning (Schacter & Szpunar, 2015; Vural, 2013). Most online quiz programs will allow the insertion of video clips. This enables instructors to use video clips of a practice sequence as a learning focus and then use quiz questions requiring students to apply their knowledge to the practice example. Multiple-choice items can require students to identify skills, mistakes, options for intervention, and other competence-based content in the videos.

On-Campus Learning Activities

Each on-campus session begins by exploring the student experiences with the online learning activities. In particular, instructors focus on the challenges inherent in the performance activities. Often a brief revisiting of some sections of the quizzes takes place in class, reinforcing the knowledge and applications of knowledge they were envisioned to highlight. These discussions reactivate knowledge and challenge students to better apply and expand on their current conceptual foundation.

A contextual framework guiding the on-campus discussions is a highlighting of the tension/difference between socialized habits and professional competencies. As such, students were challenged to scan situations, listen, and respond using professional, rather than habitual, understandings and skills. When discussing the online learning activities, students were assisted in identifying how habitual responses can emerge as a pathway of least resistance. Discussions further explore how some professional skills and responses may feel awkward at times, and even rude in comparison to past socialization.

Knowledge Application Scaffolds

Following the discussion of online learning, in-class exercises are used to reinforce and extend the online learning. Typically, the exercises use a client statement, or a series of statements, to engage students in identifying salient content and using this content to build their professional responses.

Demonstration Scaffolds

After the exercises, additional video examples were used to illustrate specific challenging areas associated with the skill applications. The use of video demonstrations often leads to student skill-related questions and struggles, frequently resulting in impromptu role plays between the instructor and the students with a view to really hone in on the illustration of specific skills and generate discussion. The impromptu role plays are followed up with summarizing the application challenges and reinforcement of the practice concepts.

Performance Scaffolds

The class discussion culminates in breaking the class into smaller groups and engaging students in simulation role plays. The group role plays are videotaped to allow for observation and feedback, which is a common practice in competence-based practice teaching (Asakura et al., 2018). Given the time and space concerns on many campuses, it provides an effective method to capture skill performances for viewing and feedback.

The second on-campus session was broken into time-blocks for each student group to meet with the instructor, review the videotaped role plays, and receive feedback on how to progress toward professional standards of practice. These two activities, observation and feedback provision, are critical activities inherent in formative feedback (Shand & Farrelly, 2018; Smith et al., 2017), which is concurrently considered a critical element in competence-based learning (Armson et al., 2019; Warhuss et al., 2018).

In regard to the provision of feedback, findings suggest the use of a structured handout standardizes the feedback, enabling students to identify and understand the gap between personal and professional standards, a critical element in guiding their adjustment to acquiring professional competencies (Wagner et al., 2019). As such, skillsets associated with the professional competency were operationalized and formed into a checklist system. When viewing each skill performance, the instructor used the checklist and gave it to the student.

ORIGINAL DATA

Implementation of the flipped-course model began with the selection of an undergraduate group work course that generated student feedback and continuous improvements over a 2-year period. The competency outcomes provided through the professional regulatory body (Council on Social Work Education) were operationalized into competency checklists. The checklists were organized into six rows, each focused on one of the required competencies. There were also four columns; two located on the left capturing the use of habitually used skills and two on the right capturing the use of skills identified in the professional literature as necessary for effective practice. These competency checklists were used to compare the face-to-face traditionally taught courses using face-to-face lecture pedagogies with the flipped format. This evaluation found that the average competency scores increased from 92.8 for traditionally taught classes to 96.5 ($t = -5.125/p = .000$) in the flipped condition.

The institutional student evaluations were also used to assess the implementation of flipped-format classes. These evaluations were administered at the end of the semester to all students. The evaluations contained an item asking students to evaluate the effectiveness of the class in promoting learning. The mean evaluation scores for students enrolled in the flipped condition were compared to the courses taught by the same instructor using the face-to-face pedagogy. The evaluation scores on this item improved from a mean score of 4.1 to 4.5 ($t = -3.106/p = .002$) on a 5-point scale.

The promising results in the undergraduate courses informed the flipped pedagogy when the foundation practice courses in the Master of Social Work curriculum were changed to include courses on individual, family, and group work practice. These 2 credit-hour courses were delivered using flipped course teaching strategies, and the design integrated FPI and modularization principles.

During the first 2 years, the flipped courses were given an additional evaluation to monitor student experiences. Evaluation items were structured into a 4-point scale of satisfaction, which was collapsed into dichotomous results to allow course developers to assess general acceptability (Table 6-1). A review of Table 6-1 indicates that the online components reflected that the majority of students found the course elements helpful in promoting learning, particularly online practice examples and the on-campus use of role-play and feedback were highly endorsed.

TABLE 6-1

Satisfaction With Flipped-Course Elements

	LEARNING ENVIRONMENT	HELPED SKILL DEVELOPMENT	HINDERED SKILL DEVELOPMENT
Online Presentations	Online	90%	10%
Online Exercises	Online	87%	13%
Video Examples	Online	96.8%	3.2%
Doing Role Plays	On campus	96.8%	3.2%
Getting Feedback	On campus	96.8%	3.2%
Small Group Work	On campus	90%	10%

To assess the effect of the flipped pedagogy, the average scores on the competency checklists were compared before and after flipped pedagogy implementation for students in the individual practice course. This was possible because the same instructor taught the previous face-to-face courses and the flipped pedagogy courses. The competency checklists were compared across both conditions because they are the strongest indicator of competence development and are based on an assessment of 5- to 8-minute videotaped role plays. Every role play results in a checklist as part of the formative feedback. At the end of the semester, students provide the checklist from their best skill performance for inclusion in their grade. The results of the comparison (Table 6-2) indicate a significant increase in the average score on the feedback sheets.

Qualitative feedback during the evaluation period identified that feedback in the on-campus face-to-face sessions frequently felt rushed. Given that the courses were now using flipped pedagogy, online feedback was structured into all practice courses (individual, family, and group) to enable timely and more specific feedback. Online feedback involved the instructor using screen-capture software to view student role plays and verbally superimpose feedback onto the recaptured video. The new annotated video was then posted to a secure online site and students were sent links to their feedback. Student evaluations of this change to the flipped pedagogy courses indicated that it effectively eased the time pressures, allowing for better discussion, engagement, and learning. They also identified that the online feedback was more convenient, allowed for repeated viewing, and was more specific in focus.

To assess the effect of adding digital feedback to the courses, the average competency checklist scores before and after the addition of online feedback were compared (Table 6-3). While there were no significant improvements in the individual practice course outcomes, the family and group courses did appear to benefit from the change. The courses seek to develop highly complex skill sets used in family and group treatment. The ability to play and replay the feedback, increased specificity, and decreased time pressures may have allowed students to better understand the skills and apply the feedback.

APPLICATION TO CROSS-DISCIPLINARY CONTEXTS

The transition to the flipped format using modularization and FPI appears to be an effective solution to the challenges of competence-based learning in a professional social work program. Perhaps most importantly, the transition provides increased options for delivery enabling instructors to better apply class time toward competence development.

TABLE 6-2

Student Outcome Differences Between On-Campus and Flipped Delivery

	COHORT	MEAN SCORE	SD	t VALUE	SIGNIFICANCE
Individual Practice (Graduate)	Face-to-face n = 57	93.23	3.97	-2.280	0.025
	Flipped n = 21	95.76	5.28		
SD = standard deviation.					

TABLE 6-3

Outcome Comparison Before and After the Inclusion of Digital Feedback

	MEAN OUTCOME ON CAMPUS ONLY (SD)	MEAN OUTCOME DIGITAL AND ON CAMPUS (SD)	t VALUE	SIGNIFICANCE
Individual Practice	n = 33 95.606 (4.892)	n = 27 96.407 (6.594)	-0.540	0.591
Family Practice	n = 32 86.969 (10.177)	n = 28 95.821 (9.518)	-3.464	0.001
Group Practice	n = 45 96.578 (3.817)	n = 32 98.656 (3.279)	-2.494	0.015
SD = standard deviation.				

The modularization enabled the courses to be structured in a manner that maintained focus. Each new module began with online materials to be completed prior to students attending the two on-campus sessions. This sequencing introduced the new content, even as students were integrating the skills from the last module. There was no wasted time in the course. With the introduction of digital feedback into the modularization, every student received feedback prior to engaging in the subsequent role plays.

A second benefit of modularization is that all knowledge was activated and expanded prior to attending the on-campus sessions. The discussions and expansion of knowledge in the on-campus are applied toward preparing students for role-played skill performances. This was a more efficient use of the on-campus time, allowing students to quickly progress to demonstrating their competencies. The number of role plays possible in the semester increased from four in the traditional courses to six, and at times seven, in the flipped condition. This expansion in itself enabled more intense learning and provision of feedback.

FPI were a useful template within each module. Both the online and on-campus conditions followed the same sequence, transitioning from activating knowledge to performing the skills. The template provides a progression in both conditions that activates, expands, demonstrates, and then applies the module's content. The repetition across the two learning conditions allows for clarification and expansion in live sessions.

Lessons from this flipped-course pedagogy application in social work are applicable to other competence-based professional programs. Competence-based learning principles and the challenges of retooling the curriculum in the light of contemporary university pressures are consistent across multiple disciplines. Like social work, all helping professionals require pedagogies that develop student competencies.

With competence as a common denominator, it is possible to extend this pedagogy to more complex interprofessional learning situations. Each profession can develop unique competency-focused online modules followed by integrated interprofessional simulations. If the simulations are videotaped, each professional group can use the videos to provide feedback for their students. The pedagogy can remain consistent regardless of the unique disciplinary elements, making it possible for multiple disciplines to advance a unified approach to developing competent professionals. While at this point, learning still tends to occur in disciplinary silos, as learning principles are endorsed across disciplines, comparable approaches to competence development can provide a model for activating and expanding cross-disciplinary knowledge to advance interdisciplinary work.

ADDITIONAL RESOURCES

- This website provides information on instructional design along with an instruction toolkit using Merrill's FPI:
  - http://instructionaldesign.io/toolkit/merrill/
- The website from the Center for Teaching and Learning provides useful consideration when designing modules for a course and offers resources on modular design:
  - https://ctl.learninghouse.com/modular-course-design/
- Everything you need to know on how to apply Merrill's FPI in e-learning:
  - https://elearningindustry.com/merrills-principles-instruction-definitive-guide
- Seven trends that will define the future of online learning:
  - https://elearningindustry.com/future-of-online-learning-modular-tailored-versatile
- How to integrate classroom spaces with collaborative technology, online lectures, and the google application suite.
  - Holmes, M. R., Tracy, E. M., Painter, L. L., Oestreich, & T., Park, H. (2015). Moving from flipcharts to the flipped classroom: Using technology driven teaching methods to promote active learning in foundation and advanced masters social work courses. *Clinical Social Work Journal, 43,* 215-224. https://doi.org/10.1007/s10615-015-0521-x
- A Canvas course containing instruction and modules on FPI:
  - https://learn.canvas.net/courses/903/pages/first-principles-of-instruction
- Flipgrid, a social learning platform, is an app that permits educators and students to collaboratively create a "web" of instruction:
  - https://info.flipgrid.com/
- The use of reflective journaling as a flipped classroom technique.
  - Sage, M., & Sele, P. (2015). Reflective journaling as a flipped classroom technique to increase reading and participation with social work students. *Journal of Social Work Education, 51*(4), 668-681. https://doi.org/10.1080/10437797.2015.1076274
- Camtasia (TechSmith) is a screen recorder and video editing software program we used in the work described in this chapter.

REFERENCES

Akçayir, G., & Akçayir, M. (2018). The flipped classroom: A review of its advantages and challenges. *Computers & Education, 126*, 334-345. https://doi.org/10.1016/j.compedu.2018.07.021

Albanese, M. A., Mejicano, G., Anderson, W. M., & Gruppen, L. (2010). Building a competency-based curriculum: The agony and the ecstasy. *Advances in Health Science Education, 15*, 439-454. https://doi.org/10.1007/s10459-008-9118-2

Armson, J., Lockyer, J. M., Zetkulic, M., Könings, K. D., & Sargeant, J. (2019). Identifying coaching skills to improve feedback use in postgraduate medical education. *Medical Education, 53*, 477-493. https://doi.org/10.1111/medu.13818

Arvandi, Z., Emami, A., Zarghi, N., Alavinia, S. M., Shirazi, M., & Parikh, S. V. (2016). Linking medical faculty stress/burnout to willingness to implement medical school curriculum change: A preliminary investigation. *Journal of Evaluation in Clinical Practice, 22*, 86-92. https://doi.org/10.1111/jep.12439

Asakura, K., Bogo, M., Good, B., & Power, R. (2018) Teaching note—social work serial: Using video-recorded simulated client sessions to teach social work practice. *Journal of Social Work Education, 54*(2), 397-404. https://doi.org/10.1080/10437797.2017.1404525

Awidi, I. T., & Paynter, M. (2019). The impact of a flipped classroom approach on student learning experience. *Computers & Education, 128*, 269-283. https://doi.org/10.1016/j.compedu.2018.09.013

Ayala, J. S. (2009). Blended learning as a new approach to social work education. *Journal of Social Work Education, 45*(2), 277-288. https://doi.org/10.5175/JSWE.2009.200700112

Bogo, M., Lee, B., McKee, E., Baird, S. L., & Ramjattan, R. (2016). Field instructors' perceptions of foundation year students' readiness to engage in field education. *Social Work Education, 35*(2), 204-214. https://doi.org/10.1080/02615479.2015.1123689

Botma, Y., Van Rensburg, G. H., Coetzee, I. M., & Heyns, T. (2015). A conceptual framework for educational design at modular level to promote transfer of learning. *Innovations in Education and Teaching International, 52*(5), 499-509. https://doi.org/10.1080/14703297.2013.866051

Bracy, W. (2018). Building a competency-based curriculum in social work education. *Journal of Teaching in Social Work, 38*(1), 1-17. https://doi.org/10.1080/08841233.2017.1400496

Brewer, R., & Movahedazarhouligh, S. (2018). Successful stories and conflicts: A literature review on the effectiveness of flipped learning in higher education. *Journal of Computer Assisted Learning, 34*, 409-416. https://doi.org/10.1111/jcal.12250

Butz, N. T., & Stupnisky, R. H. (2017). Improving student relatedness through an online discussion intervention: The application of self-determination theory in synchronous hybrid programs. *Computers & Education, 114*, 117-138. https://doi.org/10.1016/j.compedu.2017.06.006

Carless, D. (2019). Feedback loops and the longer-term: Toward feedback spirals. *Assessment & Evaluation in Higher Education, 44*(5), 705-714. https://doi.org/10.1080/02602938.2018.1531108

Day, L. J. (2018). A gross anatomy flipped classroom effects performance, retention, and higher-level thinking in lower performing students. *Anatomical Sciences Education, 11*(6), 565-574. https://doi.org/10.1002/ase.1772

Desiatov, T. (2014). Training future teachers from the standpoint of implementation of modular-activity programs: International experience. *Comparative Professional Pedagogy, 4*(1), 5-11.

Ding, X., Huang, R., & Liu, D. (2012). Resource allocation for open and hidden learning in learning alliances. *Asia Pacific Journal of Management, 29*(1), 103-127. https://doi.org/10.1007/s10490-009-9189-5

Elliott, T. R. (2016). External funding and competing visions for academic counseling psychology. *The Counseling Psychologist, 44*(4), 525-535.

Fitch, D., Canada, K., Cary, S., & Freese, R. (2016). Facilitating social work role plays in online courses: The use of video conferencing. *Advances in Social Work, 17*(1), 78-92. https://doi.org/10.18060/20874

Fitzgerald, J. T., Burkhardt, J. C., Kasten, S. J., Mullan, P. B., Santen, S. A., Sheets, K. J., Tsai, A., Vasquez, J. A., & Gruppen, L. D. (2016). Assessment challenges in competency-based education: A case study in health professions education. *Medical Teacher, 38*(5), 482-490. https://doi.org/10.3109/0142159X.2015.1047754

Greener, S. (2009). e-Modeling: Helping learners to develop sound e-learning behaviors. *Electronic Journal of e-Learning, 7*(3), 265-272.

Hoogerheide, V., Loyens, S. M. M., & van Gog, T. (2014). Comparing the effects of worked examples and modeling examples on learning. *Computers in Human Behavior, 41*, 80-91. https://doi.org/10.1016/j.chb.2014.09.013

Hua, K. (2013). Online video delivery: Past, present, and future. *ACM Transactions on Multimedia Computing, Communications, and Applications, (TOMM) 9*(1s), 1-4. https://doi.org/10.1145/2502435

Hwang, G., & Chen, P. (2019). Effects of a collective problem-solving promotion-based flipped classroom on students' learning performances and interactive patterns. *Interactive Learning Environments.* https://doi.org/10.1080/10494820.2019.1568263

Jaggars, S. S., & Xu, D. (2016). How do online course design features influence student performance? *Computers & Education, 95*, 270-284. https://doi.org/10.1016/j.compedu.2016.01.014

Klotz, D. E., & Wright, T. A. (2017). A best practice modular design of a hybrid course delivery structure for an executive education program. *Decision Sciences Journal of Innovative Education, 15*(1), 25-41. https://doi.org/10.1111/dsji.12117

Liang-Yi, L., & Tsai, C. C. (2017). Accessing online learning material: Quantitative behavior patterns and their effects on motivation and learning performance. *Computers & Education, 114,* 286-297. https://doi.org/10.1016/j.compedu.2017.07.007

Lo, C. K., Lie, C. W., & Hew, K. F. (2018). Applying "first principles of instruction" as a design theory of the flipped classroom: Findings from a collective study of four secondary school subjects. *Computers & Education, 118,* 150-165. https://doi.org/10.1016/j.compedu.2017.12.003

Merrill, M. D. (2002). First principles of instruction. *Educational Technology Research & Development, 50*(3), 43-59. https://doi.org/10.1007/BF02505024

Nami, F., Marandi, S. S., & Sotoudehnama, E. (2018). Interaction in a discussion list: An exploration of cognitive, social, and teaching presence in teachers' online collaborations. *ReCALL: Journal of Eurocall, 30*(3), 375-398. https://doi.org/10.1017/S0958344017000349

Nwosu, J. C., John, H. C., & Akorede, O. J. (2018). Availability and accessibility of ICT-based instructional tools in medical colleges in Ogun State, Nigeria. *Educational Research and Reviews, 13*(11), 391-398.

Owston, R. (2018). Empowering learners through blended learning. *International Journal on E-Learning, 17*(1), 1-19.

Peng, W. (2017). Research on model of student engagement in online learning. *EURASIA Journal of Mathematics, Science, & Technology Education, 13*(7), 2869-2882. https://doi.org/10.12973/eurasia.2017.00723a

Petrovic, J., Pale, P., & Jerrin, B. (2017). Online formative assessments in a digital signal processing course: Effects of feedback type and content difficulty on students learning achievements. *Education and Information Technology, 22,* 3047-3061. https://doi.org/10.1007/s10639-016-9571-0

Reddy, S. T., Chao, J., Carter, J. L., Drucker, R., Katz, N. T., Nesbit, R., Roman, B., Wallenstein, J., & Beck, G. L. (2014). Alliance for clinical education perspective paper: Recommendations for redesigning the "final year" of medical school. *Teaching and Learning in Medicine, 26*(4), 420-427. https://doi.org/10.1080/10401334.2014.945027

Robbins, S. P., Coe Regan, J. A. R., Williams, J. H., Smyth, N. J., & Bogo, M. (2016). From the editor—the future of social work education. *Journal of Social Work Education, 52,* 387-397. https://doi.org/10.1080/10437797.2016.1218222

Rousmaniere, T., Abbass, A., & Frederickson, J. (2014). New developments in technology-assisted supervision and training: A practical overview. *Journal of Clinical Psychology, 70*(11), 1082-1093. https://doi.org/10.1002/jclp.22129

Schacter, D. L., & Szpunar, K. K. (2015). Enhancing attention and memory during video-recorded lectures. *Scholarship of Teaching and Learning in Psychology, 1*(1), 60-71.

Schuman, S. (2014). Profit, productivity, and honors. *Journal of the National Collegiate Honors Council, 15*(1), 41-44.

Shand, K., & Farrelly, S. G. (2018). The art of blending: Benefits and challenges of a blended course for preservice teachers. *Journal of Educators Online, 15*(1), 1-15.

Smith, T. L., Landes, S. J., Lester-Williams, K., Day, K. T., Batdorf, W., Brown, G. K., Trockel, M., Smith, B. N., Chard, K. M., Healy, E. T., & Weingardt, K. R. (2017). Developing alternative training delivery methods to improve psychotherapy implementation in the U.S. Department of Veterans Affairs. *Training and Education in Professional Psychology, 11*(4), 266-275. https://doi.org/10.1037/tep0000156

Toetenel, L., & Rienties, B. (2016). Learning Design—Creative design to visualise learning activities. *Open Learning: The Journal of Open and Distance Learning, 31*(3), 233-244. https://doi.org/10.1080/02680513.2016.1213626

Toste, J. R., Bloom, E. L., & Heath, N. L. (2014). The differential role of classroom working alliance in predicting school-related outcomes for students with and without high-incidence disabilities. *Journal of Special Education, 48*(2), 135-148. https://doi.org/10.1177/0022466912458156

Trief, E., & Rosenblum, L. P. (2016). The use of the library of video excerpts (L.O.V.E.) in personnel preparation programs. *Journal of Visual Impairment & Blindness, 110*(2), 123-128.

Vural, Ö. F. (2013). The impact of a question-embedded video-based learning tool on e-learning. *Educational Sciences: Theory & Practice, 13*(2), 1315-1323.

Wagner, N., Acai, A., McQueen, S. A., McCarthy, C., McQuire, A., Petrisor, B., & Sonnadara, R. R. (2019). Enhancing formative feedback in orthopaedic training: Development and implementation of a competency-assessment framework. *Journal of Surgical Education, 76*(5), 1376-1401. https://doi.org/10.1016/j.jsurg.2019.03.015

Warhuss, J. P., Blenker, P., & Emholdt, S. T. (2018). Feedback and assessment in higher-education, practice-based entrepreneurship courses: How can we build legitimacy. *Industry and Higher Education, 32*(1), 23-32.

Wilkoning, G. L., Gannon, J. M., Ross, C., Brennan, J. L., Fablan, T. J., Marcisin, M. J., & Benedict, N. J. (2017). Evaluation of branched-narrative virtual patients for interprofessional education of psychiatry residents. *Academic Psychiatry, 41,* 71-75. https://doi.org/10.1007/s40596-016-0531-1

Windale, M. (2010). How science works: Bringing the world of science into the classroom through innovative blended media approaches. *Education in Science,* (236), 16-17.

7

THE FLIPPED CLASSROOM MODEL
Empowering Future Clinicians

Eric J. Sanders, PhD, CCC-SLP; Mary Culshaw, PhD, OTR/L;
and Louise C. Keegan, PhD, CCC-SLP, BC-ANCDS

DESCRIPTION OF TEACHING/LEARNING CONTEXT

The flipped classroom model (FCM) has recently received attention as an andragogical approach across the health sciences (Sattar et al., 2019). In the FCM an instructor provides lecture material prior to class with class time dedicated to activities that solidify the learned content. In health sciences education, there has also been a movement toward increased interdisciplinary opportunities for students in the health sciences in order to encourage early development of collaboration and cooperation among clinical providers (Interprofessional Education Collaborative [IPEC], 2016).

Research methods are an inherently challenging topic, especially for undergraduate students who have had limited exposure to research. Based on the authors' experiences, students often have difficulty engaging with the complex content and typically do not retain the information throughout their respective health sciences graduate programs. Research methods are often taught in a discipline-specific, traditional lecture format. The authors hypothesized that an interdisciplinary course presented in a FCM format would enhance not only engagement but also retention of the information and enthusiasm for the topic among students.

This chapter reviews how a FCM was implemented in an introductory, interdisciplinary research methods course for undergraduate health sciences majors. Qualitative analysis of interviews of students who participated in this model revealed several themes that are subsequently described and discussed relative to the course structure and extant literature.

Friberg, J. C., Visconti, C. F., & Ginsberg, S. M. (Eds.). *Evidence-Based Education in the Classroom: Examples From Clinical Disciplines* (pp. 59-68).
© 2021 Taylor & Francis Group.

REVIEW OF LITERATURE

Theoretical Background

While the term *flipped classroom* may be relatively new, the premise of the concept is not. The FCM is grounded in constructivist theories, where the application of information facilitates the learning process and allows for the assimilation and integration of content (Harrington et al., 2015). This model is "flipped" from the traditional approach in which the instructor uses face-to-face time to deliver the specific content and may assign homework to reinforce the learning. Rather, the instructor provides lecture material for review outside of class and class time is spent on activities that review this information. The purpose of the flipped classroom is to improve synthesis of learning, reasoning skills, and problem solving, and to increase student engagement, thus improving the educational experience (Tattersall, 2015).

The FCM has the potential to be a particularly powerful approach for health sciences students because it encourages clinical skills, such as reasoning and problem solving (Dehghanzadeha & Jafaraghaee, 2018). Additionally, this type of learning context may help teach students important skills, such as self-sufficiency and working collaboratively (Sergis et al., 2018). For these reasons, the FCM has been implemented within a variety of health-related fields, including medicine, nursing, speech-language pathology, audiology, and physical therapy (Berg et al., 2015; Depry, 2018; Missildine et al., 2013; Sharma et al., 2015; Tattersall, 2015).

McNally and colleagues (2017) discussed how learner outcomes are supported by increasing student participation through the use of technology. They also emphasized that students appreciate the inclusion of technology in the learning process. Online teaching and expanded use of online applications continue to grow within the educational arena, appealing to students who are comfortable in the online world (O'Flaherty & Phillips, 2015). The increase in web-based teaching resources has allowed instructors more opportunities to implement the FCM and encourage student interactions (McNally et al., 2017). Inclusion of online polls, quizzes, and discussion boards outside the classroom setting can give instructors valuable information prior to class. This allows the instructor the opportunity to tailor in-class learning and address student understanding "in the moment."

While the FCM embraces the development of professional skills, the structure of the model and the technology that supports it facilitate learning of content (Harrington et al., 2015; Sergis et al., 2018). Measuring learning outcomes related to content suggests the FCM has had positive results and is similar in effectiveness to the traditional class model (Gillette et al., 2018; Whillier & Lystad, 2015). Both knowledge and professional skills are vitally important for individuals entering clinical professions.

The FCM does not suit all students, and some students have reported that it requires more work, leading them to prefer the traditional classroom (McNally et al., 2017; Missildine et al., 2013). McNally and colleagues (2017) surmise that this is possibly because these students are not motivated to complete the required independent assignments. The FCM provides students with opportunities to independently master content on their own time. Some studies report increased student engagement in the learning process through the FCM (Sergis et al., 2018; Tattersall, 2015). This engagement may be, in part, attributable to the requirement for students to assume a more active role in their learning (Sattar et al., 2019). Nevertheless, self-motivation affects whether the student takes advantage of the opportunity (Gillette et al., 2018).

Unfortunately, there is limited qualitative data to aid in understanding students' perceptions of specific aspects of the FCM. In order for educational organizations to continue to adapt to student needs and provide effective learning environments, it is crucial to understand more about the student experience of the FCM. The following study aimed to identify aspects of the FCM that influenced student experiences.

Applying the Flipped Classroom Model Theory

The purpose of the course investigated in this chapter was to introduce students to basic concepts related to evidence-based medicine. This included learning how to frame clinical and research questions, search research databases, select and analyze research designs to best answer a question, and interpret research results. Twenty-four upper-level health sciences undergraduate students, intending to study areas as diverse as athletic training, physical therapy, occupational therapy, and speech-language pathology, were enrolled in this course.

As stated previously, the FCM is implemented by having students complete tasks outside of class that would traditionally be the focus of in-class work (e.g., watching a lecture). Then, in class, students would complete activities related to the topics presented before the class period (Moffett, 2015; Sharma et al., 2015). In this course, students completed assigned readings and watched recorded online lectures about a topic (e.g., writing a patient/population, intervention, comparison, and outcomes [PICO] question) outside of class. Typically, there were multiple videos per topic that were approximately 10 to 15 minutes in length. Students were provided with a list of guided reading/watching topics that functioned as a study guide to facilitate note taking as they read the text and watched the lectures. Additionally, different learning checks (e.g., online quizzes) were used to ensure student completion and understanding of the out-of-classroom work.

In a FCM, the work that is completed in class is often collaborative and allows for an in-depth understanding of the concepts presented outside of class (Bergmann & Sams, 2012). In this course, class group activities were designed to align with the learning objectives of the topic area. Students in the course were split into interdisciplinary groups in which they were presented with materials, such as cases, scenarios, and research articles, and were asked to answer questions or develop a product related to the topic. These timed activities were often completed using technology, such as Google Forms. As students worked, the instructor visited the groups, scaffolding and facilitating their understanding of the related core concepts. At the conclusion of a particular activity, students from each group would present their work and a classroom discussion would commence.

ORIGINAL DATA

As described in the literature review, there is limited information on students' perceptions of the FCM. Thus, six of the 24 upper-level health sciences students who participated in the FCM were interviewed about their experiences. Participants were all traditional undergraduate students pursuing graduate study in diverse health care fields—athletic training, occupational therapy, physical therapy, and speech-language pathology. Interviews were 15 to 30 minutes long and assumed a semi-structured format (see Appendix), where researchers asked the participants to describe their experiences of the FCM. Interviews were conducted by the second and third authors, as the first author was also the teacher of the course, and it was important that participants felt comfortable expressing their true opinions and perspectives of the course. The interviewers used a phenomenological approach to interviewing, asking questions in a conversational style that allowed the interviewer to support the interviewee in exploring their personal lived experiences of the phenomenon (Crotty, 1998).

Interviews were transcribed, and the transcripts were qualitatively analyzed using a framework of interpretative phenomenological analysis (Smith & Osborn, 2003). This strategy of inquiry is especially useful when investigating participants' perspectives, as it allows the researchers to describe how the participants make sense of their personal and social experiences (Keegan, 2012). As is typical of qualitative research, the authors assumed an inductive approach to data description, and no predetermined hypotheses were formed (Creswell & Poth, 2018). Triangulation of the data was ensured as each of the three investigators independently completed a detailed analysis of the transcripts with the goal of identifying key ideas and then clustering such ideas into themes, using NVivo qualitative coding software (Version 12, 2018; QSR International Pty Ltd., 2012). Once initial themes had been created, the investigators compared their independent analyses and came to a consensus about the overarching themes that presented as common to all analyses. Investigators then collaboratively developed an interpretive model of the participants' experiences and perspectives of the flipped classroom.

Analysis of the interviews with the participants revealed three major themes composed of seven subthemes. The three major themes included impact on learning, reference to structure, and emotional response. Further details on these themes, subthemes, relation to participant experiences, and literature are described in subsequent paragraphs.

Impact on Learning

One major theme that emerged from the data was reference to the impact of the methods used in this particular FCM on learning. Here, the subthemes included reference to learning style, cognitive processes, engagement, and development of self-sufficiency.

Learning Style

As participants spoke about the course, many referenced the impact of the FCM in relation to their own particular learning style. Participants mentioned specific strategies related to the flipped classroom approach and increased learning. Regarding lectures occurring outside of class, some participants appreciated that they were able to learn at their own pace and rewatch them if they felt as though they did not understand the content. Some participants found that the use of Google Forms during the in-person activities was helpful for learning. Additionally, the hands-on, engaging approach of the activities was reported to be beneficial in solidifying understanding for some of the participants. These results are similar to findings from Tattersall (2015), where graduate and undergraduate students also noted that the in-class activities solidified their learning and aided in comprehension. One student reflected:

> I did like the activities a lot because again, it helped me dive more into detail with what's learned because if you just sit in a lecture, you don't really absorb everything, but if you go through a lecture and then do an activity, it helps you put what you just learned into action.

Cognitive Processes

Participants also referenced cognitive processes, such as problem solving and remembering, as they spoke about the course. Remarks included how aspects of the class, such as the videos and activities, supported comprehension and facilitated memory of important concepts. In particular, one participant stated that even if he did not understand a concept when watching a video, he knew he would have an opportunity to increase his comprehension through the in-class activities that reviewed the specified topics. Relatedly, one participant found that the collaborative act of doing the activities "together as a class really helped me kind of grasp the material a little bit better." Sattar and colleagues (2019) highlighted that a strength of the FCM is that in-class activities support the student in solidifying learning of concepts that were introduced in the "pre-class" time, at the students' own pace.

Engagement

Closely related to cognitive processes, many participants mentioned engagement (e.g., attention, gaining and losing interest) when discussing the course. A few participants noted that the short length of the videos (15 minutes or less) helped them stay engaged. Additionally, the use of the study guide was reported to be "very helpful in focusing on the content that was most important." Some participants also found that the interactive nature of the in-class activities resulted in increased attention and engagement during the in-class portions. One student noted, "We had more time to spend on discussion and less on lecture. So, I was able to pay attention more easily."

However, some participants mentioned that watching the videos at home could be challenging because there were more distractions than in a traditional classroom lecture. Related to this, one participant remarked that "outside of class, I'm not going to be as engaged with those lectures as I will be in class." This speaks to the need of students to be self-motivated as described by McNally and colleagues (2017). Engagement in the material outside of class can be challenging for students who prefer passive learning within the traditional class (Sattar et al., 2019).

Another concept to consider is student comfort with online resources, on which this research class relied. Yilmaz (2017) found that student readiness for e-learning platforms significantly affected their motivation and engagement in the FCM. Students demonstrated increased motivation in learning within a FCM environment when they were comfortable using the online resources (O'Flaherty & Phillips, 2015). This course was taught at a college where all students are provided with laptops and have previous experience using the Google suite of tools. This previous experience with such platforms and tools may have contributed to their engagement.

Development of Self-Sufficiency

The final subtheme that emerged in relation to impact on learning was in the area of self-sufficiency. In particular, several participants remarked that the FCM required them to be more independent than traditional classes did. These participants appreciated the independence and resulting responsibility that the FCM accords. These findings are similar to those from a number of studies, where key outcomes of the FCM were found to be development of reasoning, self-sufficiency, self-responsibility, and motivation (McNally et al., 2017; Sattar et al., 2019; Sergis et al., 2018, Yilmaz, 2017). One participant responded, "It allows you to learn on your own, but also if you have any questions or concerns, you can go right to the professor because you have class time with them."

Reference to Structure

During the interviews, many participants referenced different structural aspects of the course. This included mentioning the tools and resources, group work, and the workload outside of class.

Tools and Resources

Participants referenced the tools and resources used in the course. Here, they consistently discussed the use of Google Forms for in-class activities and for assessing student learning. Additionally, participants indicated that they valued supportive resources that the professor provided, such as take-home quizzes and study guides: "I really liked it, the tools. I thought that it gave a nice twist to the classroom instead of the standard, 'I have a question, what's the answer?'"

Yilmaz (2017) suggests that online resources like these play an important part in the success of the FCM and student satisfaction. Instructors should be aware of the value of online resources used in the class and ensure that students have the knowledge to efficiently access and utilize online resources.

Group Work

Another subtheme related to structure was reference to the group work during class. Participants underscored the importance and effectiveness of the use of groups for the in-class activities as well as for some of the major assignments in the course. Two participants referenced the interdisciplinary nature of the groups. They appreciated that they were able to view and interpret the content from the perspective of other disciplines. The importance of group work is highlighted by others who have investigated the FCM (Griffith et al., 2019; Sattar et al., 2019; Tattersall, 2015). "We were able to work with groups to answer those questions too. So, I thought that helped me participate more."

Workload Outside of Class

The final subtheme related to structure was references to the work completed outside of class. Some participants mentioned feeling increased pressure with this particular type of model because of the amount of work they were required to complete. Participants mentioned a preference for watching shorter videos that were more "to the point" as opposed to ones that were longer. However, the reference to workload was also connected to the independence and self-sufficiency that some participants enjoyed about the FCM.

Sharma and colleagues (2015) warned that students can perceive the workload outside the classroom as unnecessary and emphasize the need to get students "on board" with the concept of the FCM. While students may believe that they have more work, this may not necessarily be the case. It may be that they now feel more compelled to do the recommended work, so they are prepared for class discussions. Missildine and colleagues (2013) also noted that students may not see the value in the interactive and collaborative nature of the FCM and how that links to workload. The traditional class model allows for passive learning in which the student absorbs the learning in the classroom with little action outside of the classroom, whereas the FCM favors the student who is internally motivated to learn and willing to work outside of class.

Emotional Response

The final major theme that emerged was participant appraisal. Both positive and negative emotional words were used to describe the FCM. Several participants repeatedly used words such as "enjoyed" and "liked" when referring to the videos and in-class activities. One student responded, "[This course] was the first time I ever, like, had that approach. And, like I said, I really liked it."

In contrast, one of the participants established a strong preference for traditional lecture classes as opposed to flipped classrooms as a whole. In this case, she remarked that she would "rather be taught in person rather than listening to a lecture (online)."

Another participant indicated that she was more confident when contributing in the online setting. She felt the use of Google Forms allowed everyone to participate, without the risk of being publicly called out as wrong. Flynn (2015) explained that the college atmosphere sets expectations for students' behaviors and level of independence. Within the classroom, students are expected to ask for clarification, maintain appropriate eye contact, and participate in discussions. Students may feel shame or other negative feelings when they cannot perform to expectations, or they may limit participation to avoid these feelings. The FCM mitigates these potential feelings of inadequacy.

APPLICATION OF LITERATURE/DATA

The results of this project informed subsequent iterations of the research methods course, other courses within the department and college, and other instructors in the Lehigh Valley Association of Independent Colleges system. Specifically related to this research methods course, results confirmed that continued use of the FCM would be beneficial for students. New instructors at the institution were trained in FCM, and additional sections of this course were offered, with trained instructors, in subsequent semesters. The fact that the flipped classroom content was already developed aided in consistency between sections and instructors.

Although the course remained mostly the same in structure, based on the data, efforts were made to improve the course in targeted areas. For example, to bolster the interdisciplinary advantages highlighted in the data, there were more interdisciplinary group activities and more opportunities for students to work in different groups. Furthermore, to address the challenges some students experienced with independent work, quizzes were substituted with reflective questions on the independent learning, which required students to critically evaluate the outside-of-class material.

The authors have shared this data within their local communities, for example, at college-wide teaching and learning seminars and regional events on the scholarship of teaching and learning (e.g., Lehigh Valley Association of Independent Colleges), and among other instructors within the department. In fact, multiple faculty within the authors' department have adopted this FCM framework in their teaching. Three graduate-level occupational therapy courses and two undergraduate communication sciences and disorders courses, as well as a graduate level speech-language pathology course, have all adopted this approach at this time. Additional instructors have expressed interest in this model, and many have incorporated aspects of the FCM into their teaching of both independently and co-taught courses. For example, these changes include group work utilizing Google Forms, hands-on activities, and an emphasis on multimodal presentation of information.

The authors have been collecting ongoing data from this course, across multiple sections and instructors, and plan to publish this once analyzed. Future research on this course design will also examine the applicability of the FCM framework to the Universal Design for Learning framework in order to support students with diverse learning needs (CAST, 2018). Furthermore, future directions should examine the effectiveness of this model on professional knowledge, attitudes, and skills, as these students move into clinical situations.

APPLICATION TO CROSS-DISCIPLINARY CONTEXTS

Interdisciplinarity is increasingly emphasized as an important component of education. The IPEC (2016) argues that interdisciplinary practice is necessary for safe, high-quality, accessible, person-centered care and improved population health outcomes. Furthermore, as an organization, it emphasizes how interdisciplinary and interprofessional education serves as an important foundation for practice (IPEC, 2016). The accrediting organizations of entry-level certification programs for health care professions require that interprofessional competencies (related to teamwork, values and ethics, communication, and roles and responsibilities) be met (IPEC, 2016). The flipped classroom approach can provide an avenue for meeting these competencies.

From a broader educational perspective, the American Association of Colleges and Universities' Valid Assessment of Learning in Undergraduate Education rubric for liberal arts education identifies the importance of understanding the different perspectives of various disciplines as part of the process of integrative learning (Rhodes, 2010). Thus, regardless of profession, a perspective wider than one's own discipline is very important for successful participation in society. The unique aspects of the FCM provide students with opportunities to participate in group classroom discussions that expose them to other perspectives and disciplines and create opportunities for them to integrate this knowledge. The primary purpose of the FCM is to integrate knowledge within an active learning environment through student engagement. The results of this study emphasize that students find value in learning about other disciplines and appreciate exposure to other perspectives in a FCM.

This particular course, however, appeared to provide students with additional interdisciplinary knowledge beyond the target content. The group discussions and Google Forms required students to reflect on their learning and discuss this learning with interdisciplinary peers, providing them with opportunities to develop their communication and reflection skills with those from other disciplines and view things from varying perspectives (e.g., "[I] wasn't just looking at the views from my own track"). Finally, the FCM emphasizes self-sufficiency and responsibility, as students are expected to work independently and subsequently contribute information about what they learned to the class group. Students even acknowledged that this approach "allows students to be self-sufficient" and develop the professional skills of independence and responsibility.

Health care education requires not only knowledge of content but also professional skills. As described in the literature review, FCM provides an avenue for the development of these professional skills when presented in an interprofessional context. Most undergraduate and graduate programs include coursework that addresses evidence-based practice or research methodologies. Such courses include concepts applicable to all professions and so lend themselves to interdisciplinary opportunities. Professional skills that are highly valued in health care professionals include knowledge, reflection on personal learning, self-sufficiency, and ability to communicate effectively with a variety of individuals. The participants in this study highlighted how the FCM allowed them to develop skills in each of these areas.

ADDITIONAL RESOURCES

- Association for Supervision and Curriculum Development—12 resources on flipped learning:
  - https://inservice.ascd.org/12-resources-on-flipped-learning/
- The University of Washington—Center for Teaching and Learning:
  - https://www.washington.edu/teaching/topics/engaging-students-in-learning/flipping-the-classroom/
- Harvard School of Engineering—Erik Mazur interview:
  - https://www.seas.harvard.edu/news/2013/03/flipped-classroom-will-redefine-role-educators
- Google for Education, Teacher Center—tutorial on using Google Forms:
  - https://teachercenter.withgoogle.com/first-day-trainings/welcome-to-google-forms
- Screencast-O-Matic—free screen recorder used to create online lectures:
  - https://screencast-o-matic.com/

REFERENCES

Berg, A. L., Ibrahim, H., Magaster, S., & Salbod, S. (2015). Flipping over the flipped classroom. *Contemporary Issues in Communication Science Disorders, 42,* 16-25.

Bergmann, J., & Sams, A. (2012). *Flip your classroom: Reach every student in every class every day.* International Society for Technology in Education.

CAST. (2018). Universal design for learning guidelines version 2.2. http://udlguidelines.cast.org

Creswell, J. W., & Poth, C. N. (2018). *Qualitative inquiry and research design: Choosing among five approaches* (4th ed.). SAGE Publications.

Crotty, M. (1998). *The foundations of social research: Meaning and perspective in the research process.* SAGE Publications.

Dehghanzadeha, S., & Jafaraghaee, F. (2018). Comparing the effects of traditional lecture and flipped classroom on nursing students' critical thinking disposition: A quasi-experimental study. *Nurse Education Today, 71,* 151-156.

Depry, S. M. (2018). Outcomes of flipped classroom instruction in an entry-level physical therapy course. *Journal of Physical Therapy Education, 32*(3), 289-294.

Flynn, E. E. (2015). It's all about saving face: Working with the urban college student. *College Student Journal, 49*(2), 187-194.

Gillette, C., Rudolph, M., Kimble, R. W. N., Smith, L., & Broedel-Zaugg, K. (2018). A meta-analysis of outcomes comparing flipped classroom and lecture. *American Journal of Pharmaceutical Education, 82*(5), 6898.

Griffith, J., Vercellotti, M. L., & Folkers, H. (2019). What's in a question? A comparison of student questions in two learning spaces. *Teaching and Learning in Communication Sciences and Disorders, 3*(1), Article 7.

Harrington, S. A., Bosch, M. V., Schoofs, N., Beel-Bates, C., & Anderson, K. (2015). Quantitative outcomes for nursing students in a flipped classroom. *Nursing Education Perspectives, 36*(3), 179-181.

Interprofessional Education Collaborative. (2016). *Core competencies for interprofessional collaborative practice: 2016 update.* Author.

Keegan, L. C. (2012). Review of research methods in speech and language pathology. *Contemporary Issues in Communication Science and Disorders, 39,* 98-104.

McNally, B., Chipperfield, J., Dorsett, P., Del Fabbro, L., Frommolt, V., Goetz, S., Lewohl, J., Molineux, M., Pearson, A., Reddan, G., Roiko, A., & Rung, A. (2017). Flipped classroom experiences: Student preferences and flip strategy in a higher education context. *Higher Education, 73*, 281-298.

Missildine, K., Fountain, R., Summers, L., & Gosselin, K. (2013). Flipping the classroom to improve student performance and satisfaction. *Journal of Nursing Education, 52*(10), 597-599.

Moffett, J. (2015). Twelve tips for "flipping" the classroom. *Medical Teacher, 37*(4), 331-336.

QSR International Pty Ltd. (2012). NVivo qualitative data analysis software.

O'Flaherty, J., & Phillips, C. (2015). The use of flipped classrooms in higher education: A scoping review. *Internet and Higher Education, 25*, 85-95.

Rhodes, T. (2010). *Assessing outcomes and improving achievement: Tips and tools for using rubrics.* Association of American Colleges and Universities.

Sattar, K., Sethi, A., Akram, A., Ahmad, T., John, J., & Yusoff, M. S. B. (2019). Flipped classroom teaching modality: Key concepts and practice endorsements. *Education in Medicine Journal, 11*(1), 1-10.

Sergis, S., Sampson, D. G., & Pelliccione, L. (2018). Investigating the impact of flipped classroom on students' learning experiences: A self-determination theory approach. *Computers in Human Behavior, 78*, 368-378.

Sharma, N., Lau, C. S., Doherty, I., & Harbutt, D. (2015). How we flipped the classroom. *Medical Teacher, 37*(4), 327-330.

Smith, J. A., & Osborn, M. (2003). Interpretative phenomenological analysis. In J. A. Smith (Ed.), *Qualitative psychology* (pp. 51-80). SAGE Publications.

Tattersall, P. J. (2015). "Flipped" classroom: Benefits versus challenges for communicative sciences and disorders faculty and students. *Perspectives on Issues in Higher Education, 18*(1), 4-15.

Whillier, S., & Lystad, R. P. (2015). No differences in grades or level of satisfaction in a flipped classroom for neuroanatomy. *Journal of Chiropractic Education, 29*(2), 127-133.

Yilmaz, R. (2017). Exploring the role of e-learning readiness on student satisfaction and motivation in flipped classroom. *Computers in Human Behavior, 70*, 251-260.

APPENDIX: SEMI-STRUCTURED INTERVIEW PROTOCOL

The purpose of this interview is to explore and learn about your experiences as a student in a flipped classroom.

(Note: Due to the phenomenological nature of this interview and the conversational style required, the questions are not necessarily asked in this order or with this wording, but all topics are covered in every interview. Additional follow-up and clarification questions were also used to reiterate and confirm the interviewees' experiences.)

Questions

- How was your general experience of the flipped classroom?
- How was your experience of activities and tools used (including online lectures)?
- Can you compare the flipped classroom with traditional courses you have taken?
- How did this model facilitate or hinder your general learning experience?

8

INTENSIVE COURSE DELIVERY DESIGN IN A GRADUATE SPEECH-LANGUAGE PATHOLOGY CURRICULUM

Kaitlyn P. Wilson, PhD, CCC-SLP
and Christina Y. Pelatti, PhD, CCC-SLP

DESCRIPTION OF TEACHING/LEARNING CONTEXT

The context of this research report is the master's level classroom within a speech-language pathology graduate program at a public, mid-Atlantic university. The goal of this classroom-based research study was to examine the self-reported learning and attitudes of graduate students enrolled in two required didactic courses when the courses were delivered through an intensive course design. The two courses were previously delivered simultaneously through a traditional, semester-long format, with each course meeting once per week for 3 hours. The intensive course design format allowed students to focus on one course at a time, with each course meeting once per week for 6 hours for 7 weeks (i.e., half the length of a full semester).

The course design shift reflected the instructors' understanding of current literature suggesting multiple benefits of intensive course design, as well as students' busy schedules that combine coursework and clinical experiences. Both courses are clinical in nature and include clinically applicable skills and knowledge. The instructors hypothesized that allowing students to focus on one content area at a time, in combination with their clinical placements, might result in students feeling more focused and better able to apply the content.

Friberg, J. C., Visconti, C. F., & Ginsberg, S. M. (Eds.). *Evidence-Based Education in the Classroom: Examples From Clinical Disciplines* (pp. 69-77).
© 2021 Taylor & Francis Group.

REVIEW OF LITERATURE

The means by which instructors impart knowledge to future professionals in clinical fields, such as speech-language pathology, may have an effect on their short- and long-term academic gains and overall attitudes about the course material. The effects are likely to cascade into students' eventual professional work environments as well. Over the last decade, there has been increased focus on innovative teaching practices that may increase learning and student attitudes in the field of speech-language pathology. A number of strategies have been investigated, with problem-based learning (Mok et al., 2009), interprofessional education (Myers & O'Brien, 2015), and online education (Myers & O'Brien, 2015) most prominent. Intensive course design has also been examined, albeit in a preliminary manner. Also referred to as *block design*, *compressed course design*, or *accelerated course design*, this course format can be defined as longer than usual class meetings, which allow for greater flexibility and depth in instruction, delivered over a shorter period of time than a traditional semester (Davies, 2006).

Intensive course design has been studied across fields over the past few decades in high school and college settings, and studies support positive effects on student performance and satisfaction equivalent to (Adams & Salvaterra, 1997; Anatasi, 2007) or better than traditional full-semester course design (Anderson & Anderson, 2012; DeVeney et al., 2015; Vlachopoulos et al., 2019). Specifically, intensive course design has been found to increase convenience of attendance, enhance student focus, improve relationships between students and instructor, and augment overall learning (Scott, 1995). The longer class meetings allow for greater continuity through presentation of material, activities, and discussion on topics that may be broken up across days, or even weeks, using semester-long course designs (Benton-Kupper, 1999). In addition, instructors have expressed positive reactions to teaching fewer days per class and to their increased opportunities to engage students in content more fully during each class meeting (Jenkins et al., 2002).

Alongside the many positives documented for intensive course design, downsides have been noted as well. Limitations to the course design have included increased student stress and decreased knowledge retention (Daniel, 2000), as well as the potential for decreased rigor compared to traditional, full-semester courses (Lutes & Davies, 2013). In addition, some researchers have noted students' preference for a less intensive course design that meets more often for shorter periods of time (Reardon et al., 2008). Furthermore, research suggests that the greater short-term learning resulting from intensive course design may not be retained long-term any more than learning resulting from traditional course design (Seamon, 2004). As detailed in Huelskamp's (2014) thorough review of the relevant literature, there is still limited evidence to prove the effectiveness or clear limitations of intensive course design, which remains true, especially in the health sciences. Importantly, aspects of instructors' style, methods, and engagement with students have an effect on course effectiveness regardless of course design format (Scott, 2003), and prior studies should be examined with this caveat in mind.

Instructors in the field of speech-language pathology have just begun to investigate whether and how an intensive course design affects their students' outcomes. Initial inquiries have shown positive effects on course satisfaction but not on students' feelings of clinical competency (DeVeney et al., 2015). Based on research across academic fields, the increased opportunity for engagement and practice allowed by intensive course design appears to suit the complex clinical learning needs of speech-language pathology graduate students. However, examination of the effect of this course design in graduate speech-language pathology programs is still in its infancy. Thus, this study was an initial step in addressing a key gap in the scholarship of teaching and learning research in the field of speech-language pathology. The aim of this study was to investigate student perceptions of an intensive course design format in two graduate courses.

ORIGINAL DATA

Sample and Procedures

This study took place during the second semester of the participating students' first year in their speech-language pathology graduate program at an accredited, public university in the mid-Atlantic region of the United States. All participating students provided informed consent to participate in the study, and all procedures were approved by the university's institutional review board. Students' responses to study measures were made anonymous by using identification numbers. Participating students ($n = 48$) were 22 to 40 years of age (mean = 24 years), all were female, and the group was 98% White and non-Hispanic. All participating students held bachelor's degrees in relevant fields (e.g., communication sciences and disorders, linguistics), and their mean prior GPA (grade point average) was 3.77.

As part of their course load, and in addition to clinical internship placements, participating students were enrolled in two required graduate courses using an intensive course design format (i.e., 6 hours per week for 7 weeks). The two 3-credit courses were School-Age Language Development and Disorders and Autism Spectrum Disorders in Speech-Language Pathology. Importantly, the students did not choose the intensive course design format (i.e., it was prescribed), which reduces the likelihood that their perceptions of the format were skewed by initial preference for or against intensive course design.

The school-age language course was taught during the first 7 weeks of the semester and the autism course during the second 7 weeks of the semester. The courses were similar in format, with didactic elements, interactive activities and discussion, and assessment of learning throughout. Both instructors were tenure-track junior faculty members with expertise in their respective course content areas; however, inherent differences in teaching style and internal format existed, as expected. The purpose of including both courses was not to compare students' responses to the two courses, but to begin to examine whether students' responses to the intensive course design format were due to the course design itself and were consistent across courses and instructors.

Measures

For the purposes of this study, three measures are reported. Following each course, participating students completed the Student Evaluation of Education Quality survey (SEEQ; Marsh, 1982), a reliable and valid tool (al-Muslim & Arfin, 2015) designed to evaluate teaching effectiveness and quality. The SEEQ survey includes 35 closed-ended questions and uses a 5-point Likert scale indicating responses ranging from "very poor" to "very good." The questions tap into a number of predetermined teaching dimensions (referred to as *scales* in the upcoming Study Outcomes section) that include academic value or learning, organization, instructor enthusiasm, rapport, breadth, assignments, examinations, and overall impressions. Readers may refer to the tool itself for more information about the specific questions that align with each dimension, or scale.

In addition to the SEEQ survey, at the end of the two courses, students were asked to complete a brief, study-specific written survey that asked open-ended questions about students' perceptions related to advantages and disadvantages of the intensive course design format. This survey also asked students whether they would or would not recommend continuation of the use of intensive course design for the courses.

Lastly, participating students completed the university's online course evaluation questionnaires at the end of each course. For this study, students' narrative responses to three open-ended questions about each course were used to better describe student learning and satisfaction, as well as to offer solutions to problems identified by the participating students. These open-ended questions asked students what they liked about the course, what could be improved, and whether they would recommend the course and why.

Data Analysis

The study used a mixed methods data analysis procedure. Simple quantitative methods were used to descriptively analyze the SEEQ survey numeric responses. Qualitative analysis methods were used to analyze the study survey responses and the narrative components of the university course evaluation questionnaires. For analysis of the narrative responses on both study surveys, two study team staff trained in thematic analysis qualitative coding methods independently coded the same narrative responses to identify recurrent themes using a thematic analysis approach (Braun & Clarke, 2006). In order to increase the rigor and decrease the subjectivity of the qualitative analysis methods used (as suggested by Barbour, 2001), the two independent coders compared codes as a means of inter-rater reliability and came to a consensus about themes that emerged from the data. The coders achieved 95% reliability before coming to a consensus. For narrative responses on course evaluations, themes were determined through instructors' review and reporting of these data at the departmental level.

Study Outcomes

As previously described, study outcomes were determined through examination of the three types of data collected: SEEQ quantitative data, study survey qualitative data, and qualitative data from the university's course evaluations. Results derived from each measure are presented in this section, along with interpretations of the findings.

Student Evaluation of Education Quality Results and Interpretation

Student responses to the Likert scale items on the SEEQ survey are presented in Table 8-1 with means presented by scale and averaged across the two courses. Individual course means are provided to indicate any discrepancy between courses, when appropriate. These results highlight students' satisfaction across elements of the two courses, delivered through an intensive course design format, and indicate any differences that may stem from the different course's content or instructional strategies.

SEEQ quantitative results show overall student satisfaction (defined for this study as ratings of "agree" or "strongly agree") with their learning in the two courses, as well as with course components and instructor attributes. There was minimal discrepancy between the two courses' results. For scales with overall scores that fell below 90% satisfaction for one course, individual items within that scale are further examined later in this chapter to determine specific issues.

Within the learning scale, one item was rated below 90% satisfaction in one of the courses. The item asked whether students' interest in the subject matter had increased because of the course—20% of students responded "neutral" and 16% "disagree." These responses may be due to students' inherent interest in certain topics or to the instructional strategies used. In the examinations scale, analysis of individual items showed lower than 90% satisfaction across items in one course, with 15% of students concerned about the appropriateness of the examinations and the feedback provided. This concern may be addressed by simple changes to the examination content and instructor feedback style. Perhaps fewer examinations would be appropriate due to the short length of the semester, with creative assessment strategies used to ensure knowledge transfer.

Overall, results of the SEEQ survey suggest student satisfaction. Results also suggest the possibility of variable difficulty capturing students' interest in subject matter in a short period of time, as well as difficulty with assessment and feedback procedures that may or may not be tied to the course design format. High-engagement activities (e.g., case studies, simulations) and decreased density of examinations may address some of these difficulties.

TABLE 8-1

Student Evaluation of Education Quality Quantitative Results

STUDENT EVALUATION OF EDUCATION QUALITY SCALE	% "AGREE" OR "STRONGLY AGREE" ON SCALE'S ITEMS MEAN *(% for each course, if discrepancy)*
Learning	92% (87%, 98%)
Instructor enthusiasm	98% (97%, 98%)
Organization	99%
Individual rapport	98% (96%, 100%)
Breadth	95% (91%, 98%)
Examinations	92% (85%, 100%)
Assignments	94% (92%, 96%)
Overall	99%

Study-Specific Survey Findings and Interpretation

In response to the study survey question, "Do you recommend that an intensive course design format continue in the future?", 37% of students did recommend continuation of this design. In line with this recommendation, a number of advantages of intensive course design were noted by the participating students. The most prominent advantages noted were the ability for students to focus on fewer courses at once, the course length being reduced to only 7 weeks, and greater feelings of immersion in the topics. Additional themes included greater feelings of information retention and increased time for discussion and clinical application. Additionally, some students reported reduced stress.

Despite students' citing of positive aspects of the format on this survey, 63% of students did not recommend continuation of its use. Accordingly, qualitative findings from the students' post-course study surveys indicate a number of specific disadvantages of the intensive course design format. The most prominent disadvantages identified by the students were that the length of the class meetings led to increased difficulty maintaining focus, and that the courses covered too much information over a short period of time. In addition to those main themes, additional minor themes emerged, such as the quick succession of due dates for assignments and readings, feelings of fatigue and being overwhelmed, and concern about keeping up with the faster pace of the course.

The word clouds in Figures 8-1 and 8-2 are provided to help readers visualize and compare the disadvantages and advantages to intensive course design, as reported by the graduate students who participated in this study. Larger font in the word clouds indicates greater frequency of that response, or theme, in the data, while smaller font indicates only a few students endorsed that idea.

Course Evaluation Results and Interpretation

To build upon and/or reinforce results of the SEEQ and study survey, students' responses to the open-ended questions on the online university course evaluations were reviewed by each instructor to examine students' perceptions of the course design, including positive aspects of the schedule and activities it allows and disadvantages to the format. This measure also allowed students to propose solutions to issues raised. Themes within these categories of feedback are summarized in the following sections.

Figure 8-1. Word cloud for advantages associated with intensive course design.

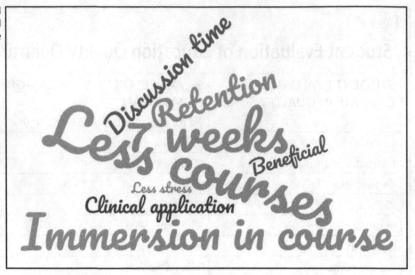

Figure 8-2. Word cloud for disadvantages associated with intensive course design.

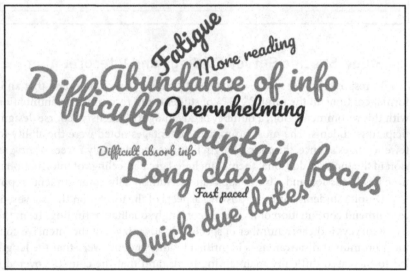

Positive Feedback

- Class activities helped cement what was learned in a hands-on manner.
- Weekly quizzes (versus one to two exams) helped students keep up with the fast pace of the information/course.
- Guest speakers provided several different viewpoints on the population.
- Group collaboration (e.g., case studies, activities) helped break up lengthy lectures and provided time to talk through concepts in a group to deepen understanding.

Constructive Feedback

- Course format made it difficult to retain material and knowledge because of the extensive class periods (i.e., a lot of information to learn in a short amount of time).
- Many assignments were given back to back or multiple were due at the same time.

Proposed Solutions to Issues

- Longer breaks for lunch would help students maintain engagement.
- Holding more regular review sessions would aid with retention of material.
- Modifying assignments to reflect the turnaround time allowed would ease stress.

This specific feedback about what made the intensive course design format effective for some and difficult for others is instructive. The positive and constructive feedback reflects many of the themes determined through coding of the study surveys, but interestingly, the course evaluation comments noted more positives than negatives, pointing to the potential of the course design. In terms of solutions to issues related to the course design format, students suggested only a few solutions. One suggestion was longer breaks to ease the fatigue induced by the longer class meetings, and another was more frequent review sessions to ease the burden of large quantities of information provided in each class meeting. A final suggestion was modification of large projects given the short time frame/turnaround. Perhaps smaller assignments that tap into the same learning outcomes would be more appropriate, as discussed later in this chapter. In addition, the instructors should be intentional about selecting due dates (e.g., midterm) to ensure "high stakes" assignments do not coincide with other intense events (e.g., start of clinical internships).

APPLICATION OF LITERATURE/DATA

The measures used in this study allowed students to report their perceptions through multiple instruments and modalities (i.e., closed-ended standardized written survey instrument questions, open-ended written study survey questions, and open-ended online course evaluation questions). Taken together, results indicate the potential for enhanced learning opportunities in intensive course design and show overall student satisfaction with the courses based on the SEEQ numeric data. However, the qualitative feedback highlights both positives and potential limitations based on student perceptions. The students directly offered several solutions to issues raised, such as longer breaks as a means of alleviating fatigue and difficulty maintaining focus. Students' noted disadvantages, such as quick succession of due dates and too much information, imply solutions indirectly as well.

Specifically, instructors trialing the use of an intensive course design format should carefully plan their assignment and reading schedule so as not to overwhelm students and inhibit learning. Assignments could also be adapted to include more group collaboration and presentations, which can reduce time constraints but maintain learning. In addition, instructors can leverage the extended class time to engage students through in-class learning and assessment. For example, a case study activity could involve a group presentation during class, which can be graded to assess learning using pre-stated criteria.

In the context of this case, a traditional course delivery format was chosen moving forward for the two courses based on student concerns. However, the instructors are in the process of completing a comparison group study to more directly compare students' perceptions of intensive versus traditional course design and to brainstorm methods for addressing the concerns raised by students. The intensive format is also being trialed within the department for courses worth fewer than 3 credits, with positive preliminary results. In the end, additional research is needed on this topic to determine if the long term, clinical benefits differ based on a traditional or intensive course design.

APPLICATION TO CROSS-DISCIPLINARY CONTEXTS

There is potential for application of the information gained from this study in several other clinically based disciplines, including occupational therapy, physical therapy, and nursing, among others. Many clinical disciplines attract nontraditional or second-career students who may appreciate a flexible schedule or shortened semester. In addition, the clinical nature of these fields is well suited to the format's longer class meetings, which allow for increased exploration of content and opportunity for deeper understanding through practice and discussion. The recommendations noted earlier are applicable to all disciplines, as they are not specific to the content but relate primarily to students' knowledge retention, engagement, and comfort.

ADDITIONAL RESOURCES

Designing Accelerated Courses

- Rochester Institute of Technology tips:
  ○ https://www.rit.edu/academicaffairs/tls/course-design/tiger-terms/designing-accel-courses

Transitioning to an Intensive Course Design

- McDonald, P. L., Harwood, K. J., Butler, J. T., Schlumpf, K. S., Eschmann, C. W., & Drago, D. (2018). Design for success: Identifying a process for transitioning to an intensive online course delivery model in health professions education. *Medical Education Online, 23*(1), 1415617.

REFERENCES

Adams, D. C., & Salvaterra, M. E. (1997). Structural and teacher changes: Necessities for successful block schedule. *The High School Journal, 81*(2), 98-105.

al-Muslim, M., & Arfin, Z. (2015). The usability of the SEEQ in quality evaluation of Arabic secondary education in Malaysia. *International Education Studies, 8*(3), 202-211.

Anatasi, J. S. (2007). Full-semester and abbreviated summer courses: An evaluation of student performance. *Teaching of Psychology, 34*(1), 19-22.

Anderson, T. I., & Anderson, R. J. (2012). Time compressed delivery for quantitative college courses: The key to student success. *Academy of Educational Leadership Journal, 16*(S1), 1655-1662.

Barbour, R. S. (2001). Checklists for improving rigour in qualitative research: A case of the tail wagging the dog? *British Medical Journal, 322*(7294), 1115-1117. https://doi.org/10.1136/bmj.322.7294.1115

Benton-Kupper, J. (1999). Teaching in the block: Perceptions from within. *The High School Journal, 83*(1), 26-34.

Braun, V., & Clarke, V. (2006). Using thematic analysis in psychology. *Qualitative Research in Psychology, 3*(2), 77-101.

Daniel, E. L. (2000). A review of time-shortened courses across disciplines. *College Student Journal, 34*(2).

Davies, W. M. (2006). Intensive teaching formats: A review. *Issues in Educational Research, 16*(1), 1-20.

DeVeney, S. L., Teten, A. F., & Friehe, M. J. (2015). Full-semester and time-compressed fluency disorders course: An evaluation of student perceptions of competence, satisfaction, and workload. *Social Welfare: An Interdisciplinary Approach, 2*(5).

Huelskamp, D. (2014). Block Scheduling and its effects on long-term student achievement: A review of the research. *Global Education Journal, 2014*(3), 122-126.

Jenkins, E., Queen, A., & Algozzine, B. (2002). To block or not to block: That's not the question. *Journal of Educational Research, 95*(4), 196-202. https://doi.org/10.1080/00220670209596592

Lutes, L., & Davies, R. (2013). Comparing the rigor of compressed format courses to their regular semester counterparts. *Innovative Higher Education, 38*(1), 19-29. https://doi.org/10.1007/s10755-012-9226-z

Marsh, H. (1982). SEEQ: A reliable, valid, and useful instrument in collecting students' evaluations of university teaching. *British Journal of Educational Psychology, 52*, 77-95.

Mok, C. K., Dodd, B., & Whitehill, T. L. (2009). Speech-language pathology students' approaches to learning in a problem-based learning curriculum. *International Journal of Speech-Language Pathology, 11*(6), 472-481. https://doi.org/10.3109/17549500903003052

Myers, C. T., & O'Brien, S. P. (2015). Teaching interprofessional collaboration: Using online education across institutions. *Occupational Therapy in Health Care, 29*(2), 178-185. https://doi.org/10.3109/07380577.2015.1017789

Reardon, J., Payan, J., Miller, C., & Alexander, J. (2008). Optimal class length in marketing undergraduate classes: An examination of preference, instructor evaluations, and student performance. *Journal of Marketing Education, 30*(1), 12-20. https://doi.org/10.1177/0273475307312193

Scott, P. A. (1995). Learning experiences in intensive and semester-length classes: Student voices and experiences. *College Student Journal, 29*, 207-207.

Scott, P. A. (2003). Attributes of high-quality intensive courses. *New Directions for Adult and Continuing Education, 97*, 29-38.

Seamon, M. (2004.) Short and long-term differences in instructional effectiveness between intensive and semester-length courses. *Teachers College Record, 106*, 852-874.

Vlachopoulos, P., Kan, S. K., & Lockyer, L. (2019). A comparative study on the traditional and intensive delivery of an online course: Design and facilitation recommendations. *Research in Learning Technology, 27*, 2196. https://doi.org/10.25304/rlt.v27.2196

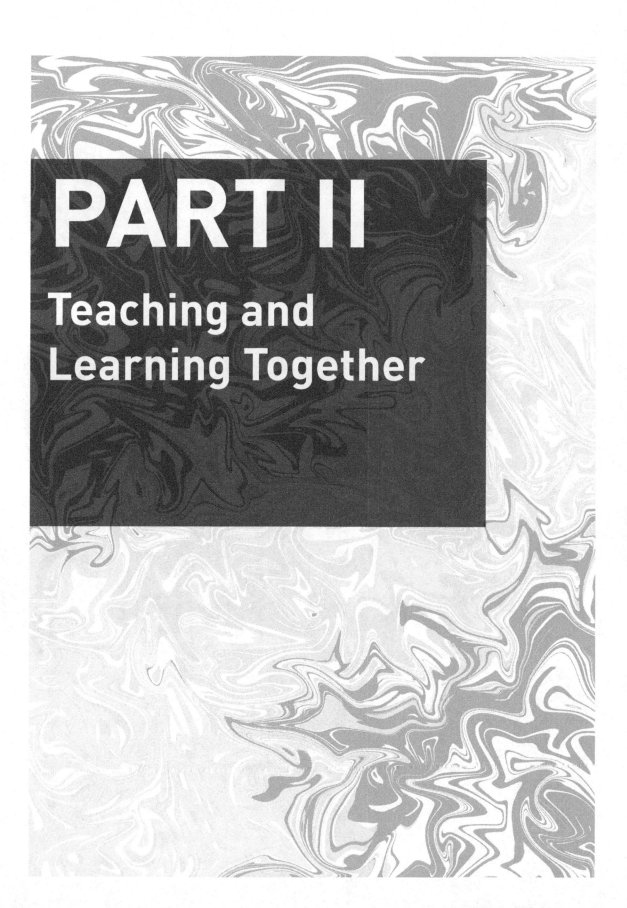

PART II
Teaching and Learning Together

ASSIGNED GROUPS AS LEARNING COMMUNITIES IN AND BEYOND THE CLASSROOM

*Cassandra Barragan, PhD, MSW
and Stephanie P. Wladkowski, PhD, LMSW, APHSW-C*

DESCRIPTION OF TEACHING/LEARNING CONTEXT

As part of a required undergraduate course—Social Work Practice with Women and Girls—social work students were given a list of books to complete a full biopsychosocial assessment (BPA) to prepare them for social work practice. A BPA is a comprehensive framework for understanding the biological, psychological, social-emotional, spiritual, and cultural elements of a person and their environment. The client assessment assignment is based on reading a book that focuses on at least one issue of importance to women/girls, and selecting a self-identified female character from the book that will be designated as the fictional client, which will be the focus of their research and critical assessment, planning, and analysis. Students are provided a list of fiction and nonfiction books to choose from. Within the social work program, the client assessment assignment has been designated as the "signature assignment" for all students taking this specific course to demonstrate learned professional social work competencies.

The assignment is constructed for students to complete in four separate sections over the semester: (1) background and presenting problem, (2) social history, (3) recommendations, and (4) the final assignment bringing all sections together for the full BPA. Students were given the opportunity for their drafts to be reviewed by the instructor at the first three points to ensure the final assessment was comprehensive and demonstrated quality synthesis of information.

In previous semesters, students had struggled to successfully complete the assignment. We identified two specific areas where students seemed to have had the most problems. First, the assignment provided upwards of 15 choices of books, which prevented students from connecting with other students who were reading the same book. This inability to connect negatively affected

Friberg, J. C., Visconti, C. F., & Ginsberg, S. M. (Eds.). *Evidence-Based Education in the Classroom: Examples From Clinical Disciplines* (pp. 81-88). © 2021 Taylor & Francis Group.

class discussions, as they were relating concepts to their specific book without opportunity to process with other students. Having a wide range of choices also placed the responsibility of discussion solely on the instructor. Second, despite having opportunity for ongoing feedback, only a few students utilized professor feedback to revise their assignment. The results were poorly constructed assignments and a lack of depth in content or demonstration of assessment skill development.

We needed to revise the assignment. Our goal was to restructure both the content delivery and the in-class application to better facilitate learning how to apply assessment skills that had been learned throughout the program curriculum. We chose to apply writing across the curriculum (WAC) principles (Bean, 2011) for the client assessment assignment combined with the high-impact practice of team-based learning (Kuh, 2007).

This chapter describes how a critical review of student performance on an assignment and teaching methods resulted in the use of group assigned learning communities to support WAC concepts to facilitate student skill development.

REVIEW OF LITERATURE

Writing Across the Curriculum

WAC is a student-centered approach to learning to write in the discipline that uses specific strategies to enable successful writing. Four specific strategies are described in the following three sections.

Scaffolded Assignments

Applying principles of WAC, such as scaffolding, helps students think about the goals of their writing and to understand writing as a process (Rutz & Grawe, 2017) that happens over the course of their education and training (Zygmont & Schaefer, 2006). Writing assignments are more impactful if students learn a new way of writing related to writing they expect to do in the future (Eodice et al., 2016). This transferability of skills gives students a new intention and purpose when challenged to redefine the meaning of an assignment (Lindenman, 2015). In essence, when writing is meaningful to a student, it facilitates the learning process by making it personal.

High- and Low-Stakes Writing

High-stakes writing is formal and is more attached to an outcome, such as a course grade or following a specific assignment format. Low-stakes writing is informal and intended to practice skills in a safe environment (e.g., "free writes," in-class reflections). A data-provided assignment (Bean, 2011) combines high- and low-stakes writing and is a strategy wherein students are provided with the information needed to complete an assignment. Data-provided assignments can be structured so students write one section at a time as low-stakes assignments that scaffold to the final, high-stakes assignment.

Peer and Instructor Feedback

Instructors often fall into the pattern of providing feedback that is in the form of unmitigated direct criticism of student work. The purpose of instructor feedback should be to facilitate improvement on low-stakes assignments offering opportunity for improvement and skill development. Instructor feedback can also be more meaningful on a late-stage draft after peer review (Bean, 2011) since the student has already had an opportunity to revise their writing. Peer-review feedback can be highly valuable to students as they have the opportunity to improve and reflect on their own writing through the evaluation of other students' work (Fosmire, 2010; Mulder et al., 2012). Students also find that peer review can help them determine if their writing is aligned with the rest of the class (Ruggiero & Harbor, 2013).

Application of Discipline-Specific Writing

When WAC strategies are used, students gain a better understanding of the application of writing in their specific field of study (Colorado State University, 2014; Luthy et al., 2009), and because learning to write in the discipline is also a skill that must be developed (Oermann & Hays, 2016), applying WAC strategies helps students to recognize writing assignments as meaningful and applicable to their field of study. While WAC strategies have been used extensively in medical sciences, specifically nursing (Hawks et al., 2016), they also improved writing in the discipline for social work students (Luna et al., 2014).

Team-Based/Collaborative Learning

Collaboration is a high-impact practice that is a key element to students feeling a writing assignment is meaningful (Eodice et al., 2016). Approaching problems with a collaborative approach helps students develop a sense of involvement and investment in learning and is most beneficial when students all share similar knowledge (Retnowati et al., 2018). Through peer interaction, students have an opportunity to connect newly learned information in a meaningful way and then practice this new knowledge with a process that makes sense to them (Council of Writing Program Administrators, 2011). This new approach is key in developing competency-related skills while also developing a personal sense of efficacy in helping resolve complex problems (Siegel, 2010).

APPLICATION OF LITERATURE/DATA

After teaching the course, we found that students struggled with the assignment and that we needed to evaluate the student work, assignment, and approach. Critical evaluation involved reviewing the rubric used to score the assignment and determining where students did well and where there were challenges. Specifically, this process entailed identifying what excellent, good, and poor examples looked like and considering what it would take for students to reach the level of competence expected at this point in their academic program. This review revealed two distinct areas that posed the greatest challenges for students: (1) the ability to practically apply concepts they had learned in other courses, and (2) taking the time necessary to complete the assignment well and thus, learn the skill. The end result was that we recognized the value of the assignment to teach necessary application of assessment skills, but students were not consistently able to make a meaningful connection to practical skills.

To address the first issue identified, we began by scaffolding the assignments, assigning high- and low-stakes values, and creating opportunities to provide meaningful feedback in a way that students could write to learn in order to apply the feedback. Using these WAC approaches also addressed the second issue identified, ensuring students were taking the time necessary to complete the assignment. To synthesize work being done in the scaffolded portions of the assignments, we created mini learning communities based on a condensed choice of books. Students could self-select into these mini learning communities based on the chosen book. Along with using a peer-review process for the scaffolded portions of the assignment, we also used these groups during class activities. This enabled them to develop a sense of safety in and out of the classroom, with the added opportunity for peer support.

Several changes were implemented using the WAC principles and collaborative learning opportunities and these include the following:

- Renamed assignment BPA: We aimed for students to utilize social work terminology with a goal to feel more connected to the developing skills and less about course task completion.
- Low-stakes submission for feedback with a three-step process: (1) Peer review for feedback, (2) revise based on feedback, and (3) submit revised assignment to instructor. For students who chose to submit for feedback, the submission was considered low-stakes as the grade was not

final and we provided ample time to respond to any feedback to improve the grade received on the draft. However, if students did not respond to feedback, the assignment became high-stakes, as this draft, in some cases, was their final grade.

- Scaffolded approach: The BPA was submitted first in three drafts following the low-stakes submission process for peer review and instructor feedback. Intentional in-class activities and writing exercises gave opportunity to practice skills demonstrated in the BPA.

- Mini learning community: Each instructor independently chose to either assign books and/or groups or have students self-select books from a small list, which would determine the group. A Google Drive was set up for groups to communicate with each other outside of class time, and time was given in class to work together on not only the final BPA but also other team-based learning in class related to course content.

- Peer review process: Mini learning communities allowed opportunity for both individual learning and collaborative learning.

An outline of the BPA client assessment assignment can be seen in Appendix.

Evaluation of Assignment

When comparing grades for the original assignment and the revised assignment with improved classroom structure, we saw an increase in final scores from 86.54% to 91.38% (Table 9-1). These scores demonstrated competency in developing skills to complete a BPA and the synthesis needed to complete the full BPA assignment.

There are limitations to our analysis that must be noted. First, we built in additional opportunities for both feedback and hands-on practice of the required skills between the course sections. Therefore, it would be assumed that the class with additional time and resources would score higher on the final assignment. Additionally, each instructor teaches and evaluates their work differently, even when using the same grading rubric. Plus, the instructors had more practice in teaching course content, revised teaching methods, and placed more emphasis in areas that differed between sections, making it a challenge to compare scores across sections. Finally, we are unable to ascertain the effect of prior instruction around the specific skills students may have obtained in previous courses.

Reflection on Assignment and Outcomes

Evaluating assignments and the role of the instructor is a critical component to this process. We were pleasantly surprised to see students not only complete the assignment more fully, but also with more confidence. Students demonstrated a sense of ownership of this process as it was explicitly applicable to the profession. Also, grouping the students by books created a cohort effect, where students could test out their thoughts and approaches in a low-stakes format without penalty.

Both authors combined experience with the course, knowledge of the program curriculum, and interest in writing pedagogy, which certainly helped revise this assignment. There was also a commitment to the scaffolding process because it is a constant and ongoing feedback loop throughout the semester. Each instructor found the scaffolded assignment schedule coupled with the small group activities improved what students submitted, and thus, reduced time spent in the final grading process. Specifically, students had more time to flesh out drafts of their work and, because of this, submitted more thought-out and edited versions. This made evaluating more efficient and more pleasurable (or at least less frustrating). This gave us more confidence that students were more prepared moving through the curriculum.

The investment of time and commitment to increasing our workload on the front end of designing this scaffolded assignment did result in positive outcomes. However, each course did present learning opportunities for future semesters. For example, students did not always see the value of submitting additional drafts (even if low stakes), and some struggled to construct several drafts of work prior to the final product. This presented teaching challenges in sustaining morale for

TABLE 9-1

Biopsychosocial Assessment Student Scores
Pre- and Post-Course Revision

	PRE-COURSE REVISION				POST-COURSE REVISION				
Semester and Class Size	Fall 2016 ($n = 21$)		Fall 2017 ($n = 16$)		Summer 2018 ($n = 24$)		Fall 2018 ($n = 11$)		Fall 2018 ($n = 14$)	
Score	n	%	n	%	n	%	n	%	n	%
90 to 100	12	57	8	50	11	46	9	82	10	71
80 to 89	3	14	4	25	10	42	0	0	2	14
70 to 79	1	5	3	19	3	13	1	9	1	7
69 and below	5	24	1	6	0	0	1	9	1	7

Note: $n = 86$ (n varies per class).

undergraduate students who are challenged by effective time management and worked to balance the workload of several courses in one semester. Also, not all students utilized these drafts to further their work and improve their writing in a way they could reap the full benefits of a satisfactory grade. However, those that did use the opportunity for multiple drafts appreciated the opportunity to do work earlier in the semester rather than the final "push" typically experienced at the end of the semester. Finally, we cannot control the attendance of students to be present for all in-class activities focused on their writing assignments. These challenges have informed future approaches, which include intentional transparency of the course pedagogy and more emphasis on the value of participating at all points in the semester.

APPLICATION TO CROSS-DISCIPLINARY CONTEXTS

The use of assigned groups as a learning community to support a scaffolded approach to learning could be used by any discipline where practice involves the synthesizing of skills. For example:

- An instructor in counseling, psychology, or psychiatry (or any other discipline requiring a mental health diagnosis) might use this approach to simulate an evaluation. This would include opportunity to apply clinical skills to diagnose a patient and use assigned groups to review the written reports through a process of writing and revisions.
- Using WAC strategies to augment the benefit of learning communities by intentionally designing assignments to teach the writing genres most appropriate for various learner populations, including undergraduate, graduate, advanced practice, and English as a second language students.
- The opportunity for interprofessional education adds value to the approaches of scaffolding. Integrated health models are interdisciplinary in nature and scaffolding enables students to be successful in fundamental skill building. This same method could be applied to interprofessional exercises, such as simulated experiences and co-taught courses.

ADDITIONAL RESOURCES

- The WAC Clearinghouse website provides resources, including books, journals, databases, resources, community organizations, and news that support the use of writing in courses across the curriculum; all materials are open access:
  - https://wac.colostate.edu/
- The Framework for Success in Postsecondary Writing from the Council of Writing Program Administrators provides a foundational understanding of the habits of mind and how they apply to writing, reading, and critical analysis:
  - http://wpacouncil.org/aws/CWPA/asset_manager/get_file/350201?ver=284
- An essential reference tool when designing scaffolded assignments, this book includes examples across disciplines and walks through the process of integrating WAC principles in your courses:
  - Bean, J. C. (2011). *Engaging ideas: The professor's guide to integrating writing, critical thinking, and active learning in the classroom* (2nd ed.). Jossey-Bass Inc.

Suggested Readings

- Eodice, M., Geller, A. E., & Lerner, N. (2016). *The meaningful writing project: Learning, teaching, and writing in higher education.* University Press of Colorado
- Kuh, G. (2007). What student engagement data tell us about college readiness. *Peer Review, 9*(1), 4-8.
- Retnowati, E., Ayres, P., & Sweller, J. (2018). Collaborative learning effects when students have complete or incomplete knowledge. *Applied Cognitive Psychology, 32*(6), 681-692. http://dx.doi.org/10.1002/acp.3444

REFERENCES

Bean, J. C. (2011). *Engaging ideas: The professor's guide to integrating writing, critical thinking, and active learning in the classroom* (2nd ed.). Jossey-Bass Inc.

Colorado State University. (2014). What is writing in the disciplines? *WAC Clearinghouse.* https://wac.colostate.edu/

Council of Writing Program Administrators. (2011). Framework for success in postsecondary writing. http://wpacouncil.org/aws/CWPA/asset_manager/get_file/350201?ver=7548

Eodice, M., Geller, A. E., & Lerner, N. (2016). *The meaningful writing project: Learning, teaching, & writing in higher education.* University Press of Colorado

Fosmire, M. (2010). Calibrated peer review: A new tool for integrating information literacy skills in writing-intensive large classroom settings. *Libraries and the Academy, 10*(2), 147-163.

Hawks, S., Turner, K., Derouin, A., Hueckel, R., Leonardelli, A., & Oermann, M. (2016). Writing across the curriculum: Strategies to improve the writing skills of nursing students. *Nursing Forum, 51*(4), 261-267.

Kuh, G. (2007). What student engagement data tell us about college readiness. *Peer Review, 9*(1), 4-8.

Lindenman, J. (2015). Inventing metagenres: How four college seniors connect writing across domains. *Composition Forum, 31.* https://files.eric.ed.gov/fulltext/EJ1061560.pdf

Luna, N., Horton, E. G., & Galin, J. (2014). The effectiveness of writing across the curriculum in a baccalaureate social work program: Students' perceptions. *Advances in Social Work, 15*(2), 390-408.

Luthy, K. E., Peterson, N. E., Lassetter, J. H., & Callister, L. C. (2009). Successfully incorporating writing across the curriculum with advanced writing in nursing. *Journal of Nursing Education, 48*(1), 54-59.

Mulder, R. A., Elgar, M. A., & Brady, D. (2012, October). APRES: Electronically managed student feedback via peer review. In Proceedings of *The Australian Conference on Science and Mathematics Education* (formerly UniServe Science Conference) (Vol. 11).

Oermann, M. H., & Hays, J. C. (2016). *Writing for publication in nursing* (3rd ed.). Springer.

Retnowati, E., Ayres, P., & Sweller, J. (2018). Collaborative learning effects when students have complete or incomplete knowledge. *Applied Cognitive Psychology, 32*(6), 681-692. http://dx.doi.org/10.1002/acp.3444

Ruggiero, D., & Harbor, J. (2013). Using writing assignments with calibrated peer review to increase engagement and improve learning in an undergraduate environmental science course. *International Journal for the Scholarship of Teaching and Learning, 7*(2), 1-15.

Rutz, C., & Grawe, N. D. (2017). How writing program best practices have transformed Carleton College. *Peer Review, 19*(1), 13-16.

Siegel, D. (2010). *The new science of personal transformation.* Random House.

Zygmont, D. M., & Schaefer, K. M. (2006). Writing across the nursing curriculum project. *Annual Review of Nursing Education, 4,* 275-290.

APPENDIX: ASSIGNMENT DESCRIPTION

The paper outline is as follows:

1. Assessment (Part I): Minimum of three pages. Provide a thorough assessment of the client and what has brought her to your agency. Also discuss the background of the client. In assessing the client and the context of her life, articulate how gender plays a role in coping, strengths, and supports.

2. Intervention (Part II): Minimum of three pages. Discuss goals of intervention, theory or theories (e.g., feminist theory, strengths perspective, empowerment, systems, crisis intervention) used and why. Research three articles from three separate professional social work journals that discuss the specific issue (e.g., rape, incest, racism, poverty, adoption, mental illness, addiction) that your client brought to you. From these articles, you will cite how they suggest you work with clients that face or deal with these issues. Use American Psychological Association style for citing articles. A bibliography or reference list must be given listing all references used. The reference list will be placed on the last page of your final submission.

3. Resources (Part III): Minimum of two pages. What actual resources are in the community that might help your client? List at least three resources that you have found in the community that could help this woman with the problems that she presented. The three resources must be different types of services. An example of a resource is a homeless shelter or a substance abuse treatment program. Do **not** use the same services with different names. For example, Catholic Social Services for counseling and (City) Counseling Center for Counseling are essentially the same service.

4. Full Client Assessment: A synthesis of Parts I, II, and III will be submitted. ***This will not be the three previous versions stapled together, as many new details and insights will shape the ongoing evolution of this paper.***

5. Final Analysis (included in the full BPA): Minimum of two pages. Included in your final client paper (Parts I, II, and III) is this short reflection: After taking this course, what specific ways might you modify or change your work with this client? What are some of the conflicts (internal or external) **you** (not your client) might confront in working from a woman-centered/feminist model with this woman? What will you do about these conflicts?

6. This paper should be a minimum of 10 pages and a maximum of 12. This does **not** include the title page, where you write your name and the name of the book, and the last page, which lists references.

10

TRAINING FUTURE HEALTH PROFESSIONALS USING AN INTERDISCIPLINARY APPROACH

Judi Brooks, PhD, RD; Diane Fenske, LMSW;
Lydia McBurrows, DNP, RN, CPNP-PC;
and Andrea Gossett Zakrajsek, OTD, OTRL, FNAP

It has been my observation that there is nothing more efficient or dynamic than an experienced and functioning interdisciplinary health care team. —Survey respondent

DESCRIPTION OF TEACHING/LEARNING CONTEXT

After teaching in professional programs for many years, the authors have observed that students do not fully comprehend the roles and responsibilities of their own intended discipline or those of multiple other disciplines. The aim of the project was to create a learning experience that enhanced both students' understanding of professional roles and responsibilities as well as their understanding of interdisciplinary teams and practices prior to entering their professional programs. The goal of this chapter is to describe the development of learning activities in a preprofessional interdisciplinary course based on a study of practitioners using survey methodology. These learning activities were designed to cultivate an awareness of the roles and responsibilities of the different health care disciplines, increase knowledge of interdisciplinary teams and teaming, and improve attitudes regarding teamwork.

The course—Aging to Infancy: A Life Course Retrospective—was planned in 2000 by a team of four faculty representing the disciplines of social work gerontology, occupational therapy, nursing, and dietetics and human nutrition. The team worked together for more than a year before the first offering of the course in January 2002. The course is unique in multiple ways:

Friberg, J. C., Visconti, C. F., & Ginsberg, S. M. (Eds.). *Evidence-Based Education in the Classroom: Examples From Clinical Disciplines* (pp. 89-95).
© 2021 Taylor & Francis Group.

- It uses a retrospective approach, starting with an older adult and working backward.
- It uses the life course perspective, which calls attention to human development and aging as a lifelong process, emphasizing the interweave of personal biography and social history (Settersten, 2002).
- It is taught in a highly integrated interdisciplinary manner by a team of three to four faculty from different health care disciplines, all of whom are in the classroom every class period as a means of modeling the health care team to the students (Schuster et al., 2003).
- It requires the students to work in faculty-assigned interdisciplinary teams to build rapport, identify important team-based skills, and complete both activities and assignments over the course of the semester.
- It is a prerequisite human growth and development course required for application to most health professions programs in the university.

Almost 20 years after its first offering, this course remains a model of both interdisciplinary education in preprofessional courses and demonstrates evidence-driven course design, content, and instruction.

REVIEW OF LITERATURE

Increasingly, it has become apparent to course instructors of Aging to Infancy: A Life Course Retrospective that future health professional practitioners require education preparation to learn with, from, and about each other in order to collaboratively practice in health care teams and ultimately improve health outcomes (O'Keefe et al., 2017; Thistlethwaite et al., 2014). One way to achieve this is through interprofessional education (IPE), where students from two or more professions learn together. This learning can occur during practice, as part of a professional program, or prior to admission to a professional program. Per the Interprofessional Education Collaborative (IPEC, 2016), the Core Competencies for Interprofessional Collaborative Practice include four domains that are vital for the learning continuum of professionals: interprofessional communication practices, roles and responsibilities for collaborative practice, values/ethics for interprofessional practice, and interprofessional teamwork and team-based practice.

According to Leipzig and colleagues (2002), there is a recognition that IPE needs to occur early on in training of students in health care professions. Because future practitioners are typically trained in isolation, it is critical that students have opportunities to collaborate and understand the roles and responsibilities of others early on in their education. The development of content in this course drew from the interdisciplinary and IPE literature that recognized the importance of construction and boundaries of roles and responsibilities of health disciplines (Drinka & Clark, 2016; MacNaughton et al., 2013; Maharajan et al., 2017). As noted in the Geriatric Interdisciplinary Team Training Core Curriculum (Long et al., 2001), it is important that each member of the health care team understands the knowledge and expertise contributed by all other professional members of the team. The focus of this chapter is on the preprofessional end of the continuum with the recommendation that IPE occur prior to entering a professional program.

Not only is the knowledge and understanding of other professionals important, but the development of professional behaviors is crucial to the success of future interdisciplinary health care teams (O'Keefe et al., 2017). These behaviors, such as respect, patience, and conflict management, are necessary in developing competence for effective collaboration in health care teams. Per Weaver and colleagues (2014), "patients are safer and receive higher quality care when providers work as a highly effective team" (p. 259). Furthermore, actively training future health care professionals in teams in the classroom improves team performance. A systematic review and meta-analysis of teamwork interventions (McEwan et al., 2017) found experiential activities, with active learning components, are the most effective in developing teamwork skills.

ORIGINAL DATA

To better prepare students to work in interdisciplinary teams, we surveyed approximately 1,800 practitioners in the disciplines represented by students' majors in the course Aging to Infancy: A Life Course Retrospective (e.g., dietetics, social work, nursing, occupational therapy, health administration). The study was approved by the university's institutional review board. The survey examined the following: (1) how practitioners understand their own discipline's roles and responsibilities on an interdisciplinary team, (2) how practitioners understand the roles and responsibilities of other disciplines, and (3) what practitioners wished they had learned as students regarding the knowledge and skills of interdisciplinary teams.

Participants were recruited through a purchased email list of professionals from a digital marketing service provider. The email lists included the following nine disciplines: dietetics, medicine, nursing, occupational therapy, pharmacy, physical therapy, respiratory therapy, social work, and speech-language pathology. Participants were sent the online survey, designed in Qualtrics (Qualtrics International Inc.) software (Qualtrics, 2019), via email. Of those surveyed, 341 practitioners responded (19%). Data were analyzed using descriptive statistics and qualitative content analysis.

Respondents identified a number of knowledge areas, skills, and values that are important to effective interdisciplinary teams. Of those who responded, 95.7% indicated knowledge regarding roles and responsibilities of their own discipline as important, and 91.9% indicated that knowledge regarding roles and responsibilities of other disciplines is important to effective interdisciplinary team collaboration. As one respondent indicated, "We all work together to provide the needs of [the] resident we take care of. Every department is essential and we must collaborate for their wellbeing."

Furthermore, the professional behaviors that respondents indicated as important included: resolving conflict (93.6%), effective communication (97.2%), leadership skills (82%), creating an environment of openness and respect (95.1%), and valuing the contributions of others (94.7%). In the open-ended survey comments, several respondents reinforced and expanded upon the importance of the above professional behaviors. For example, one respondent stated, "Experiencing good teams in action first hand … discussing strategies for team conflict resolution and how to manage team input in respectful ways … is invaluable." Another respondent noted the importance of good leadership skills, such as "knowing how to facilitate the team, effectively move[ing] people to problem solving and planning versus rehashing the problems." In addition, several respondents indicated the importance of *listening* to one another and creating opportunities to hear one another. One respondent specifically defined this as "inquiry before judgment." Several respondents also discussed the importance of respect for others on an interdisciplinary team; one stated, "Everyone's position is important."

APPLICATION OF LITERATURE/DATA

These results were applied to the course Aging to Infancy: A Life Course Retrospective. Using the findings from the surveyed practitioners, the teaching team revised an existing lecture on the interdisciplinary health care team (IHCT 1) and created three new lectures: an additional lecture on the IHCT (IHCT 2), a lecture on conflict resolution, and a lecture on the application of life course perspective. We also developed four new learning activities related to team building and group dynamics, engaging students in both small and large group discussions. The following sections discuss the course changes.

Interdisciplinary Health Care Team 1

The first lecture in the series covered development of IHCT and foundational knowledge of each of the health care disciplines. The goal of the lecture was to prepare students to work in interdisciplinary teams. Within this lecture, we defined interdisciplinary teams, the challenges and objectives, the core set of values of teaming (Mitchell et al., 2012), the mechanism of teams, the roles and responsibilities, and how teams are developed and maintained. Activities included Team Bus Stop ice breaker (David P. Weikart Center for Youth Program Quality, 2012) and creating Team Ground Rules (see Additional Resources section for activity descriptions). At the end of the class session, students were provided note cards and given 2 minutes to write a reflection on the lecture content and activities. Students also engaged in an online threaded discussion regarding the purpose of teams in the course and why faculty formed these teams as part of the students' experience. Following the last team-based assignment, students were asked, in an online journal entry, to reflect on their experience in teams throughout the semester and compare their experience to the article, "The Steps to Developing and Maintaining Effective Work Teams" (Sidler & Lifton, 1999).

Interdisciplinary Health Care Team 2

The second lecture in the series covered specific knowledge areas, skills, and values important to effective team experiences. The goal of the lecture was to build on the content covered in the IHCT 1 lecture and address professional behaviors identified through our survey as important to team development (i.e., communication and active listening, respect, accountability, and leadership; Arnold & Stern, 2006; Nancarrow et al., 2013). We used the activity "What Color Am I?" adapted from the True Colors Personality Test (www.truecolorsintl.com) to support students' understanding of self and how to interact with others so that students would have the best possible teaming experience. At the end of the class session, students were provided note cards and given 2 minutes to write a reflection on the lecture content and activities.

Conflict Resolution

The third lecture in the series focused on conflict resolution skills. The goal of the lecture was to prepare students to manage any conflict arising as part of their team interactions. Within the lecture, conflict resolution, the outcomes of conflict in teams, and strategies for reducing counterproductive conflict were described. At the end of the class session, students were provided note cards and given 2 minutes to write a reflection on past conflict resolution experiences and application of strategies for reducing conflict.

Application of Life Course Perspective

During the last class session, students were given an opportunity to discuss their teaming experience and their understanding of the roles and responsibilities of health care disciplines using a Team Bus Stop activity (David P. Weikart Center for Youth Program Quality, 2012). The Team Bus Stop questions included: What did you learn about a health care discipline, other than your chosen major, that you did not know before? and Following the "What Color Am I?" exercise, how did knowledge of your team's color makeup affect team building?

APPLICATION TO CROSS-DISCIPLINARY CONTEXTS

The work discussed in this chapter has implications for all students intending to work in a health care career. For example, skills for effective conflict resolution are necessary for effective interdisciplinary teams and can be included, not just in courses within discipline-specific programs of study, but in any preprofessional course. We recognize students only begin to understand the roles and responsibilities of other disciplines in a preprofessional class, such as Aging to Infancy: A Life Course Retrospective. The work required in their professional programs does not always allow for experiences with other disciplines. Issues of isolation occur and communication skills across disciplines are not always emphasized. We must assist students in developing a shared appreciation and respect for the multiple disciplines in their work environment early on (Leipzig et al., 2002). These team skills, the understanding of roles and responsibilities, and valuing of others are prerequisites regardless of the student's intended profession.

Findings from the study briefly described earlier suggest that an interdisciplinary teamwork course developed for preprofessional health care students from multiple disciplines (e.g., dietetics, nursing, occupational therapy, social work) is beneficial. Topics, such as team development and maintenance, professional behaviors (e.g., communication and active listening, respect, accountability, and leadership), conflict resolution, mutual respect, and collaboration, could be explored by various methods and approaches. Students would understand that failure to learn these skills and work using an interdisciplinary team approach will cause lost opportunities for patient care (IPEC, 2016). In a course with this emphasis, students would gain knowledge regarding all roles, and what each profession brings to the team. This learning can then be taken into their discipline-specific programs of study to foster successful interdisciplinary practice now and in the future.

Additional Resources

Interdisciplinary Health Care Team 1 Lecture Activities

Team Bus Stop (Ice Breaker) Activity Description

Break into color group teams. Stand by the sheet that corresponds with your color and team number. Discuss the topic listed until the timer rings, then move to the next sheet and topic. Discuss each topic within your color group team. After the five topics are discussed as a team, the whole class comes together, and faculty facilitate a large group discussion to share a summary of discussions at each bus stop. Team Bus Stop topics addressed:

1. Describe a positive experience you have had working as part of a team.
2. Describe a negative experience you have had working as part of a team.
3. Describe your expectations or goals for your team experience this semester.
4. Describe the strengths you bring to the team.
5. Describe yourself using three adjectives.

Interdisciplinary Team Ground Rules Criteria

Ground rules are statements of values and guidelines that a group establishes to help individual members decide how to behave. To be effective, ground rules must be clear, consistent, agreed-to, and followed. Team ground rules are guiding principles that address how individuals treat each other, communicate, participate, cooperate, support each other, and coordinate joint activity. When ground rules are well-thought-out, the chance that a team will function as a cohesive unit, instead of as a group of individuals, increases. Ideally, team ground rules should be created, documented, and adopted within the first few team meetings. To create the ground rules, follow these steps:

1. Each interdisciplinary team will come up with a list of five or more ground rules.
2. The ground rules must be clear, well-thought-out, and relevant to the group's work.
3. Begin by brainstorming. Ask each team member to consider what is important to them when working on a team. What expectations do they have of one another throughout the team process?
4. Combine and clarify suggestions.
5. Arrive at a consensus on the set of ground rules that you will use to govern your team.

6. Document your ground rules so that you have a written record.

7. Each team member must agree with the documented ground rules. Agreement will be demonstrated by each team member signing the ground rules document.

8. Scan or take a picture of this document and upload it into the appropriate assignment module.

Examples of ground rules:
- Work is done on time
- Everyone contributes equally
- There must be consensus on decisions
- Confront issues directly and promptly
- Be candid but respectful
- Be on time and prepared for meetings

Interdisciplinary Health Care Team 2 Lecture Activities

"What Color Am I?" Activity Description

The "What Color Am I?" activity (adapted from True Colors [www.truecolorsintl.com]; all worksheets and handouts discussed are available) is an easy and fun way to help you understand yourself and others based on your personality temperament. Each color (Blue, Gold, Green, Orange) is reflective of your personality. Each person is a unique blend of the four colors, with one color being most prominent. This activity will help you understand your personality type and provide you with tools to help you work with others with different personality types. Our hope is by understanding yourself and your team members better, you will have the best possible team experience.

- Discover your color personality by completing the color personality quiz worksheet.
- Explore your color personality attributes and styles. Read your color style's explanation, attributes, leadership style, strengths, and weaknesses.
- Review how your color personality relates to other color personalities. Think about how you may see other colors and how you can reframe those thoughts.
- Share your color and discuss its characteristics with your team members. Discuss how your colors relate to each other and your leadership style. Also discuss what you can do to eliminate conflict that may occur between the color personalities, and how you can overcome your own strengths and weaknesses, to work with each other.

Application of Life Course Perspective

Team Bus Stop (Team Experience Reflection) Activity Description

Break into color group teams. Stand by the sheet that corresponds with your color and team number. Discuss the topic listed on the sheet until the timer rings, then move to the next sheet and topic. Discuss each topic within your team. After the five topics are discussed as a team, the whole class comes together, and the faculty facilitates a large group discussion to share a summary of discussions at each bus stop. Team Bus Stop topics addressed include the following:

1. How can you see yourself utilizing the life course principles in your chosen discipline?

2. In what stage do you place yourself in either Maslow's hierarchy or Erikson's stages of psychosocial development? Why?

3. What did you learn about a health care discipline, other than your chosen major, that you did not know before?

4. Following the "What Color Am I?" exercise, how did knowledge of your team's color makeup affect team building?

5. In one or two words, or a short phrase, how would you describe this course? Why?

REFERENCES

Arnold, L., & Stern, D. T. (2006). What is medical professionalism? In D.T. Stern (Ed.), *Measuring medical professionalism* (pp. 15-38), Oxford University Press.

David P. Weikart Center for Youth Program Quality. (2012). *The forum for youth investment: Building community.* The Weikert Center.

Drinka, T. J. K., & Clark, P. G. (2016). *Healthcare teamwork: Interprofessional practice and education* (2nd ed.). Praeger.

Interprofessional Education Collaborative. (2016). *Core competencies for interprofessional collaborative practice: 2016 update.* Author.

Leipzig, R. M., Hyer, K., Ek, K., Wallenstein, S., Vezina, M. L., Fairchild, S., Cassel, C. K., & Howe, J. L. (2002). Attitudes toward working on interdisciplinary healthcare teams: A comparison by discipline. *Journal of the American Geriatric Society, 50,* 1141-1148.

Long, D. M., Fay, V., & Wilson, N. L. (2001). Interdisciplinary teams—members and their roles. In D. M. Long, & N. L. Wilson (Eds.), *Houston geriatric interdisciplinary team training curriculum.* Baylor College of Medicine's Huffington Center on Aging.

MacNaughton, K., Chreim, S., & Bourgeault, I. L. (2013). Role construction and boundaries in interprofessional primary health care teams: A qualitative study. *Biomedical Central Health Services Research, 13,* 486-499.

Maharajan, M. K., Rajiah, K., Khoo, S. P., Chellappan, D. K., Alwis, R. D., Chui, H. C., Tan, L. L., Tan, Y. N., & Lau, S. Y. (2017). Attitudes and readiness of students of healthcare professions towards interprofessional learning. *PLoS ONE, 12*(1), e0168863. https://doi.org/10.1371/journal.pone.0168863

McEwan, D., Ruissen, G. R., Eys, M. A., Zumbo, B. D., & Beauchamp, M. R. (2017). The effectiveness of teamwork training on teamwork behaviors and team performance: A systematic review and meta-analysis of controlled interventions. *PLoS ONE, 12*(1). https://doi.org/10.1371/journal.pone.0169604

Mitchell, P., Wynia, M., Golden, R., McNellis, B., Okun, S., Webb, C.E., Rohrbach, V. & Von Kohorn, I. (2012). Core principles & values of effective team-based health care. Discussion Paper, Institute of Medicine, Washington, DC. https://doi.org/10.31478/201210c

Nancarrow, S. A., Booth, A., Ariss, S., Smith, T., Enderby, P., & Roots, A. (2013). Ten principles of good interdisciplinary team work. *Human Resources for Health, 11*(19), 1-11.

O'Keefe, M., Henderson, A., & Chick, R. (2017). Defining a set of common interprofessional learning competencies for health profession students. *Medical Teacher, 39,* 463-468.

Qualtrics. (2019). Qualtrics Software. *Qualtrics.* https://www.qualtrics.com

Schuster, E. O., Francis-Connolly, E., Alford-Trewn, P., & Brooks, J. (2003). The conceptualization and development of the course aging to infancy: A life course retrospective. *Educational Gerontology, 29,* 841-850.

Settersten, R. A. (Ed.). (2002). *Invitation to the life course: Toward new understandings of later life.* Baywood Publishing Company.

Sidler, G., & Lifton, H. (1999). The steps to developing and maintaining effective work teams. *Forum, 200,* 17-20.

Thistlethwaite, J. E., Forman, D., Matthews, L. R., Rogers, G. D., Steketee, C., & Yassine, T. (2014). *Academic Medicine, 89,* 869-875.

Weaver, S. J., Dy, S. M., & Rosen, M. A. (2014). Team-training in healthcare: A narrative synthesis of the literature. *BMJ Quality & Safety, 23,* 359-372. http://dx.doi.org/10.1136/bmjqs-2013-001848

11

COMMUNITIES OF PRACTICE
Addressing Faculty Frustrations as Teachers

Susan L. Caulfield, PhD
and Lisa R. Singleterry, PhD, RN, CNE

DESCRIPTION OF TEACHING/LEARNING CONTEXT

Examining the practice of teaching future health care professionals is especially important when working with those who have clinical expertise who transition to teach in an academic setting. Professional practice of clinical faculty is not necessarily well aligned with what is needed in teaching the next generation of practitioners because clinical expertise does not necessarily translate into teaching expertise. Our research has found that this is true across multiple health care disciplines, such as blindness and low vision studies, nursing, occupational therapy, and social work, which is also supported by the findings of Irby and O'Sullivan (2018). The key is that faculty who previously worked as health care practitioners have not been oriented to work as faculty. Current health care practice expertise is highly valued, but at what cost when those experts are novice educators. Importantly, assessment of student learning outcomes is a crucial part of creating a context that is effective in terms of both teaching and learning. Likewise, students who are just entering a professional health-related program have vastly different needs than those in their final semester before graduation. Knowing how we, as instructors, create learning opportunities that move our students forward in their acquisition of knowledge, skills, and attitudes (KSAs) is central to creating good learning environments.

Our college assessment committee included representatives from all departments in the college (college units consisted of blindness and low vision studies, interdisciplinary health, nursing, occupational therapy, physician assistant, social work, and speech, language, and hearing sciences). In 2015, a subset of the committee, representing four of the seven units (interdisciplinary health, nursing, occupational therapy, and holistic health, which represented physician assistant) chose to

Friberg, J. C., Visconti, C. F., & Ginsberg, S. M. (Eds.). *Evidence-Based Education in the Classroom: Examples From Clinical Disciplines* (pp. 97-106).
© 2021 Taylor & Francis Group.

focus its efforts on the assessment of core competencies within the college. While there were 10 such competencies, the members of the assessment committee chose written communication as its focus, knowing this was an area of much discussion and frustration among both faculty and students. The goal of the assessment committee was to assess potential roadblocks in meeting written communication competency for our students. This led to three internal grants. The first grant supported a research process to meet with faculty and learn more about potential roadblocks and, later, a faculty-led series of workshops on addressing those roadblocks, which would come to be known as *frustrations*. The second grant supported the development of a faculty learning community (FLC), with a continued focus on writing-related issues. The third supported a faculty community of practice (CoP), focused on seeking excellence in teaching and learning.

This chapter describes the process by which we discovered faculty frustrations regarding student writing may be related to lack of andragogic preparation of faculty. We used what we learned to build a process of faculty support and development that included workshops, a FLC, and, finally, a CoP. One problem facing faculty is that we teach alone. The nature of teaching is that one person imparts specialized KSAs to a group of students. Specialized knowledge is important, which is why we seek clinical experts to teach in clinically based programs. However, specialized knowledge is not always enough (Irby & O'Sullivan, 2018).

The practice of teaching is a unique specialty; whole colleges are devoted to the andragogy of teaching. Interestingly, university faculty represent various specialties outside of education to meet a goal of higher learning, but few universities require teacher certification (Irby & O'Sullivan, 2018) and therefore faculty may lack teaching specialty as a preparation. For example, a professor may possess highly specialized KSAs in nursing without the KSAs for andragogy. Therefore, the overall objective of the chapter is to link data to the development of a CoP for specialized faculty to be socialized to teaching and acquire KSAs consistent with evidence-based teaching strategies that improve student learning outcomes. While our work initially focused on writing-related instruction, we found it applicable to all aspects of teaching and learning.

REVIEW OF LITERATURE

A CoP is well suited to socialize clinical faculty to teaching. In health care, a CoP is commonly used to create change through enhancement of evidenced-based practice knowledge focused on patient safety (Seibert, 2015). Wenger and colleagues (2002) define a CoP as "groups of people who share a concern, a set of problems, and a passion about a topic, and who deepen their knowledge and expertise in this area by interacting on an ongoing basis" (p. 4). Buckley and colleagues (2019) describe the purpose of a CoP as socialization of novice health care practitioners. Indeed, orientation methods used for health care institutions are a "situated process of participation" (Buckley et al., 2019, p. 763) to socialize and teach new people about the work culture. Buckley and colleagues (2019) go on to discuss the idea of deliberate group cultivation in a CoP. Given this example and definition, a CoP is well suited and familiar to clinically prepared faculty. A CoP offers a participatory social process using situated learning, discussion, and support versus formal instruction. Our experience working with faculty who have a clinical specialty with no formal preparation to teach is that they desire a CoP because it is a familiar, nonthreatening format to focus on teaching strategies.

Communication is important in academia. Effective communication can take on many different forms: verbal, nonverbal, informatics, and written. Student learning outcomes are often based on communication assignments, with the most common assessment method being written work in the form of essay and prose (Oermann et al., 2015). Given the importance of communication for evaluation in academia and patient-safety in the health field, multiple experiences to develop clear and effective writing skills are necessary throughout each professional health-related program's core curriculum, not just those focused on writing (Oermann et al., 2015). To succeed as professionals, health care students need to be adept at various forms of analysis, and written communication is an essential tool to evaluate in such endeavors.

The choice to focus on communication for this research also aligns with the call from the Institute of Medicine (2003) that encourages health profession educators to be innovative and improve health education practices. The Institute of Medicine identifies patient-centered care, interdisciplinary teams, evidence-based practice, and quality improvement and informatics as focal points for education reform. Communication is a thread within these five core competencies and the cornerstone of effective teamwork and patient safety. Today, researchers have continued to search for tools (Rehim et al., 2017; Russ et al., 2013), training (Omura et al., 2017), or skills (Mardis et al., 2016) that might improve communication in health care.

Given the importance of written communication in health care and academia mentioned earlier, faculty preparation to teach and evaluate writing also seems important. Faculty development is one way to address the needed changes. For example, in some European countries, teacher certification is required in higher education (Irby & O'Sullivan, 2018). Another change agent may be from health professional organizations, such as the National League for Nursing (2019), who promote the certification of nurse educators and academic clinical nurse educators with a certifying exam. While that may seem a stretch to some, intermediate interventions seem called for as frustrations are present for both faculty and students, and we are learning that to reduce those frustrations will require a targeted form of change. It seems that we might strive to view faculty development as an important tool for those commonalities we have as faculty. Regardless of our discipline and to meet the needs of the classroom and students, there must be some attention given to the development of tools and skills that support teaching. No matter how skilled one is at their discipline, if they have not had any introduction to creating effective writing assignments, we (in higher education) have done a disservice to them and their students.

ORIGINAL DATA

Using an interpretive research process (Koch, 1999), we first sought to learn from instructors what they viewed as student writing-related frustrations. In the spring and summer of 2016, we conducted three focus groups to explore faculty frustrations with student work on writing assignments and present insights gained from the original data. Recruitment flyers inviting faculty to attend workshops addressing frustrations with students' writing were posted, and emails detailing the workshop were sent to all full- and part-time faculty in our college, thus resulting in a convenience sample. Focus groups were chosen to gather information from other faculty, and the facilitators took an observation only role during the focus groups. Three focus groups, each 1.5 hours in length, were held with faculty members representing four of the seven teaching departments in the college (interdisciplinary health, nursing, occupational therapy, and physician assistant). The total number of participants was 17, including the three facilitators. This research was approved by the university human subjects institutional review board.

For the focus groups, we used the interpretive research approach of asking a question to learn about the participants' experiences. The focus groups centered on four sections:

1. Participants were asked to describe their frustrations with students' writing in less than 10 words in an open format. Facilitators simultaneously transcribed those frustrations on a large piece of flip chart paper.

2. Next, participants were asked to help "group" the frustrations into themes.

3. After the participants created theme areas, the facilitators wrote their three *a priori* themes on the paper and asked the group to discuss the "fit" of these three themes to those they identified. Participants' responses to the *a priori* themes were also recorded on large flip chart paper.

4. The participants were asked to brainstorm potential interventions for the frustrations and then classify the interventions into categories.

After each focus group, the written record of the discussion was organized by the lead facilitator into themes. Data verification was completed using member checks (Guba & Lincoln, 1989). Member checks consisted of focus group participants being asked by either a follow-up meeting or via a written list of themes sent via email to them to verify what was discussed during the focus group meeting and to add any other information to the list that they had thought of after the focus group meeting. Based on member check responses, a final frustration theme sheet was developed. While each focus group provided new insights into the topic, by the third group there were predictable common themes and data saturation was reached (Guest et al., 2006).

As an academic committee, the college assessment committee might have moved forward on addressing writing in the college based on its own three themes of writing, critical thinking, and American Psychological Association style. However, the outcomes from the focus groups led the work in a somewhat different direction. Indeed, after the first focus group, while there was agreement that all faculty wanted students, through writing, to take content and demonstrate how it can be used, there was no agreement on or alignment with the three themes identified by the facilitators.

The first focus group identified 14 frustrations. These were translated by participants into four general themes: logic, argument, drawing conclusions, and looking for a mature level of expression (including content/substance/ideas; as well as critical thinking shown by organization, supportive statements, and intellectual integrity).

From the second focus group, 18 frustrations were identified. From those, four themes were identified: composition, critical thinking, missing links, and system issues. The third focus group identified six frustrations. Because of the low number of frustrations, this focus group was not asked to look for themes across the listed frustrations. By the end of the third focus group, the overall themes had evolved to six categories of frustration.

These six categories of frustrations are listed in Table 11-1, along with an explanation of each category. Specific examples of faculty verbiage that was used to develop the categories can be found in Appendix.

APPLICATION OF LITERATURE/DATA

What we learned from the focus groups in terms of the frustrations is important. Indeed, the list of frustrations became a checklist tool for faculty to use to assess students' errors and reflect on their writing assignments. If they compared the checklist to all student papers and found common themes in the student errors, this could point to areas for improvement within the assignment design. For example, one faculty member was frustrated that no one was citing a nursing journal; yet, when they reviewed the assignment, they noted that they did not specify such a requirement. The checklist tool helped the faculty rectify an element of the assignment design that reduced their frustration with student outcomes in the next semester. The importance of the work, however, goes beyond the checklist of identified frustrations. Indeed, the greatest learning outcome of this work was when the shift of focus happened.

While workshop sessions, held subsequent to what was learned from the focus groups, were cathartic in that faculty were able to voice their frustrations, some sessions searched for causes outside the student, such as lack of secondary school preparation, prediscipline general education courses that lack a focus on specifics (i.e., American Psychological Association formatting), or transferring in from community colleges. The conversation for ownership eventually came back to faculty members themselves. Some voiced concern that they, as discipline-specific faculty, lacked preparation in teaching grammar, mechanics, and formatting. Others voiced concern that, although they earned terminal degrees in their clinical discipline, they lacked educational preparation in assignment, course, and curriculum development.

TABLE 11-1

Six Categories of Frustrations

CATEGORY	EXPLANATION OF FRUSTRATION CATEGORY
1. Lack of	This category represents what faculty consider to be basic elements of good writing. Expectations varied by faculty but did include organization, logical structure, use of paragraphs, or even following an assigned format. This was considered descriptive or objective in nature.
2. Poor use of	Faculty reported expecting students to come to their classes already having mastered proper use of grammar, spelling, and a professional tone. This category represented frustration with what many would consider to be minimal expectations for good writing. One faculty member reported giving a paper a score of zero if it had numerous spelling or grammatical errors, without quantification of errors or attention to the content itself.
3. Misunderstanding of	The intent of the assignment is not met in this case. Faculty describe this as a disconnect between what was assigned and what was produced by the student. However, we would later learn that misunderstanding may be based on the lack of assignment clarity by faculty.
4. Focus misplaced	A central focus or intent of assignments for faculty was to increase clinical reasoning in their students. However, faculty found the students focused on aspects within the assignment not considered most important by faculty. Examples include students worrying about the number of pages rather than focusing on substance or simply regurgitating facts rather than providing a thoughtful response. Faculty were frustrated to find a list of answers, rather than a synthesis of the issue at hand.
5. Missing relevance	Faculty reported this in response to student papers that did not recognize the importance of extant research or the importance of linking their knowledge to that which has already occurred. Faculty see this when students do not demonstrate the importance of using research or citing others for their work and would rather simply state their own opinion on the issue. Faculty desire students to see how important it is to use writing as a means of communication or to better their profession. When students do not use citations or proper format, they weaken their ability to make a persuasive argument, which they will need to be able to make to help others in health care.
6. Perceived laziness	This category was unique in that, while it contains some of the same examples found in other categories, it reflects faculty feelings or perceptions more than what might be in the paper itself. "Perceived" was added after conversation among the members of the focus group that laziness might not be an accurate representation of the students' work but a reaction of the faculty member.

As the shift unfolded, the facilitators began to see that not all frustrations had the same locus of control. Indeed, when the faculty first attended the focus groups, what they told us focused on the actions of students. For example, faculty told us that students did not care about writing or were ill-equipped to write. By the end of the three focus groups, the facilitators saw a different pattern emerging, which led to the questions: What are we asking of students? and What are we telling them to do in writing assignments?

Our findings align with Oermann and colleagues (2015), who said that "planned instructional strategies that enable students to learn to write effectively in their courses are critical for student success" (p. 28). After the shift, it became clear that faculty played as much of a role as students did in the writing-related frustrations from course assignments. Attention to planning assignments using evidence-based teaching strategies would be necessary to address student writing.

Results of this study arose in four different ways. First, the facilitators used the information to develop a writing frustration checklist (see Appendix). Second, faculty identified that student writing outcomes (seen as frustrations) could be the result of the system or structure of assignment development. Third, faculty began to trust one another and a quasi-FLC developed. Fourth, faculty learned that what they most desired was a CoP focused on teaching and learning.

First, in addition to assignment development, the writing frustration checklist was explored as a quality improvement tool to identify areas that may need clarity in assignment development to reduce frustration in the next iteration of the assignment. With this tool, faculty could track the type of frustrations encountered in reading student papers and use this information to assess if the frustrations were due to only a couple of students, or if there was a pattern suggesting either student or instructor lack of clarity. There is a certain familiarity in using a checklist or tool to guide practice for health care practitioners who are accustomed to finding and fixing problems. The tool was a bridge of communication, helping clinical faculty use pedagogical strategies that impact student outcomes.

Second, through examination of patterns in frustrations, faculty came to realize that some of the frustrations were a function of assignment development itself. Indeed, at a follow-up meeting that partially focused on a member check of the data, one of the facilitators projected an assignment on the screen. Right away, a participant asked for clarification on the intention of the assignment. Over the next year, a small group of 12 faculty members—dubbed the writing assessment group (WAG)—met a couple of times a month to explore teaching strategies and solutions in the form of semi-structured workshops guided by three facilitators. An instructional design framework was developed to guide clinical faculty in assignment development using the acronym PODE (Singleterry & Caulfield, 2020). Faculty were encouraged to describe the purpose (P) of the assignment, write clear objectives (O) and directions (D), and to communicate the evaluation (E) or grading logic for the assignment. Facilitators felt the workshops were successful and participants voiced interest in continuing them.

Third, the next major result of this study was the development of a FLC focused on writing assignment development. In addition to some members of the WAG, we opened the FLC up to all faculty in the university. In addition to faculty from health sciences, the FLC included faculty from the humanities and business. Supported by a faculty development grant, a small faculty cohort formed, and we met every 2 to 3 weeks, as recommended by Cox (2004), and focused on producing an outcome. While we tried to align with all recommendations of a formal FLC, which includes an outcome, such as a new curriculum or sharing of data, we found the group was more interested in exchanging knowledge on teaching practices. Ultimately, the eight-member group decided the outcome of the FLC would be development of a CoP. We did have consistent attendance and good movement around the topic of developing effective writing assignments, but we realized we were not a FLC. Indeed, we more closely resembled a CoP. One distinction between a FLC and a CoP is that the former is focused on academia and the generation of a product, while the latter can apply to any group of like-minded individuals. According to Wenger-Trayner and Wenger-Trayner (2015), "Communities of practice are groups of people who share a concern or passion for something they do and learn how to do it better as they interact regularly" (para. 5).

Fourth, this study led to the development of a CoP. The members of the FLC mentioned earlier decided that the outcome of the FLC would be to form a CoP that would be open to all faculty at our institution. What we learned from the FLC was that faculty were not looking for a process that also included a product (such deliverables are key to the structure of a FLC), but instead, wished to have a community of like-minded professionals who would help each other to seek excellence in teaching and learning. Wenger and colleagues (2002) described the purpose of a CoP as a way "to create, expand, and exchange knowledge, and to develop individual capabilities" (p. 42). With a CoP, there is less focus on a shared discipline, with greater focus on a shared concern. We developed a plan to alternate meetings with a common read and reflection to explore evidence-based teaching practices.

APPLICATION TO CROSS-DISCIPLINARY CONTEXTS

We see our research and development of a CoP as relevant to any discipline, whether clinically based or not. We entered this work curious to learn how faculty viewed student writing-related frustrations. What we learned aligns well with the literature. Faculty in our focus groups learned that they play an important and often unobserved role in frustrations related to student writing. What we have presented here are data that support changes that need to occur for both faculty and students to experience fewer frustrations when it comes to writing assignments. Indeed, specialized faculty need an opportunity to develop teaching skills just as they needed an opportunity to develop clinical skills. A CoP is well-suited for this task and is familiar to clinically based faculty. A CoP can be assembled within a department, but we found interdisciplinary collaboration helpful in exploring teaching and learning strategies across multiple contexts.

As noted earlier, faculty who participated in the focus groups represented four of the seven teaching departments in the college. When we expanded to a FLC, members represented seven unique disciplines. The conversations within the FLC demonstrated the applicability of this work to cross-disciplinary contexts, as there were common themes found throughout the conversations.

Based on our experiences, we recommend that faculty create a CoP. As we have documented previously, once faculty realized that some of their frustrations were based on a lack of preparation, they were hungry for some type of programming. We first addressed this need with our WAG workshops, followed by the development of a FLC. However, what faculty most wanted is what can be found in a CoP.

One limitation of this study may be that only one college was included in the data collection part of the project. Another is that there were a limited number of health science–focused faculty. Indeed, in the first year, 17 of 138 faculty were involved in this project. However, the consistency across responses from the participants and the ensuing data saturation speak to the authenticity of the findings for health science–focused educators. As we continued our work with faculty from other disciplines and colleges, we found consistency with the focus group findings.

ADDITIONAL RESOURCES

- Annells, M. (1999). Evaluating phenomenology: Usefulness, quality and philosophical foundations. *Nurse Researcher, 6,* 5-19.
- Ashworth, P. (1990). Nurses now read more, what about writing too? *Intensive and Clinical Care Nursing, 14,* 107.
- Borglin, G., & Fagerström, C. (2012). Nursing students' understanding of critical thinking and appraisal and academic writing: A descriptive, qualitative study. *Nurse Education in Practice, 12,* 356-360.
- Byrne, M. M. (2001). Understanding life experiences through a phenomenological approach to research. *AORN Journal, 73,* 830-832.

- Hawks, S. J., Turner, K. M., Derouin, A. L., Hueckel, R. M., Leonardelli, A. K., & Oermann, M. H. (2015). Writing across the curriculum: Strategies to improve the writing skills of nursing students. *Nursing Forum, 51*(4), 261-267. https://doi.org/10.1111/nuf.12151
- Whitehead, D. (2002). The academic writing experiences of a group of student nurses: A phenomenological study. *Journal of Advanced Nursing, 38*(5), 498-506.
- Wimpenny, P., & Gass, J. (2000). Interviewing in phenomenology and grounded theory: Is there a difference? *Journal of Advanced Nursing, 31*, 1485-1492.

References

Buckley, H., Steinert, Y., Regehr, G., & Nimmon, L. (2019). When I say…community of practice. *Medical Education, 53*(8), 763-765. https://doi.org/10.1111/medu.13823

Cox, M. (2004). Introduction to faculty learning communities. *New Directions for Teaching and Learning, 97*, 5-23.

Guba, E. G., & Lincoln, Y. S. (1989). *Fourth generation evaluation.* SAGE Publications.

Guest, G., Bunce, A., & Johnson, L. (2006). How many interviews are enough? An experiment with data saturation and variability. *Field Methods, 18*(1), 59-82.

Institute of Medicine. (2003). Health professions education: A bridge to quality. *National Academies Press (US).* http://www.ncbi.nlm.nih.gov/books/NBK221528/

Irby, D. M., & O'Sullivan, P. S. (2018). Developing and rewarding teachers as educators and scholars: Remarkable progress and daunting challenges. *Medical Education, 52*(1), 58-67.

Koch, T. (1999). An interpretive research process: revisiting phenomenological and hermeneutical approaches. *Nurse Researcher, 6*, 20-34.

Mardis, T., Mardis, M., Davis, J., Justice, E. M., Riley Holdinsky, S., Donnelly, J., Ragozine-Bush, H., & Riesenberg, L. A. (2016). Bedside shift-to-shift handoffs: A systematic review of the literature. *Journal of Nursing Care Quality, 31*(1), 54-60.

National League for Nursing (2019). Certification for nurse educators. http://www.nln.org/Certification-for-Nurse-Educators

Oermann, M. H., Leonardelli, A. K., Turner, K. M., Hawks, S. J., Derouin, A. L., & Hueckel, R. M. (2015). Systematic review of educational programs and strategies for developing students' and nurses' writing skills. *Journal of Nursing Education, 54*(1), 28-34. https://doi.org/10.3928/01484834-20141224-01

Omura, M., Maguire, J., Levett-Jones, T., & Stone, T. E. (2017). The effectiveness of assertiveness communication training programs for healthcare professionals and students: A systematic review. *International Journal of Nursing Studies, 76*, 120-128. https://doi.org/10.1016/j.ijnurstu.2017.09.001

Rehim, S. A., DeMoor, S., Olmsted, R., Dent, D. L., & Parker-Raley, J. (2017). Tools for assessment of communication skills of hospital action teams: A systematic review. *Journal of Surgical Education, 74*(2), 341-351. https://doi.org/10.1016/j.jsurg.2016.09.008

Russ, S., Rout, S., Sevdalis, N., Moorthy, K., Darzi, A., & Vincent, C. (2013). Do safety checklists improve teamwork and communication in the operating room? A systematic review. *Annals of Surgery, 258*(6), 856-871.

Seibert, S. (2015). The meaning of a healthcare community of practice. *Nursing Forum, 50*(2), 69-74. https://doi.org/10.1111/nuf.12065

Singleterry, L., & Caulfield, S. L. (2020). Continuous quality improvement of assignments: A process for faculty development. *Nursing Education Perspectives, 42*(2), 122-123.

Wenger, E., McDermott, R., & Snyder, W. M. (2002). *Cultivating communities of practice.* Harvard Business School Press.

Wenger-Trayner, E., & Wenger-Trayner, B. (2015). Introduction to communities of practice. https://wenger-trayner.com/introduction-to-communities-of-practice/

APPENDIX: TRACKING WRITING-RELATED FRUSTRATIONS FOR QUALITY IMPROVEMENT

IDENTIFIED FRUSTRATIONS TO TRACK		COLUMNS FOR USE BY ASSIGNMENT OR STUDENT						
1. Lack of	Argument							
	Coherence							
	Logical flow							
	Organization/structure							
	Critical thinking							
	Use of substance to support content							
	Integration of feedback							
	Asking for clarification							
	Proofreading							
	Utilization of assigned format/template							
2. Poor use of	Grammar							
	Spelling							
	Professional tone							
3. Misunderstanding of	Content							
	Assignment							
	Directions							
	Expectations							
	Words used in directions							
	Shift in focus (first 5, then 1)							
4. Focus misplaced	Number of pages versus substance							
	Black/white response versus thoughtfulness							
	Focus on the irrelevant							
5. Missing relevance	Citations							
	Formatting style							
	Writing as professional tool/skill							
	Planning and drafting work							

(continued)

(CONTINUED)

IDENTIFIED FRUSTRATIONS TO TRACK		COLUMNS FOR USE BY ASSIGNMENT OR STUDENT							
6. Perceived laziness	Unintentional plagiarism								
	Improper citations								
	Lack of proofreading								
	Mind dump								
	Declarative versus elaboration								
	Use of abbreviations								
	Write as they talk								
	Word salad								
	Text/shorthand/images seen as acceptable								
7. Other frustrations									

12

IMPROVING DENTAL ASSISTING AND RADIOLOGIC TECHNOLOGY EDUCATION THROUGH INTERPROFESSIONAL EXPERIENCES

Amy Egli, MHA, LDH, CDA, EFDA; Heather Schmuck, MS, RT(R); and Amanda Reddington, LDH, MHA, CDA, EFDA

DESCRIPTION OF TEACHING/LEARNING CONTEXT

Interprofessional collaboration is becoming the standard for allied health care providers in both clinical and educational settings. That said, many non–bachelor-level programs struggle to incorporate or provide opportunities for interprofessional education (IPE) experience into their curricula. As the call for IPE continues to grow, the importance for all allied health professionals to participate in IPE early in their educational programs becomes important for the success of the entire health care team (Oandasan & Reeves, 2005).

The idea for the study presented in this chapter spawned from an on-campus event held each year at our university to showcase undergraduate students' scholarship. The radiologic technology program had several students in attendance who were presenting a poster from a recent professional conference. The poster had radiographic images that were of interest to the dental assisting students, prompting them to engage in discussions around the similarities and differences in their radiographic knowledge with the radiologic technology students. During this discussion, one of the authors (a radiologic technology instructor) was listening to this dialogue and inquired about the type of equipment that dental students worked with in their dental lab. It was discovered that they regularly worked with a digital panoramic machine. The radiologic technology students listening to this discussion were excited to realize that there was a panoramic unit that they could potentially practice with prior to attempting this type of exam on a real patient in the hospital setting. The radiologic technology instructor reached out to the dental assisting program chair who put her into contact with the other two authors of this chapter, each of whom have primary teaching responsibilities with the dental assisting students. The three authors met to discuss how they could potentially

Friberg, J. C., Visconti, C. F., & Ginsberg, S. M. (Eds.). *Evidence-Based Education in the Classroom: Examples From Clinical Disciplines* (pp. 107-116).

bring their students together to learn and apply their skills for panoramic imaging through an interprofessional activity. After thoughtful planning, the authors successfully implemented an IPE experience for their dental assisting and radiologic technology students in a university setting.

At the university where this study took place, the dental assisting program is an associate degree program and the radiologic technology program is a bachelor degree program, which differentiates this IPE experience from many others described in the literature. The intention of this endeavor was two-fold: to study student perceptions of IPE as it relates to both programs and to examine whether bachelor and associate degree–seeking programs could successfully collaborate to learn from one another. This chapter describes the evidence-based outcomes from the first 3 years of this IPE collaboration, as well as changes implemented each year.

Review of Literature

To prepare for this activity, current IPE practices from graduate, bachelor, and associate degree programs were researched through a review of relevant literature. The results from this review demonstrated that IPE opportunities were abundant in graduate degree programs and in nursing, prepharmacy, premedicine, and pretherapy undergraduate programs (Olson & Bialocerkowski, 2014). However, there was limited information about incorporating IPE into non-nursing bachelor's programs and even less for associate degree health professions programs.

In addition to utilizing available IPE studies, we also reviewed the benefits of live patient experiences compared to simulations. For the purpose of our study, we considered live patients to be actual patients encountered in a clinical environment with a prescribed physician order for imaging. A review completed by Hicks and colleagues (2009) compared simulation types as they relate to student learning and IPE activities. Munshi and colleagues (2015) concluded that both low- and high-fidelity simulations provide meaningful learning experiences for students at various stages in their education. Low-fidelity simulations involving case studies or mannequins are best incorporated early in students' education and should progress to high-fidelity simulations as their clinical skills and confidence grows. High-fidelity simulations involving actors or computerized mannequins help replicate the live patient experience and are most efficient when students need to demonstrate and practice skills in a monitored low-risk environment (Munshi et al., 2015). Weller and colleagues (2012) compared simulations to live patient experiences and concluded that while simulations are necessary and effective for novice clinicians, they may not accurately portray clinical situations and can feel staged.

Original Data

A mixed-methods study design was used that included a combination of pre- and post-IPE experience surveys, researchers' observations, and researcher-led group discussions to determine the effectiveness of our IPE activities around the use of panoramic imaging. Participants were drawn from a convenience sample, with all students enrolled full-time in the university dental assisting and radiologic technology programs invited to participate.

Pre-Interprofessional Education Experience Preparation

Prior to this activity, each student received didactic instruction on panoramic imaging techniques and acquisition. Radiologic technology students completed this course work in the weeks leading up to this IPE activity. Dental assisting students completed relevant didactic coursework during the semester immediately preceding the semester when the IPE activity occurred. For the dental assisting students, during years 1 and 2 of this activity, their previous instruction included low-fidelity simulations on a mannequin, and during year 3, a live patient panoramic image exposure. Radiologic technology students received no simulation activity related to panoramic imaging.

Students completed a modified form of McFadyen and colleagues' (2007) Interdisciplinary Education Perception Scale (IEPS). This survey is used to examine IPE participant perceptions of other professions compared to their held beliefs about their profession. The IEPS survey is designed with a 6-point Likert-type scale of agreement for various survey statements (refer to the Additional Resources section for a copy of this instrument).

Interprofessional Education Experience

While the design of the IPE activity remained similar each year, there was a substantial change in the format of the IPE experience from year 1 to years 2 and 3. During the first year of this IPE activity, student participants were required to find a person who qualified for a panoramic image based upon the practice standards for panoramic image requisition for the dental profession, and who also agreed to serve as a live patient for one of the groups of students for the activity. During years 2 and 3, a radiologic technology student mimicked the live patient role, while the other students in the group completed the necessary steps to assess and position the simulated live patient for a panoramic image. For all years, group sizes were kept small, with instructors aiming for no more than four students in a group, which resulted in seven or eight small groups with a balanced composition of radiologic technology and dental assisting participants. Each group was then assigned a live patient volunteer (year 1) or an imaging procedure time (years 2 and 3).

The live patient volunteers submitted a completed health history form to the supervising dentist of the on-campus dental clinic prior to the day of the activity. On the day of the activity, each participant group completed necessary steps to assess and acquire a panoramic image on the live patient assigned to the group. Specifically, each group brought back their patient to the university dental clinic where each group completed a patient assessment, including a detailed medical history, vital signs (blood pressure, temperature, respiration, pulse), and oral radiographic history. Students then completed patient-informed consent and spoke with the dentist who verified and prescribed the panoramic image to be captured.

After arriving in the panoramic imaging area, each group discussed the differences between panoramic machines utilized in each profession and general procedural and positioning steps involved in image acquisition. Following this discussion, image acquisition took place and positioning of the live patient (in year 1) or a radiographic phantom (in years 2 and 3). Students remained in their small groups after image acquisition and were given a private area to analyze their image. They also completed associated image evaluation forms created by their course instructor.

After each group had completed the panoramic evaluation form, all participants met in a didactic classroom for a large group discussion and presentation of produced images for critique. As a large group, students discussed normal and abnormal patient anatomy, technique errors, and similarities and differences between programs and professional roles. To help encourage student discussion and to gain qualitative data on the activity, students were asked three questions:

1. What did you learn from the activity?
2. What did you like most about the activity?
3. What would you change about the activity?

Following completion of the activity, students were surveyed again using the same adapted IEPS survey, and years 2 and 3 students also completed an adapted Student Evaluation of Educational Quality (SEEQ; see Additional Resources at end of chapter) survey that assessed the activity itself.

Study Methods and Outcomes

Researchers utilized paired t-test to examine differences in the pre and postaggregate survey responses of study participants between the utilization of a live patient experience versus a high-fidelity simulation experience (Table 12-1). With a live patient experience, multiple survey items yielded significant results ($p < .05$), including student perceptions both within and across disciplines. When utilizing a simulated experience, many of the significant findings from year 1

TABLE 12-1

Paired *t* Test Between Pre- and Post-Surveys Across Simulation Experience

Question	Survey	LIVE CLIENT				SIMULATED CLIENT			
		n	m	SD	p *value*	n	m	SD	p *value*
1. Individuals in my profession are well trained.	Pre	25	5.48	0.65	.420	58	5.466	0.78	.340
	Post	25	5.60	0.5		58	5.379	0.95	
2. Individuals in my profession are able to work closely with individuals in other professions.	Pre	25	5.36	0.81	.230	58	5.310	0.86	.727
	Post	25	5.56	0.65		58	5.345	0.87	
3. Individuals in my profession are very positive about their goals and objectives.	Pre	25	5.16	0.85	.010	58	5.138	0.90	.008
	Post	25	5.68	0.48		58	5.362	0.87	
4. Individuals in my profession need to cooperate with other professions.	Pre	24	5.58	0.65	.790	58	5.707	0.56	.008
	Post	24	5.54	0.66		58	5.397	0.94	
5. Individuals in my profession are very positive about their contributions and accomplishments.	Pre	25	5.28	0.84	.030	58	5.190	0.78	.241
	Post	25	5.64	0.49		58	5.328	0.87	
6. Individuals in my profession must depend on the work of people in other professions.	Pre	25	4.36	1.08	.010	58	4.897	1.15	.301
	Post	25	4.92	1.38		58	5.069	1.01	
7. Individuals in my profession trust each other's professional judgment.	Pre	25	4.76	0.78	.001	58	5.155	0.83	.243
	Post	25	5.36	0.76		58	5.259	1.02	
8. Individuals in my profession are extremely competent.	Pre	25	5.16	0.69	.005	58	5.138	0.96	.761
	Post	25	5.60	0.5		58	5.103	1.22	

(continued)

TABLE 12-1 (CONTINUED)

Paired *t* Test Between Pre- and Post-Surveys Across Simulation Experience

Question	Survey	LIVE CLIENT				SIMULATED CLIENT			
		n	m	SD	p value	n	m	SD	p value
9. Individuals in my profession are willing to share information and resources with other professionals.	Pre	25	5.20	0.71	.010	58	5.293	0.92	.070
	Post	25	5.60	0.65		58	5.483	0.90	
10. Individuals in my profession have good relations with people in other professions.	Pre	24	4.88	0.95	.002	58	5.155	0.83	.020
	Post	24	5.58	0.5		58	5.345	0.87	
11. Individuals in my profession think highly of other related professions.	Pre	25	4.92	0.91	.002	58	5.052	0.93	.146
	Post	25	5.56	0.51		58	5.190	1.05	
12. Individuals in my profession work well with each other.	Pre	25	5.20	0.87	.009	58	5.362	0.78	.322
	Post	25	5.72	0.46		58	5.276	1.01	

Note: Survey questions were adapted from McFayden, A. K., Maclaren, W. M., & Webster, V. S. (2007). The Interdisciplinary Education Perception Scale (IEPS): An alternative remodelled sub-scale structure and its reliability. *Journal of Interprofessional Care, 21*(4), 433-443.

SD = standard deviation.

no longer manifested in the participant responses for years 2 and 3 in the aggregate data, but still produced mostly positive perceptions regarding interprofessional practice. A surprising result with the simulated experience was the significant decrease in student perceptions with the simulated experience when questioned on the need to cooperate with other professions ($p = .008$). However, this same question had a decrease in overall mean response even with the live patient experience, though not significant.

Examining these significant differences between pre- and post-survey responses by program also yielded interesting findings (Table 12-2). When utilizing a live patient experience, significant differences in perceptions among radiologic technology students were found for six survey questions, while dental assistant students only had four questions where significant differences were noted. Radiologic technology students' perceptions ($n = 13$) increased in the areas of intraprofessional positive outlook on goals and objectives ($p = .002$), contributions and accomplishments ($p = .03$), and working well with others in the profession ($p = .01$). Interprofessionally, radiologic technology students expressed increases in willingness to share information and resources with other professions ($p = .03$) and had an increased perception of thinking highly of other professions ($p = .01$). Dental assistant students' perceptions ($n = 12$) increased in questions related specifically to

TABLE 12-2

Individual Program Paired *t* Tests

Question	n	YEAR 1 LIVE CLIENT EXPERIENCE		n	YEARS 2 AND 3 SIMULATED CLIENT EXPERIENCE	
		Discipline	p value		Discipline	p value
1. Individuals in my profession are well trained.	13	RADT	1.00	33	RADT	.23
	12	DA	.34	25	DA	1.00
2. Individuals in my profession are able to work closely with individuals in other professions.	13	RADT	.55	33	RADT	.69
	12	DA	.27	25	DA	.16
3. Individuals in my profession are very positive about their goals and objectives.	13	RADT	.002	33	RADT	.16
	12	DA	.39	25	DA	.005
4. Individuals in my profession need to cooperate with other professions.	13	RADT	.08	33	RADT	.004
	12	DA	.55	25	DA	1.00
5. Individuals in my profession are very positive about their contributions and accomplishments.	13	RADT	.03	33	RADT	.57
	12	DA	.44	25	DA	.26
6. Individuals in my profession must depend upon the work of people in other professions.	13	RADT	.24	33	RADT	.88
	12	DA	.01	25	DA	.12
7. Individuals in my profession trust each other's professional judgment.	13	RADT	.08	33	RADT	.63
	12	DA	.005	25	DA	.01
8. Individuals in my profession are extremely competent.	13	RADT	.046	33	RADT	.07
	12	DA	.04	25	DA	.02
9. Individuals in my profession are willing to share information and resources with other professionals.	13	RADT	.03	33	RADT	.36
	12	DA	.19	25	DA	.03
10. Individuals in my profession have good relations with people in other professions.	13	RADT	.11	33	RADT	.23
	12	DA	.01	25	DA	.01
11. Individuals in my profession think highly of other related professions.	13	RADT	.02	33	RADT	.33
	12	DA	.052	25	DA	.19
12. Individuals in my profession work well with each other.	13	RADT	.01	33	RADT	.044
	12	DA	.44	25	DA	.33

DA = dental assisting; RADT = radiologic technology.

interprofessional practice including having good relationships with other professions ($p = .01$) and dependence on other professions ($p = .01$). Within their profession, dental assistant students had an increase in perceptions regarding trust of each other's professional judgment ($p = .005$). Both groups of students in radiologic technology and dental assisting expressed increased perceptions related to competency within their profession ($p = .046$ and $p = .04$, respectively).

In years 2 and 3 with the simulated experience, changes in responses between pre- and post-surveys yielded a significant change related to working well within the profession for radiologic technology students ($p = .044$). Dental assistant students had several significant changes including both intraprofessional and interprofessional items. Within the profession, dental assistant students reported increases in positive outlook about goals and objectives ($p = .005$), competency within the profession ($p = .02$), and trust in professional judgment ($p = .01$). Interprofessionally, dental assistant students reported significant increases in the area of willingness to share information and resources with other professions ($p = .03$) and having good relationships with other professions ($p = .01$).

Overall, radiologic technology students were more positively affected intraprofessionally with the live patient experience. Dental assistant students were equally affected both intraprofessional and interprofessionally during the same experience. With the simulated experience, both radiologic technology and dental assistant students reported a more positive impact interprofessionally with only dental students having a positive perception impact for interprofessional collaboration and teamwork. Together with year 1 data, these findings suggest students perceptions are positively affected about their profession and other professions when interprofessional activities are implemented into the curriculum.

Researchers combined the data from years 2 and 3 for the SEEQ tool into a single spreadsheet to evaluate mean responses for each surveyed item (Table 12-3). By implementing this tool in later years, feedback about the specific activity was quantitatively assessed to determine effectiveness and student agreement with the various surveyed items. This evaluation allowed for discussion on potential changes for future offerings of the activity and moved beyond simply evaluating changes in student perceptions about IPE. Students generally agreed that the activity was beneficial to their learning with higher mean responses for items associated directly with the instructors influence on the activity, such as enthusiasm and rapport. Students did not report a strong agreement ($m = 3.52$) with the activity being stimulating and challenging. However, students did agree that they learned and understood the material relevant to the IPE activity ($m = 4.29$).

APPLICATION OF LITERATURE/DATA

Our initial pilot results corresponded with published literature and showed a statistically significant increase in students' perceptions ($p = < .05$; Reddington et al., 2018). We used our initial results as a positive indicator to repeat the activity in future years. When planning for our subsequent activities in years 2 and 3, we encountered unforeseen barriers with attracting volunteer live patients. We decided to modify the activity for years 2 and 3 whereby students completed a high-fidelity simulation. Other modifications from year 1 to years 2 and 3 included adding an additional student survey to evaluate the activity itself and slight modifications to the dental assisting radiology course curriculum. The pilot year results showed positive outcomes of student's perceptions of each other's disciplines (Reddington et al., 2018), but all data collected about student perceptions of the activity itself were gathered through informal student feedback. This made it difficult to objectively evaluate the effectiveness of the IPE activity design. To help meet this need, we researched how other IPE activities measured student perceptions and the effectiveness of the activity. For years 2 and 3, we implemented a modified SEEQ survey. Since beginning this IPE panoramic activity, it was noted on end of program reviews (conducted by the program and not associated with the project) that students were requesting even more opportunities with panoramic imaging. From year 2 to year 3, the oral radiology curriculum was modified to increase panoramic imaging lecture time and require each student to acquire and expose one panoramic image on a live patient in a laboratory setting.

Table 12-3

Student Evaluation of Educational Quality of an Interprofessional Education Activity

	n	MEAN RESPONSE[a]
Learning		
This IPE activity was stimulating and challenging.	58	3.52
I learned something valuable from this IPE activity.	58	4.10
My interest in IPE has increased as a result of this activity.	58	3.81
I have learned and understood the material relevant to this IPE activity.	58	4.29
Enthusiasm		
Instructors were enthusiastic about the IPE activity.	58	4.72
Instructors were dynamic and energetic in conducting the IPE activity.	58	4.67
Organization		
Explanation of the IPE activity was clear.	58	3.98
Materials for the IPE activity were well prepared and explained.	58	4.07
Objectives for the IPE activity aligned with what was actually covered.	58	4.28
Group Interaction		
Instructors encouraged student participation in group discussion.	58	4.67
Students were able to openly express ideas and share knowledge or ask questions throughout the activity.	58	4.66
I learned valuable information or perspective from working with different students in this IPE activity.	58	4.38
Individual Rapport		
Instructors were friendly with students participating in the IPE activity.	58	4.74
Instructors made students feel welcome in asking for help during the IPE activity.	58	4.67
Breadth		
Instructors provided enough background on concepts covered in the IPE activity in class prior to the activity.	58	4.29
Instructors adequately discussed current concepts related to the IPE activity pertinent to each field.	58	4.45
Overall[b]		
Compared with other class activities, this IPE activity is	58	4.28
Compared with other instructors, these instructors are	58	4.57
As an overall rating, these instructors are	58	4.62

Note: Survey adapted from Student Evaluation of Educational Quality (SEEQ) standardized instrument at the U of S. (n.d.). https://teaching.usask.ca/documents/seeq/Standardized_SEEQ_Instrument_at_UofS.pdf
[a]Surveyed item responses were Likert-scale options from 5 = Strongly Agree to 1 = Strongly Disagree.
[b]Overall item responses were based upon 5 = Very Good, 4 = Good, 3 = Average, 2 = Poor, and 1 = Very Poor.

APPLICATION TO CROSS-DISCIPLINARY CONTEXTS

The activity used in our study design is simple and easily replicable. The design does not need any additional financial support and is easy to incorporate into an already existing curriculum. Collaborations could include diagnostic medical sonography programs performing carotid doppler screenings in collaboration with gerontology program students to understand the effects of aging on the cardiovascular system. Occupational therapy, nursing, and respiratory students could use this type of activity to assess "code blue" simulations. These interdisciplinary simulations foster real-world crisis moments and encourage learning as a health care team.

This IPE experience gave students the opportunity to learn about other roles that a health care provider may play in providing patient care. The students also learned that there are many different approaches to some of the same tasks associated with the care of a patient.

The health care environment is evolving and challenging health care providers to work more collaboratively (Brame et al., 2015). IPE is one way to create this collaboration and improve quality of care to the patient and is beneficial for any clinical collaboration focused on understanding the perspective between two or more programs. Another benefit of this IPE activity is that it encourages teamwork and professional growth, which is beneficial for all professions. For example, a nutrition program may use a similar structure with a dental hygiene program to establish collaboration between nutrition and the condition of the oral cavity. Students could collaborate to assess a patient's current oral and nutritional health either through a live patient or high-fidelity simulation. Based on the findings, students could work together to make treatment and diet modifications.

Our study showed that programs traditionally not included in IPE opportunities can also benefit from these types of experiences, highlighting the importance for educators to think outside of the box and investigate other potential collaborations that ultimately seek the goal of preparing future professionals for the ever-changing health care world. Due to the increasing call for IPE collaborations, it is vital that allied health curricula provide interdisciplinary approaches to instruction (Oandason & Reeves, 2005).

ADDITIONAL RESOURCES

- Activity involving three disciplines (nursing, physical therapy, and radiologic technology). Communication and role discernment were highlights of the study:
  - Karnish, K., Shustack, L., Brogan, L., Capitano, G., & Cunfer, A. (2019). Interprofessional socialization through acute-care simulation. *Radiologic Technology, 90*(6), 552-562.
- IPE importance before students move into a clinical environment:
  - Iverson, L., Bredenkamp, N., Carrico, C., Connelly, S., Hawkins, K., Monaghan, M., & Malesker, M. (2018). Development and assessment of an interprofessional education simulation to promote collaborative learning and practice. *Journal of Nursing Education, 57*(7), 426-429. https://doi.org/10.3928/01484834-20180618-08
- Developing high-fidelity simulations:
  - Alinier, G. (2010). Developing high-fidelity health care simulation scenarios: A guide for educators and professionals. *Simulation & Gaming, 42*(1), 9-26. https://doi.org/10.1177/1046878109355683
- Step-by-step consideration for designing IPE:
  - El-Awaisi, A., Anderson, E., Barr, H., Wilby, K. J., Wilbur, K., & Bainbridge, L. (2016). Important steps for introducing interprofessional education into health professional education. *Journal of Taibah University Medical Sciences, 11*(6), 546-551. https://doi.org/10.1016/j.jtumed.2016.09.004

REFERENCES

Brame, J., Mitchell, S., Wilder, R., & Sams, L. (2015). Dental and allied dental students' attitudes towards and perceptions of intraprofessional education. *Journal of Dental Education, 79*(6), 616-625. https://doi.org/10.1038/sj.bdj.2015.709

Hicks, F. D., Coke, L., & Li, S. (2009, June). *The effect of high-fidelity simulation on nursing students' knowledge and performance: A pilot study*. (NCSBN Research Brief, Volume 40). http://docplayer.net/208024-The-effect-of-high-fidelity-simulation-on-nursing-students-knowledge-and-performance-a-pilot-study.html

McFadyen, A., Maclaren, W., & Webster, V. (2007). The Interdisciplinary Education Perception Scale (IEPS): An alternative remodeled sub-scale structure and its reliability. *Journal of Interprofessional Care, 21*(4), 433-443. https://doi.org/10.1080/13561820701352531

Munshi, F., Lababidi, H., & Alyousef, S. (2015). Low- versus high-fidelity simulations in teaching and assessing clinical skills. *Journal of Taibah University Medical Sciences, 10*(1), 12-15. https://doi.org/10.1016/j.jtumed.2015.01.008

Oandasan, I., & Reeves, S. (2005). Key elements for interprofessional education. Part 1: The learner, the educator and the learning context. *Journal of Interprofessional Care, 19*(Suppl. 1), 21-38. https://doi.org/10.1080/13561820500083550

Olson, R., & Bialocerkowski, A. (2014). Interprofessional in allied health: A systematic review. *Medical Education, 48*(3), 236-246. https://doi.org/10.1111/medu.12290

Reddington, A., Egli, A., & Schmuck, H. (2018). Understanding interprofessional education perceptions of radiologic technology and dental assisting students through a live patient experience. *Journal of Dental Education, 82*(5), 462-468.

Weller, J. M., Nestel, D., Marshall, S. D., Brooks, P. M, & Conn, J. J. (2012). Simulation in clinical teaching and learning. *The Medical Journal of Australia, 196*(9), 594-598. https://doi.org/10.5694/mja10.11474

13

TRANSDISCIPLINARY COLLABORATION FOR SPEECH-LANGUAGE PATHOLOGY, SPECIAL EDUCATION, AND PSYCHOLOGY STUDENTS

Katrina Fulcher-Rood, PhD, CCC-SLP;
Pamela Schuetze, PhD; and Kathy Doody, PhD

DESCRIPTION OF TEACHING/LEARNING CONTEXT

Upon entering the workforce, students will need to collaborate successfully with individuals within and across disciplines to be effective in their chosen field. Even though collaboration is imperative in all fields, college students are rarely afforded opportunities to work with students that are not within their own discipline. To respond to this problem, three faculty members across different disciplines created a transdisciplinary applied learning project so that students could work together to conduct developmental screenings in community-based day care settings. Undergraduate seniors in a speech-language pathology class, junior-level students in a psychology class, and graduate students in a special education class were teamed together and trained to administer the Ages and Stages Questionnaire-3 (ASQ-3; Bricker et al., 1999) to children 1 month to 5.5 years of age in two different childcare centers. These students were selected to work together as these disciplines typically collaborate on assessment and treatment teams in school settings.

For this transdisciplinary applied learning project, students were first grouped together so that at a minimum one student from each discipline was in a group. After being assigned a group, students were trained in class to administer and score the ASQ-3. Another component of training was to have students watch videos that described each discipline and included the roles and responsibilities each profession had within a school setting. After training, students met with their teams to discuss their collaboration strategies and what role they would have when administering the screening (e.g., administer, score keeper, observer). Next, teams screened three children of various ages using the ASQ-3. After completing the screening, students were required to submit their scores through an online database. For assessment purposes, students completed an oral case presentation, a

Friberg, J. C., Visconti, C. F., & Ginsberg, S. M. (Eds.). *Evidence-Based Education in the Classroom: Examples From Clinical Disciplines* (pp. 117-124).

developmental assessment paper, and self-reflective journals. To assess the effectiveness of this project, pre- and post-surveys were used to collect data regarding student perceptions about transdisciplinary collaborations. These data were analyzed using both quantitative and qualitative methods.

REVIEW OF LITERATURE

Definitions of Transdisciplinary Education

In many health care professions, there is an increasing need for professionals across disciplines to work collaboratively to administer assessments and treatments (Bridges et al., 2011; Keshmiri et al., 2017; Ludwig & Kerins, 2019; Zraick et al., 2014). Given this need, students will benefit from having educational experiences that allow them to learn effective collaboration skills. A possible solution to provide this type of experience is the use of transdisciplinary education, also referred to as *interprofessional education* (IPE). Transdisciplinary education is a collaborative approach where students from a variety of disciplines work with one another (Bridges et al., 2011; Zraick et al., 2014). The World Health Organization defined IPE as "students from two or more professions learning about, from, and with each other to enable effective collaboration and improve health outcomes" (2010, p. 13). In this type of educational opportunity, it is important to distinguish the differences between multidisciplinary, interdisciplinary, and transdisciplinary (McClam & Flores-Scott, 2012). McClam and Flores-Scott (2012) describe multidisciplinary as equally dividing problems/tasks across different professionals, interdisciplinary as dividing and sharing problems/tasks, and transdisciplinary as a way to fuse and integrate knowledge from all disciplines so that all members solve problems together. Transdisciplinary work aims to go beyond collaboration and instead focuses on developing a shared skill set and collaborative decision making (Bellamy et al., 2013). Therefore, the goal of transdisciplinary education is not merely to have students divide tasks, but to learn from one another's expertise and carry out activities together that use knowledge and practices from their various professions.

Importance of Transdisciplinary Learning

In our transdisciplinary learning experience, students who would eventually search for careers in school settings worked together to complete developmental screenings. This was critically important because legislation in the public education setting mandates that children are assessed by professionals across a variety of disciplines (Myers et al., 1996). In addition, the use of transdisciplinary models for assessment and treatment is seen to be crucial for improving health care outcomes for patients (Keshmiri et al., 2017). Transdisciplinary teaching is being recognized as imperative by professional organizations as well. For example, the American Speech-Language and Hearing Association stated that including IPE experiences should be a high priority in clinical training programs (Ludwig & Kerins, 2019). The importance of the transdisciplinary model has also been well accepted by other relevant stakeholders involved in assessment and treatment procedures (Myers et al., 1996). For example, parents perceived that they received more information and that the information derived from a transdisciplinary assessment was more informative compared to traditional assessment models where professionals complete assessments individually (Myers et al., 1996). If the health care field would like best-evidence recommended practices integrated in daily decision making, specific training that goes beyond a single discipline will be needed (Bellamy et al., 2013). While transdisciplinary models are important and fields such as education and health care are pushing for IPE, many students do not get the opportunity to work across disciplines during their academic career. For example, Ludwig and Kerins (2019) found that less than 25% of the school-based speech-language pathologists they surveyed reported receiving formal training regarding collaboration or interprofessional practices.

Previous Work in Transdisciplinary Education

Transdisciplinary education and IPE has been used in a variety of fields including education, speech-language pathology, social work, and nursing. This educational approach aims to have individuals share their expertise and work toward a common goal (Bridges et al., 2011). In general, findings from research examining the outcomes of these educational experiences have found that students have an increase in positive attitudes regarding collaborative interaction and working with other professionals (Herrmann et al., 2015; Kenaszchuk et al., 2012; Silverman et al., 2010; Zraick et al., 2014). Specifically, students involved in an interprofessional educational workshop increased their ratings about the importance of collaboration, communication, and teamwork. In similar work, Herrick and colleagues (2002) created an IPE team for students learning about mental health initiatives for children with emotional disturbance. After participating, students stated that this experience fostered an interest in working collaboratively in the future. In addition, students involved in IPE are more likely to come to the job market with knowledge about the scope of practice, philosophies, and language used not only in their profession but in other disciplines as well (Herrick et al., 2002; Zraick et al., 2014). Most importantly, transdisciplinary education allows students to start developing their own professional identity (Zraick et al., 2014).

Components of Transdisciplinary Learning Experiences

Transdisciplinary learning is effective when problem-based activities are presented to students and foster collaboration among students to solve the presented problems (Zraick et al., 2014). Transdisciplinary education can be seen in many forms, including but not limited to, orientation sessions, clinical practicums, interprofessional simulations, group workshops, and fully integrated IPE curriculum (Stanley et al., 2016). No matter the structure of the transdisciplinary learning experience, the following components should be considered:

- Multiple transdisciplinary educational experiences are needed early in the learning process and should occur frequently across a student's curriculum so that they are able to learn the importance of working collaboratively on a team (Bridges et al., 2011)
- Structured experiences to understand and discuss their role as a professional, the roles of other professionals, and how roles change when on a transdisciplinary team (Bridges et al., 2011; Zraick et al., 2014)
- Guidelines/criteria so that students know their specific responsibilities and have effective ways to communicate with other team members (Bridges et al., 2011; Keshmiri et al., 2017; Zraick et al., 2014)
- Activities that provide students a way to build mutual trust and respect among their team members (Bridges et al., 2011; Keshmiri et al., 2017; Zraick et al., 2014)
- Mechanisms to show students the effect they have on their own learning, their team's learning, and the community and individuals they serve (Bridges et al., 2011; Zraick et al., 2014)
- Methods for self-reflection so that students can assess their own learning, understand their potential for bias and stereotyping, and evaluate their role on the team (Zraick et al., 2014)
- Support from administrative staff, including financial support, professional development opportunities, infrastructure, and committed faculty (Bridges et al., 2011; McClam & Flores-Scott, 2012; Stanley et al., 2016)

Another important aspect to consider when constructing transdisciplinary learning experiences is the methods used to assess the effects and outcomes of the project (Zraick et al., 2014). When developing assessment methods, five categories can be considered (Reeves et al., 2002; Zraick et al., 2014):

1. Students' reactions and perspectives about the transdisciplinary model and learning experiences
2. Change in attitudes, perceptions, or opinions regarding communication, collaboration, and teamwork
3. New knowledge or skills acquired by being exposed to a transdisciplinary experience
4. Transfer of new skills or knowledge to real-world experiences or actual professional practice
5. Clients, patients, families, or other relevant stakeholders' opinions about their participation in the learning experience

APPLICATION OF LITERATURE/DATA

Based on the earlier mentioned literature, our transdisciplinary project was constructed so that students from speech-language pathology, psychology, and exceptional education could collaborate to carry out developmental screening for children attending local child care centers. First, we devised methods to teach students about their role on a transdisciplinary team and how to complete a developmental screening. Students received in-class training from their instructors about the importance of developmental assessment, the definition of a transdisciplinary team, the ways a transdisciplinary team operates, and directions on administering the ASQ-3. Another component of training was to have students watch multiple videos of individuals administering the ASQ-3. Students also reviewed videos for ASQ-3 administration and scored the screenings on their own. Next, students were instructed about the roles and responsibilities of the other disciplines they would be collaborating with. To do this, each instructor created a 10- to 15-minute video describing their profession, including their roles and responsibilities, aspects of development that they were most concerned with, and their daily job tasks in a school setting. While watching the videos, students were required to answer questions that assessed their comprehension of the information. Next, students were given a handbook that outlined the goal of the project, the expectations for their involvement in the project, a timeline for the semester, and a description of the associated assignments. To provide a structure and mechanism for collaboration among team members, students were required to meet with their entire team before completing the developmental screening. At this meeting, students were instructed to discuss and coordinate their role on the assessment team (e.g., mentor, observer, tester). Also, students were asked to discuss a collaboration survey they completed prior to the meeting. In this survey, students were asked to reflect on their work habits, how they handle conflict, and barriers to successfully completing group work. This meeting and collaboration survey provided the space and opportunity for students to start effectively communicating with their team and begin building team morale and trust. After students met, they completed at a minimum three different developmental screenings at one of two community-based day care centers. To relate the project to other tasks or activities a student would complete in a school setting, they were required to score their screening, analyze the screening results, present to the class the findings and recommendations of the screening, and complete a paper that was tailored to their discipline and level. To ensure that students had opportunities for self-reflection, all students completed four separate self-reflection journal entries throughout the semester. The first journal assignment asked students to think about the skills they would need to be successful on a transdisciplinary team, the second journal assignment provided prompts for students to reflect on what they learned during the training period, the third journal assignment was completed after they conducted their developmental screening and required them to think about their performance during the screening, and finally, the fourth journal assignment asked students to reflect upon the ways this project would affect them in their future careers and if their perspectives about collaboration and transdisciplinary teams had changed.

The authors also constructed assessment measures to evaluate the outcomes of the transdisciplinary project. All students completed a pre- and post-survey that included Likert scale and open-ended questions regarding their perceptions and attitudes about collaboration, group projects, and their perceived competency about working with children and completing screenings. Also, the authors contacted the various community partners and teachers in the day care centers to discuss their perceptions of the project, the professionalism of the students, and suggestions for modifying the project in the future. These assessment measures not only helped the authors understand the impact and effectiveness of their transdisciplinary project but also aided in modifying future aspects of the experience.

Findings From Current Transdisciplinary Project

To date, this transdisciplinary project has taken place for 2 years. Both quantitative and qualitative assessments were used to explore the effectiveness of using an applied-learning project to enhance student interest in participating in transdisciplinary collaborations that mirror those found in professional settings.

Quantitative Findings

Quantitative measures of student perceptions to interdisciplinary collaborations and attitudes about working with young children were obtained using a survey designed by the authors. This survey consisted of six items, which were each measured using a 5-point Likert-type rating scale ranging from strongly disapprove to strongly approve, and was administered before and after the project. Separate 3 (course) X 2 (pre/post) analyses of variance were conducted for all six items. Statistically significant differences in pre- and post-testing were found regarding students' perceived comfort level in using developmental screenings and working with professionals from other disciplines ($p = .00$ and $p = .003$, respectively), suggesting that this teaching modality was successful in allowing students to gain more confidence in their future job responsibilities. Students' perceived comfort level in working with young children was only marginally statistically different after participating in the transdisciplinary learning project ($p = .054$). For students in the speech-language pathology and psychology fields, this was their first time interacting one-on-one with children in a professional capacity. It is possible that only having this one exposure was not enough to increase comfort level to a statistically significant level, suggesting that students will need repeated exposure in these types of experiences to receive more of a benefit. A statistically significant difference was found regarding students' interest level in working with people from other disciplines after participating in this learning opportunity ($p = .014$). This finding corroborates previous findings about the positive effect transdisciplinary learning has on increasing student interest in collaboration and teamwork. Interestingly, a statistical difference was not found in students' interest in working with young children in the future. This again could be due to the limited exposure students had working with children before this project. It is possible that with more experience, a student's interest could change. Finally, students were asked before and after participating in this project, "How would you assess the effectiveness of learning in authentic community-based settings?" A statistically significant difference was found after completing this project ($p = .008$), further confirming the impact of this teaching modality.

Qualitative Findings

One factor of the qualitative analysis was to analyze students' perspectives on collaborating before and after completing this project. Pre-project analysis revealed that when completing collaborative assignments, students liked being able to learn from others, having a variety of perspectives, and dividing work among group members. Scheduling time with team members, resolving disagreements, and establishing trust with group mates were cited as areas of difficulty by respondents in all three groups. Qualitative analysis from post-surveys showed that students tended to have more positive perceptions of collaborative work due to this transdisciplinary learning experience. This was evident as students provided fewer negative comments in the post-project survey. Students discussed a feeling of growing as a professional and as a student in three primary ways. First, students noted that, through collaboration, they were able to build their confidence and strengthen their learning. For example, one student said, "Hearing other people's ideas and values ... [w]orking with someone older than me and more experienced made me more confident when I was completing my screening." Similarly, another student said that her favorite aspect of this learning opportunity was "being able to help my partner find confidence and ease when doing the ASQ and helping her with strategies to help the child's attention." Second, students wrote about the ways this project helped them develop future professional skills. This theme was evident in comments similar to the reflection this student provided: "I very much enjoyed service learning. It helped to prepare me to work with children in my field someday. I am confident assessing children after taking this course." Another student stated, "It has made me hopeful in other psychology courses. It has opened my mind to actually understanding and enjoying psychology." A different student wrote that this type of class "is a great opportunity to use what you learned in the classroom and apply it to real life. It has also opened my eyes to possible career options." Finally, students discussed that this experience allowed them to connect with and understand their community more. For example, a student stated the project "got [me] more familiar with my community and what is offered." Similarly, a different student wrote that she enjoyed this project "because they are new and different ways to incorporate topics and procedures learned in class and put them to use in an environment that matters. It gets me more familiar with my community."

While most of the qualitative information provided positive perceptions of the transdisciplinary project, there were still some persistent negative opinions regarding collaborative work. Students still discussed issues with collaborating with others due to lack of equal distribution of work across team members, difficulty finding a common schedule, and disagreements among group members. These topics should be carefully considered when creating these opportunities. For example, specific roles or tasks could be assigned to group members in advance to alleviate this concern. Also, students could work together to decide in advance which tasks they will be responsible for. Once this agreement is made, students could sign agreements that list their contributions and pledge to uphold their part of the project. In addition, students with similar schedules could be grouped together to help with scheduling conflicts. In advance of completing the assignment, teams could identify and agree upon conflict resolution strategies to overcome issues surrounding disagreements and miscommunication among team members when differences arise. These strategies may help to remediate some of the concerns or areas of conflict students referenced in the post-project surveys.

Conclusion

In summary, students across three different professional fields who participated in a transdisciplinary learning experience had positive perspectives regarding this teaching modality and viewed collaboration as an important aspect of their professional practice. Students expressed that they enjoyed learning from other disciplines and stated they benefited from other's expertise to more effectively complete developmental screenings. This is important, as this is the primary goal of transdisciplinary learning models. Projects similar to the one presented here can be adapted to multiple professions.

APPLICATION TO CROSS-DISCIPLINARY CONTEXTS

Transdisciplinary learning experiences are not only for students who are studying the disciplines of speech-language pathology, psychology, or education. The concept behind this transdisciplinary project can easily be transferred to related health care and education-based fields, such as social work, nursing, physical therapy, and occupational therapy. Individual aspects of the project, such as the assessment tool utilized, the target population/client, and the composition of team members, can easily be adapted to meet professional standards in any field of study. Beyond these fields, transdisciplinary education can be applied to almost all areas, as each profession has a unique set of skills that need to be explicitly taught, and most professions will require that individuals collaborate and share responsibilities and decision making. Therefore, it is key for an instructor to plan what professional skills the students will be expected to acquire while considering what other professions their colleagues may address in an employment setting. With this in mind, the instructor will be able to design a more realistic transdisciplinary project. In addition, it is important to remember that these learning opportunities do not have to be complicated or last the entire semester—one can start small. Transdisciplinary experiences include, but are not limited to, transdisciplinary professional development seminars, workshops and/or orientation, creating a transdisciplinary virtual professional support network, constructing assignments to consider interprofessional collaboration (e.g., asking for ways a student would include other disciplines, researching what other professions would do to solve a problem), and having student or professional organizations from different backgrounds complete community or campus work together. All of these experiences are geared toward the primary goal of transdisciplinary education—to ensure students learn the necessary skills for collaboration and teamwork so they can be successful in their chosen career.

Additional Resources

- Helpful websites:
  - The State University of New York Buffalo State's Applied Learning website:
    - https://appliedlearning.buffalostate.edu/
  - The State University of New York's Applied Learning Resources, including an "Applied Learning Toolkit":
    - https://www.suny.edu/applied-learning/resources/
- Example self-reflective journal prompts:
  - What personal qualities (e.g., leadership, communication skills, empathy) have you developed through this service learning project?
  - What contribution can you make to public understanding of this issue based on your service learning experience?
  - In what ways are you finding your involvement with service learning difficult? What have you found that is helping you follow through despite the difficulties you encounter?
  - How does the service experience relate to the course material?
  - What aspects of your learning may have been due to your service experience?
  - Do you feel this service learning project has prepared you for a future career? Why or why not?

References

Bellamy, J. L., Mullen, E. J., Satterfield, J. M., Newhouse, R. P., Ferguson, M., Brownson, R. C., & Spring, B. (2013). Implementing evidence-based practice education in social work: A transdisciplinary approach. *Research on Social Work Practice, 23*(4), 426-436.

Bricker, D., Squires, J., Mounts, L., Potter, L., Nickel, R., Twombly, E., & Farrell, J. (1999). *Ages and stages questionnaire.* Paul H. Brookese.

Bridges, D. R., Davidson, R. A., Odegard, P. S., Maki, I. V., & Tomkowiak, J. (2011). Interprofessional collaboration: Three best practice models of interprofessional education. *Medical Education Online, 16*(1), 6035.

Herrick, C. A., Arbuckle, M. B., & Claes, J. A. (2002). Teaching interprofessional practice: A course on a system of care for children with severe emotional disturbance and their families. *Journal of Family Nursing, 8*(3), 264-281.

Herrmann, G., Woermann, U., & Schlegel, C. (2015). Interprofessional education in anatomy: Learning together in medical and nursing training. *Anatomical Sciences Education, 8*(4), 324-330.

Kenaszchuk, C., Rykhoff, M., Collins, L., McPhail, S., & van Soeren, M. (2012). Positive and null effects of interprofessional education on attitudes toward interprofessional learning and collaboration. *Advances in Health Sciences Education: Theory and Practice, 17*(5), 651-669.

Keshmiri, F., Rezai, M., Mosaddegh, R., Moradi, K., Hafezimoghadam, P., Zare, M. A., Tavakoli, N., Cheraghi, M. A., & Shirazi, M. (2017). Effectiveness of an interprofessional education model based on the transtheoretical model of behaviour change to improve interprofessional collaboration. *Journal of Interprofessional Care, 31*(3), 307-316.

Ludwig, D. A., & Kerins, M. R. (2019). Interprofessional education: Application of interprofessional education collaborative core competencies to school settings. *Perspectives of the ASHA Special Interest Groups, 4*(2), 269-274. https://doi.org/10.1044/2018_PERS-SIG2-2018-0009

McClam, S., & Flores-Scott, E. M. (2012). Transdisciplinary teaching and research: What is possible in higher education? *Teaching in Higher Education, 17*(3), 231-243.

Myers, C. L., McBride, S. L., & Peterson, C. A. (1996). Transdisciplinary, play-based assessment in early childhood special education: An examination of social validity. *Topics in Early Childhood Special Education, 16*(1), 102-126.

Reeves, S., Freeth, D., McCrorie, P., & Perry, D. (2002). "It teaches you what to expect in future…": Interprofessional learning on a training ward for medical, nursing, occupational therapy and physiotherapy students. *Medical Education, 36*(4), 337-344.

Silverman, K., Hong, S., & Trepanier-Street, M. (2010). Collaboration of teacher education and child disability health care: Transdisciplinary approach to inclusive practice for early childhood pre-service teachers. *Early Childhood Education Journal, 37*(6), 461-468.

Stanley, K., Dixon, K., Warner, P., & Stanley, D. (2016). Twelve possible strategies for enhancing interprofessional socialisation in higher education: Findings from an interpretive phenomenological study. *Journal of Interprofessional Care, 30*(4), 475-482.

World Health Organization. (2010). Framework for action on interprofessional education and collaborative practice. https://www.who.int/hrh/resources/framework_action/en/

Zraick, R. I., Harten, A. C., & Hagstrom, F. (2014). Interprofessional education and practice: A primer for training future clinicians. *Perspectives on Issues in Higher Education, 17*(2), 39-46. https://doi.org/10.1044/aihe17.2.39

14

SHARED MISSION: UNITE, SUPPORT, ACHIEVE
Interprofessional Education for Traumatic Brain Injury

Casey Keck, PhD, CCC-SLP; April Garrity, PhD, CCC-SLP; and Keiko Ishikawa, PhD, CCC-SLP

DESCRIPTION OF TEACHING/LEARNING CONTEXT

Shared Mission: Unite, Support, Achieve (USA) is an interprofessional training program that prepares graduate speech-language pathology students to provide collaborative rehabilitation services to military service members and veterans (SM/Vs) with traumatic brain injury (TBI). Speech-language pathology program faculty and professionals from campus units, including the Military Resource Center, Counseling Center, and the Student Accessibility Resource Center, collaboratively teach graduate speech-language pathology students (hereinafter referred to as *students*) about cognitive-linguistic intervention, military cultural competence, and counseling/support services for SM/Vs with TBI to prepare them to serve this unique population.

Shared Mission: USA was created to address a curricular need in our graduate program as well as to complement our institution's commitment to providing educational services to SM/Vs and their families. Evidence of this commitment has been widely recognized, including being named the number one 4-year institution for SM/Vs (Military Times Reboot Camp, n.d.). In addition to this institutional commitment, our program is an accredited graduate-level speech-language pathology program, which means that, among other things, faculty members are committed to providing knowledge and skills in cultural competence and cognitive-communication disorders among diverse populations. Assessment and intervention among SM/Vs with TBI is complex, often complicated by comorbidities, and requires an understanding of military culture (Working Group to Develop a Clinician's Guide to Cognitive Rehabilitation in mTBI: Application for Military Service Members and Veterans [Working Group], 2016).

Friberg, J. C., Visconti, C. F., & Ginsberg, S. M. (Eds.). *Evidence-Based Education in the Classroom: Examples From Clinical Disciplines* (pp. 125–132).

REVIEW OF LITERATURE

Understanding Traumatic Brain Injury Among Service Members/Veterans

According to the Defense and Veterans Brain Injury Center (DVBIC), between 2000 and 2018, nearly 384,000 U.S. SM/Vs sustained TBIs, most of which were caused by blast injuries. The majority of these injuries are considered mild traumatic brain injuries (mTBIs; DVBIC, 2018), as characterized by a Glasgow Coma Scale score of 13 to 15 within 30 minutes of the injury (15 is the highest score on the Glasgow Coma Scale). Individuals with mTBI may initially present with disorientation or amnesia for events that occurred around the time of the injury.

Although the initial disorientation and memory alterations of mTBI typically resolve within 24 hours of the injury (Diagnosis, 2017), individuals with mTBI may have persistent deficits, sometimes called *postconcussive symptoms*, which interfere with their activities of daily living. These can include fatigue or sluggishness; headaches; dizziness; and cognitive difficulties, such as trouble concentrating and impaired memory (U.S. Department of Health and Human Services, 2016). Recent research suggests that SM/Vs with blast-injury mTBIs suffer more severe and persistent postconcussive symptoms than civilians with mTBI (Beran & Bhaskar, 2018; Summerall, n.d.).

These differences in SM/Vs' recovery from mTBI have been attributed, in part, to the traumatic nature of the events associated with their injuries (e.g., combat-related injuries). SM/Vs who survive traumatic events may have a comorbid psychiatric diagnosis of depression, anxiety, and posttraumatic stress disorder (PTSD; Summerall, n.d.), which bring about complaints of physical pain, sleep disturbances, and attention and memory deficits (American Psychiatric Association, 2013). These complaints are similar to those associated with mTBI and some experts believe their presence may extend and complicate the presence of postconcussive symptoms for SM/Vs with mTBI (Working Group, 2016).

SM/Vs also bring a unique cultural perspective to the experience of illness, perceived disability, and recovery. The military strongly encourages its members to display characteristics such as loyalty and respect, especially to superiors. Commitment to completing the assigned mission and to always performing tasks to the best of one's ability are also principles that are central to military culture (Working Group, 2016). Furthermore, each branch of the military has its own traditions, customs, songs, nomenclature, and personnel structure that dictates how members conduct themselves. In order to best serve SM/Vs, health care professionals must possess cultural competence by learning about military culture and how it translates to caring for these individuals.

Teaching Students About Traumatic Brain Injury Among Service Members/Veterans

TBI instruction in health professions training programs focuses primarily on aspects of symptoms, treatment, and recovery in the civilian population. However, because of the unique and complex needs of SM/Vs with TBI, students should also receive specialized instruction on topics such as the differences between TBI recovery among civilians and SM/Vs; psychiatric and other comorbidities associated with SM/Vs with TBI; and cultural values and beliefs common to SM/Vs. Health professions students also need opportunities to learn during interprofessional collaborative practice experiences with this population. Evidence suggests that an interprofessional collaborative approach to TBI treatment (e.g., one including disciplines such as physical therapy, occupational therapy, nursing, counseling, neuropsychology, and speech-language pathology) leads to positive outcomes, including patient safety and overall health (World Health Organization [WHO], 2010).

While most health professions training programs recognize the responsibility to incorporate specialized content and clinical experiences, such as that of TBI among SM/Vs, this can be challenging because they are already providing students with a content- and clinical experience–heavy curriculum. Action research is well suited to addressing such a challenge.

Action Research

Action research is the process of using evidence to systematically improve a procedure/practice used in a specific situation or context (Koshy et al., 2011). Elliot's (1991) action research model describes multiple cycles within a project. Each cycle includes several steps: identify the initial idea, gather information about the idea, create a plan and action steps, implement the action steps, monitor the effects of the implementation, explain failures of implementation and their effects, revise the idea, implement the amended plan, and repeat cycles. This process allows one to continually improve the action plan based on the results of the previous plan. Action research is particularly useful in health care and educational settings because it allows practitioners to make rapid and responsive improvements to their practices. This chapter describes how we used the action research approach to address a curricular challenge, namely, providing students with an interprofessional education experience focused on TBI in SM/Vs.

ORIGINAL DATA AND APPLICATION OF LITERATURE/DATA

Cycle 1: Development and Implementation of the Piloted Program

Shared Mission: USA was funded through an institutional grant in 2016 and was piloted in 2017. The goals of the pilot program were to (1) train speech-language pathology students to serve SM/Vs with TBI- and/or PTSD-related deficits and (2) assist SM/Vs with TBI- and/or PTSD-related deficits with their transition to civilian life. These goals were targeted over two phases. Phase 1 focused on developing and implementing student training, and Phase 2 focused on clinical instruction in speech-language pathology service delivery to SM/Vs with TBI- and/or PTSD-related deficits.

Training for students was voluntary and consisted of students completing pre- and post-training assessments and attending workshops. Students from two graduate cohorts, first- ($n = 16$) and third-semester students ($n = 13$), participated; however, their participation varied. First-semester students were invited to participate in both program phases, whereas third-semester students were only invited to complete pre-training assessments. Pre- and post-training assessments were composed of two online surveys (using Google Forms) that assessed the students understanding of TBI symptoms, the recovery process, and military culture. These surveys were the Common Misconceptions About Traumatic Brain Injury–Modified Clinician Survey (CM-TBI) and Adapted Military Cultural Certificate Program Assessment Scale (MCCP).

The CM-TBI measured students' understanding of the effects of TBI and the recovery process. This survey was adapted from a TBI misconceptions questionnaire developed by Springer and colleagues (1997) and the Common Misconceptions About TBI Questionnaire–Modified developed by Schellinger (2015). The MCCP measured students' understanding of military culture and was adapted from Nedegaard and Zwilling (2017). The surveys were made up of multiple choice items and/or Likert scale items.

The CM-TBI and MCCP surveys and the students' pre-training responses on these surveys informed the content taught in the workshops, which were led by representatives from the Military Resource Center, Counseling Center, the Student Accessibility Resource Center, and speech-language pathology graduate program faculty. Shared Mission: USA representatives were provided with a list of topics addressed by the CM-TBI and MCCP surveys and asked to incorporate content related to these topics into their workshop presentations. These representatives were further asked to emphasize topics on which participants performed below competency (80%) on the pre-tests.

Student training consisted of five 1-hour workshops over 8 weeks. Each workshop was prepared and led by a different Shared Mission: USA representative. Workshop presentation topics included TBI core content, counseling in communication sciences and disorders, military and veteran resources, disability and academic resources, and counseling resources for psychosocial impairments. Each representative addressed at least the following learning objectives in their workshop presentation: the roles and responsibilities of the representative's profession, management of TBI- and/or PTSD-related impairments and/or resources for SM/Vs with these types of impairments, and SM/Vs as a culturally distinct population. Workshops were held on campus and students completed post-training surveys after completing the eight workshops.

Phase 2 of the piloted program required students to deliver speech-language pathology services to SM/Vs with TBI- and/or PTSD-related deficits through group treatment. First-semester students who attended the eight workshops and completed the pre- and post-training surveys were eligible to serve as clinicians for the group treatment sessions. Despite extensive recruitment efforts, no SM/Vs volunteered to participate; therefore, the service provision component of the program was abandoned to focus solely on student training.

However, the plan for Phase 2 was to collect information from the SM/V participants regarding their reasons for participating in Shared Mission: USA group treatment and what goals they hoped to accomplish. SM/V participants' information was going to be collected through focus groups and used to develop treatment plans.

Cycle 1: Monitor Effects and Explain Failures

Consistent with the action research approach, we evaluated and reflected on the pilot program's outcomes. Excessive student attrition was identified as a significant problem. Of the 16 first semester students that started the training program, only 4 completed all workshops and post-training surveys, resulting in a 75% attrition rate. Additionally, comparison of students' pre- and post-training survey responses revealed lower than expected student learning. Post-training survey responses suggested that the four students who completed the workshops showed evidence of improvement on the CM-TBI and MCCP surveys but continued to lack some basic knowledge of the effects of TBI and the recovery process. Students also had weaknesses in their understanding of military culture, PTSD, and their own clinical skills related to this population (Keck et al., 2017).

Potential reasons for these program failures were assessed by thoroughly reviewing the piloted program's format, students' pre- and post-survey results, and content taught in the workshops. Lack of student motivation to complete training (surveys and workshops) was identified as the primary reason for the program's failures. Student motivation was likely diminished by the inability to earn course credit for the training and/or the limited opportunity to work with SM/V participants. Additionally, students may have lost interest in training and/or had difficulty retaining the content over the 8-week time frame without review or application of content learned.

Cycle 2: Program Modifications

Several improvements were made to the Shared Mission: USA program in 2018 based on evidence gathered through the action research process, including condensing the training time frame; obtaining programmatic support for training, including instituting mandatory participation by students; and adding case-based teaching and assessment elements to training. To reduce attrition, the time frame for training was condensed to a half-day workshop. Student participation in the workshop was required as an ancillary learning module to provide students with additional information about a specific clinical population and to ensure that students met the American Speech-Language-Hearing Association's certification standards. Students' participation in the institutional review board–approved research project associated with the workshop was optional.

To improve learning and application of knowledge, problem-based learning was incorporated in the training by using clinical cases (see Albanese & Dast, 2014; Vandenhouten et al., 2017 for more information on this evidence-based pedagogy). Students were provided with pre- and post-workshop clinical case studies of two SM/Vs with TBI. The pre-workshop clinical case consisted of open-ended questions about the case that aligned with the program's learning objectives. The post-workshop clinical case consisted of multiple-choice questions that were similar to the open-ended questions presented in the pre-workshop case. The open-ended pre-workshop questions were completed in the quiz tool of our institution's learning management system prior to attending the training. The pre-workshop case and answers to the questions were reviewed as a teaching tool at the end of each representatives' workshop presentation. Questions for the post-workshop case were also available through the quiz tool of our university's learning management system. The pre- and post-training assessment surveys (CM-TBI and MCCP) that were administered in Cycle 1 were administered again in Cycle 2.

Cycle 2: Monitor Effects and Explain Failures

Efforts to improve the students' program completion rate were effective. All 20 second semester speech-language pathology students completed the training program. Student learning also improved. Wilcoxon sign-rank tests were completed to test changes in the students' basic knowledge of TBI (CM-TBI) and military cultural competence (MCCP) after training. This statistical test was selected because it examines differences in the medians of a variable for two related groups and can be used with data that is not normally distributed.

There was a statistically significant increase in the number of students who correctly answered questions on the CM-TBI post-training compared to pre-training ($w = 190$, $p = .01$). Of the 25 multiple-choice questions on the CM-TBI survey, 15 were correctly answered by more students after training than before, two were correctly answered by more students before training than after, and eight were correctly answered by an equal number of students before and after training. The two questions students correctly answered on the pre-test but incorrectly answered on the post-test were related to coma and rehabilitation.

There was a statistically significant increase in the number of students whose responses indicated military cultural competence on the MCCP survey post-training compared to pre-training ($w = 190$, $p = .02$). Of the 16 multiple-choice questions on the MCCP survey, 15 were answered in a way that indicated military cultural competence by more students after training than before. One of the 16 questions was answered in a way that indicated military cultural competence by an equal number of students before and after training. This one question was related to students' ability to effectively work with veterans.

Post-workshop case study assessment results suggested that students were able to apply some of the content learned in the workshop to a case scenario. Of the nine post-workshop assessment questions, seven were correctly answered by at least 80% of the students. The two questions that did not reach 80% accuracy were related to counseling within the discipline of speech-language pathology's scope of practice and identifying the impact of cognitive deficits on a SM/Vs quality of life.

Cycle 3: Program Modifications

The evidence gathered through the action research process suggested that the revised Shared Mission: USA program successfully trained students in the areas of cognitive-linguistic intervention, military cultural competence, and support services for SM/Vs with TBI. Also, the Shared Mission: USA format changes improved students' program completion rate and retention of content taught in the workshop. Although the results of the revised program were mostly positive, the students' performance on the post-workshop case study, 77.7% accuracy (seven out of nine questions correctly answered by 80% of students), was concerning. Specifically, the students struggled to apply the counseling and quality of life content.

The 2019 iteration of Shared Mission: USA will be modified to improve students' application of the content learned in the workshop to case studies. To achieve this goal, we plan to revise the format of the pre-workshop case from open-ended questions to multiple-choice questions. Although the open-ended questions provided valuable qualitative information on the students' application skills, assessing their responses was laborious and did not permit timely assessment of the students' skills. Changing the format of the pre-workshop case will allow us to quickly evaluate the students' pre-workshop application skills and address application concerns in the workshop while reviewing the teaching case. Additionally, aligning the format of the pre- and post-workshop case will allow us to statistically compare students' pre-workshop application skills to their post-workshop skills for evaluation purposes.

APPLICATION TO CROSS-DISCIPLINARY CONTEXTS

Shared Mission: USA's interprofessional structure and focus on the specialized population of SM/Vs with TBI is relevant to many health professions training programs. This section outlines some potential modifications to Shared Mission: USA to expand its application to other disciplines.

Interprofessional education (IPE) has become an essential component of health professions training programs and a number of professional associations have developed interprofessional practice core competencies to be instituted in higher education (Interprofessional Education Collaborative [IPEC], 2016). Additionally, Shared Mission: USA's focus on SM/Vs with TBI lends itself to IPE because this disorder can result in a multitude of cognitive, physical, sensory, and behavioral impairments (Cornis-Pop et al., 2012). TBI rehabilitation guidelines suggest that evaluation and treatment involve interprofessional collaboration (Institut National d'Excellence en Santé et en Services Sociaux–Ontario Neurotrauma Foundation, 2017; Marshall et al., 2018). The Shared Mission: USA program could be modified to meet various professional associations' criteria for IPE and expanded to include professionals and students from a variety of health professions.

WHO defines IPE as "when students from two or more professions learn about, from, and with each other to enable effective collaboration and improve health outcomes" (WHO, 2010, p. 8). IPEC has used this definition to develop interprofessional core competencies. These IPEC core competencies have been widely adopted by professional associations including occupational therapy, physical therapy, speech-language pathology, social work, and psychology (IPEC, 2016) to establish interprofessional practice competencies for each discipline.

The content of the Shared Mission: USA workshop could be expanded to include the IPEC core competencies. IPEC (2016, p. 10) developed four core competency domains of collaborative practice and team-based care: (1) values and ethics, (2) roles and responsibilities, (3) interprofessional communication, and (4) teamwork and team-based care.

Furthermore, the structure of Shared Mission: USA could be modified to meet this definition's criterion of students learning from, with, and among each other. Students from other disciplines that provide services to SM/Vs with TBI, such as nursing, psychology, occupational therapy, physical therapy, and social work, could be invited to participate in the workshop and the clinical component of Shared Mission: USA. The structure of workshop activities could be modified to include cooperative learning approaches. This might consist of having small groups of students work together to identify and develop ways to address various symptoms or problems described within the case. Modifications such as these would position Shared Mission: USA as an interprofessional clinical practice in which instructors/professionals and students from a variety of disciplines work together to coordinate and deliver health care services for SM/Vs. Ultimately, this is the type of cooperative learning experience that we strive to provide to health professions students, as it teaches about the signs and symptoms of a clinical population, focuses on cultural competence, and fosters skills needed for successful interprofessional practice.

ADDITIONAL RESOURCES

Many excellent resources (in addition to those provided in the reference list) are available for further information on the topics discussed in this chapter. A sampling of curated resources can be found below, organized by topic.

Interprofessional Education

- The American Physical Therapy Association offers a directory of organizations engaged in interprofessional education and practice. The directory contains links to each organization:
  - American Physical Therapy Association. (2019). Interprofessional Education and Collaborative Practice resources. https://www.apta.org/for-educators/interprofessional-collaboration
- An example of a professional association's position statement on interprofessional education and practice:
  - Larson, E. L., DeBasio, N. O., Mundinger, M. O., & Shoemaker, J. K. (n.d.). Interdisciplinary Education and Practice. *American Association of Colleges of Nursing.* https://www.aacnnursing.org/News-Information/Position-Statements-White-Papers/Interdisciplinary-Education-Practice
- An article explaining one counselor education program's experience with developing an interprofessional training program:
  - Okech, J., & Geroski, A. (2015). Interdisciplinary training: Preparing counselors for collaborative practice. *The Professional Counselor.* http://tpcjournal.nbcc.org/interdisciplinary-training-preparing-counselors-for-collaborative-practice/

Traumatic Brain Injury in Service Members/Veterans

- DVBIC has published a collection of clinical resources to assist clinicians serving SM/Vs and SM/Vs with persistent cognitive problems after TBI. Resources include webinars, podcasts, information sheets, and more:
  - Military Health System. (n.d.). Cognitive rehabilitation for service members and veterans following mild to moderate traumatic brain injury clinical suite. *Defense and Veterans Brain Injury Center.* https://health.mil/About-MHS/OASDHA/Defense-Health-Agency/Research-and-Development/Traumatic-Brain-Injury-Center-of-Excellence/Provider-Resources
- This book offers clinical management guidelines for concussion across a range of rehabilitation topics, including balance, vision, cognition, participation, and quality of life:
  - Weightman, M., Radomski, M., Mashima, P., & Roth, C. (Eds.). (2014). *Mild traumatic brain injury rehabilitation toolkit.* Borden Institute.

Military Culture

- The Center for Deployment Psychology offers an online course for health care professionals on military culture, in addition to other military culture resources:
  - Uniformed Services University. (n.d.). Learn about military culture. *Center for Deployment Psychology.* deploymentpsych.org/military-culture

REFERENCES

Albanese, M. A., & Dast, L. (2014). Problem-based learning: Outcomes evidence from the health professions. *Journal on Excellence in College Teaching, 25*(3-4), 239-252.

American Psychiatric Association. (2013). *Diagnostic and statistical manual of mental disorders* (5th ed.). Author.

Beran, R., & Bhaskar, S. (2018). Concussion within the military. *Journal of Military and Veterans' Health, 26,* 20-27.

Cornis-Pop, M., Mashima, P. A., Roth, C. R., MacLennan, D. L., Picon, L. M., Hammond, C. S., Goo-Yoshino, S., Isaki, E., Singson, M., & Frank, E. M. (2012). Cognitive-communication rehabilitation for combat-related mild traumatic brain injury. *Journal of Rehabilitation Research and Development, 49*(7), xi-xxxii. http://dx.doi.org/10.1682/JRRD.2012.03.0048

Diagnosis. (2017). Brainline: All about brain injury and PTSD. https://www.brainline.org/identifying-and-treating-concussionmtbi-service-members-and-veterans/diagnosis

Defense and Veterans Brain Injury Center. (2018). DoD worldwide numbers for TBI. https://dvbic.dcoe.mil/dod-worldwide-numbers-tbi

Elliot, J. (1991). *Action research for educational change.* Open University Press.

Interprofessional Education Collaborative. (2016). *Core competencies for interprofessional collaborative practice: 2016 update.* Author.

Institut national d'excellence en santé et en services sociaux-Ontario Neurotrauma Foundation. (2017). INESSS-ONF Guideline for rehabilitation of adults with moderate-to-severe TBI. https://braininjuryguidelines.org/modtosevere/

Keck, C., Garrity, A., & Bradshaw, J. L. (2017, November). Shared Mission USA: An interprofessional intervention and support group for military students with brain injury. *American Speech-Language-Hearing Association Annual Conference.* Symposium conducted at the meeting of the American Speech-Language-Hearing Association, Los Angeles, California.

Koshy, E., Koshy, V., & Waterman, H. (2011). *Action research in healthcare.* SAGE Publications.

Marshall, S., Bayley, M., McCullagh, S., Berrigan, L., Fischer, L., Ouchterlony, D., Rockwell, C., Velikonja, D., et al. (2018). Guideline for concussion/mild traumatic brain injury and persistent symptoms: 3rd edition (for adults over 18 years of age). *Ontario Neurotrauma Foundation.* https://braininjuryguidelines.org/concussion/index.php?id=154

Military Times Reboot Camp. (n.d.). Best for vets: Colleges 2019 4-year schools. https://charts.militarytimes.com/chart/9

Nedegaard, R., & Zwilling, J. (2017). Promoting military cultural competence among civilian care providers: Learning through program development. *Social Sciences, 6,* 1-11.

Schellinger, S. K. (2015). Public perceptions of traumatic brain injury: Knowledge, attitudes, and the impact of education [Doctoral dissertation, University of Minnesota]. *University of Minnesota Digital Conservancy.* http://conservancy.umn.edu/handle/11299/175326

Springer, J. A., Farmer, J. E., & Bouman, D. E. (1997). Common misconceptions about traumatic brain injury among family members of rehabilitation patients. *Journal of Head Trauma and Rehabilitation, 12*(3), 41-50.

Summerall, E. L. (n.d.). Traumatic brain injury and PTSD. *United States Department of Veterans Affairs.* https://www.ptsd.va.gov/professional/treat/cooccurring/tbi_ptsd_vets.asp

U.S. Department of Health and Human Services. (2016). What are common TBI symptoms? https://www.nichd.nih.gov/health/topics/tbi/conditioninfo/symptoms

Vandenhouten, C., Groessl, J., & Levintova, E. (2017). How do you use problem-based learning to improve interdisciplinary thinking? *New Directions for Teaching and Learning, 151,* 117-133.

Working Group to Develop a Clinician's Guide to Cognitive Rehabilitation in mTBI: Application for Military Service Members and Veterans. (2016). Clinician's guide to cognitive rehabilitation in mild traumatic brain injury: Application for military service members and veterans. *American Speech-Language-Hearing Association.* https://www.asha.org/siteassets/practice-portal/traumatic-brain-injury-adult/clinicians-guide-to-cognitive-rehabilitation-in-mild-traumatic-brain-injury.pdf

World Health Organization. (2010). Framework for action on interprofessional education and collaborative practice. https://www.who.int/hrh/resources/framework_action/en/

15

IMPROVING CLINICAL REASONING IN HEALTH PROFESSIONS STUDENTS THROUGH TEAM-BASED LEARNING

Andi Beth Mincer, PT, EdD

DESCRIPTION OF TEACHING/LEARNING CONTEXT

Today's health professionals need to demonstrate effective team behaviors in order to function as part of a health care team, apply an ever-expanding stream of information to their personal knowledge base in order to continue growing professionally and reason clinically in order to make optimal ongoing patient care decisions. Health professions curricula should include an emphasis on skill development in these three important areas. Unfortunately, most educators in the health professions struggle to balance an expanding set of important disciplinary knowledge, skills, and behaviors against the fixed number of classroom hours available, so it is critical to be able to use these hours efficiently. This chapter describes team-based learning (TBL) and the use of research and my own experiences to demonstrate that it is an extremely efficient and effective way to achieve these learning goals. This chapter also provides ideas for how it might be applied to various health professions topics and disciplines.

Prior to using TBL, my nearly 2 decades of teaching in doctoral-level physical therapy education had always been conducted with a strong emphasis on active learning, ongoing student self-assessment, and applied clinical reasoning, but I accomplished these by stitching together separate methods that were either developed by me or adapted from others. When I was first exposed to TBL several years ago, I realized immediately that I could improve my students' clinical reasoning more consistently and effectively through this single, unified approach.

Friberg, J. C., Visconti, C. F., & Ginsberg, S. M. (Eds.). *Evidence-Based Education in the Classroom: Examples From Clinical Disciplines* (pp. 133-141).
© 2021 Taylor & Francis Group.

Students in a TBL classroom spend the vast majority of class time actively applying course concepts to real-world problems instead of on acquiring knowledge. In fact, "the primary learning objective in TBL is ... to practice using course concepts" (Michaelsen, 2004, p. 28). Initial knowledge is acquired through independent, individual pre-class assignments, and after basic understanding is verified, knowledge is then advanced through specifically designed and progressive team activities that require application of those basic concepts. This structure results in several significant paradigm shifts: Emphasis is placed on applying instead of simply knowing; students are active and responsible for their own learning instead of being passive recipients of instruction; and faculty become coaches in the students' learning instead of the sole source of knowledge (Sibley & Spiridonoff, n.d.).

TBL is not, however, simply a "flipped classroom." It consists of a series of interlocking and interdependent components, each of which is supported by well-established learning theory (Michaelsen, 2012; Sibley et al., 2014). Some of the components that make TBL unique are embedded in the design of the whole course, and some affect how individual classes are run. These components are underlined in the remainder of this section.

At the macro-level, the typical semester-long course is divided into five to seven modules, and these are specifically designed and ordered to advance student skills through Bloom's taxonomy to reach higher order processing and decision making, even with the first one. Individual academic achievement is assessed at the end of each module, much as in traditional courses. Students work in permanent, teacher-created, heterogeneous five-to-seven-person teams. Teams are heterogeneous to distribute student assets, liabilities, and characteristics across teams (Michaelsen, 2004). Semester-long team membership allows students to continually evaluate and improve their team outcomes as well as their individual behaviors that impact team function. This long-term evaluation and development are significantly linked to another important aspect of TBL: formative and summative intra-team peer review. Students are assisted to recognize that the team, as well as the individual, will benefit from improving individual, interpersonal, and academic behaviors, and they are taught to provide meaningful and specific individual feedback using these reviews. This anonymous feedback increases their understanding of how their peers perceive them, which can often be more impactful than how their instructors perceive them.

On a class session micro-level, readiness assurance is important for verifying that students have independently achieved at least a superficial grasp of the basic concepts conveyed in the reading for each module; in other words, that they are ready to try applying that information. This advance student preparation is assured through specifically designed and graded individual readiness assessment tests (iRAT). This and other elements of each module are illustrated in Figure 15-1. Each team then completes the same assessment (team readiness assessment test [tRAT]). This collaboration is enhanced by the immediate feedback provided by using scratch-off cards for scoring the tRAT, which improves both student learning and team development (Michaelsen, 2004). The team readiness assurance test exposes any unprepared students, which provides built-in student accountability to the team. Teams have the option of appealing tRAT scores. Based on the individual and team readiness scores, both of which are applied to individual team members' course grades, the instructor may opt to provide a mini lecture to prepare students to engage in the next component: in-class activities.

Students in TBL spend the rest of each module's multiple class sessions working through in-class application activities designed to give them practice applying course concepts to specific problems. These activities provide opportunities for individuals and teams to engage in supervised and guided practice and development of critical thinking and decision making. Using health professions activities turns this decision making into clinical reasoning. The process of selecting a single team answer for each of these specific problems requires members to verbalize, compare, and critique the reasoning each applied. The decisions of each team are revealed so that they can be compared. Instructor-facilitated whole-class discussion then requires students to explain, compare, and critique each team's thought process and results, which further enhances the self-evaluation and development of clinical reasoning.

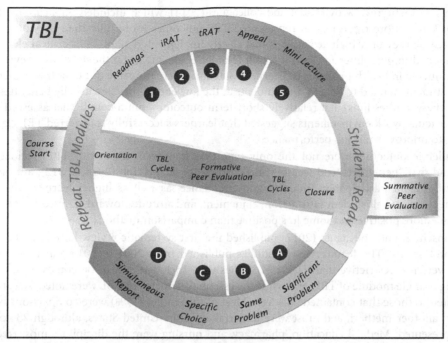

Figure 15-1. Components of learning modules. (Reproduced with permission from Jim Sibley.)

These in-class activities are always designed and conducted according to the 4S model: significant, same, specific, and simultaneous. Problems are significant, real-world applications of course content. Because they are discipline-specific, students are interested and more easily engaged. Because they are similar to problems students will face in the clinic, the practice is meaningful to students and they develop important disciplinary skills. By requiring all teams to address the same problem, teams can directly compare their reasoning and selection to that of other teams, which allows each team to self-assess and further develop. Specific problems force students and teams to make a single best choice, which requires them to weigh and debate alternatives carefully. That team's single best choice is revealed to other teams simultaneously, to force reliance on their own reasoning instead of following other teams' decisions.

REVIEW OF LITERATURE

In a meta-analysis of various approaches for teaching critical thinking skills, Abrami and colleagues (2015) identified two approaches that significantly improved the development of these skills. One was providing the opportunity for dialogue (e.g., discussion), "especially where the teacher poses questions, when there are both whole-class teacher-led discussions and teacher-led group discussions," and the other was exposing students to "authentic or situated problems and examples ... particularly when applied problem solving and role playing methods are used" (Abrami et al., 2015, p. 302). TBL clearly includes both of these and is therefore likely to be more effective for teaching critical thinking than approaches that do not.

TBL has a rapidly growing (Haidet et al., 2014; Reimschisel et al., 2017) and mature body of research evidence, including multiple systematic reviews (Haidet et al., 2014; Mincer, 2016; Reimschisel et al., 2017) and one meta-analysis (Swanson et al., 2019), which demonstrates academic outcomes at least equal to and in many cases superior to other methods. A large majority of this research (Reimschisel et al., 2017) and two of the systematic reviews (Mincer, 2016; Reimschisel et al., 2017) focused specifically on health professions education. The results of the most recent published reviews and meta-analysis are summarized here.

The systematic review by Haidet and colleagues (2014), which included publications through early 2013, was more rigorous and represented TBL outcomes more fully than previous reviews, partly because they only included studies that clearly implemented all of TBL's critical elements, as recommended in guidelines for TBL research (Haidet et al., 2012). Of the 40 studies reviewed, 28 were conducted in health professions. Learning outcomes were the same or better than other methods. All students tended to benefit, but students at the low end of the class usually benefitted more. Most of these studies looked at relatively short-term outcomes, but a couple that assessed performance in actual work environments suggested that learners successfully transferred TBL classroom learning to improve their job performance.

Academic outcomes were not the only type that improved more with TBL. Haidet's team also found that "benefits extend well beyond" knowledge acquisition (2014, p. 312), and included improved student participation, interest, and attendance, as well as higher learner self-efficacy. Assessments of overall student satisfaction, enjoyment, and attitudes toward teamwork were mixed, with some more positive and some less positive than comparison methods.

Reimschisel and colleagues (2017) published the first systematic review limited to TBL in the health professions. The team reviewed studies published from 2001 to 2016, but their selection criteria were less restrictive than Haidet's. Studies were included even if outcomes were reported following a single module of TBL, and while the essential elements of TBL were noted, selection was not limited to those that contained all seven. Most of the studies (57%) were comparisons between TBL and another method, and most were undertaken in the United States, although 23 countries were represented. Medical education, pharmacy, and nursing were the disciplines most frequently represented in their sample.

Since there was a good deal of overlap of studies included, it is not surprising that the Reimschisel team's conclusions regarding academic effectiveness in health professions paralleled those of the earlier general review: Cumulative exam scores after TBL were either better than or equal to those after lecture (Reimschisel et al., 2017). Findings reported in health professions research were usually based on short-term outcomes. Long-term outcomes were only assessed in a very limited number of studies and were similar to those following lecture. TBL had a greater positive academic effect on weaker students than on stronger ones, though in one study, it was reported that TBL helped "academically weak students, but not the weakest" (Reimschisel et al., 2017, p. 1233).

Reimschisel's team also found positive effects on nonacademic outcomes. TBL students generally enjoyed the interaction with their peers and the active nature of the TBL classroom. They also felt that they achieved a deeper understanding of course material because of having discussed and applied it. They also reported increased student engagement with TBL. "Generally speaking, learners preferred TBL to other, more traditional forms of instruction, most notably lecture" (Reimschisel et al., 2017, p. 1230). Most studies that analyzed learners' attitudes toward teams found significant improvement, and Reimschisel and colleagues noted an "overall satisfaction with (students') experience of working in a team and the quality of learning in teams," though 11% of her team's sample "illustrated that it is not rare for students to dislike TBL when it is first introduced" (Reimschisel et al., 2017, p. 1232). Student satisfaction and positive perceptions, however, increased significantly after one semester, especially with several iterations, and learners' perceptions improved significantly in the second year of using TBL over the first year. Faculty perception of TBL was also very positive, and most felt it was effective and planned to continue using it.

Swanson and colleagues (2019) conducted a synthesis ($n = 30$) and meta-analysis ($n = 17$) of experimental or quasi-experimental TBL research published 2000 to 2014. This was the first published meta-analysis of TBL outcomes. Though not limited to health professions research, it did include mostly graduate health professions students. Results demonstrated a significant moderate positive effect of TBL (mean effect size = 0.55 [SE = 0.10; $p < .001$; 95% confidence interval = 0.37, 0.74]) and an even more significant increase in the mean effect size when the TBL groups included five or fewer members.

APPLICATION OF LITERATURE/DATA

The bulk of my teaching has been focused on physical therapy content related to specific patient care skills, and I have applied TBL at multiple points and multiple topic areas of our curriculum for several years. I introduce it to each cohort of students in their second semester in a didactic (nonlabratory) course focused on clinical reasoning and introductory orthopedic examination and intervention. I use TBL again in their fifth semester for my 3-week prosthetic unit of a team-taught course. In their sixth semester, I apply TBL for all of my 12 weeks of another team-taught course; this time mostly in advanced orthopedics.

In an effort to get a more current understanding of the TBL effectiveness research, I updated the Haidet team's review (2014) using the same selection criteria, but for those published 2011 to 2015 (Mincer, 2016). Not surprisingly, my results were very similar to Haidet's. Academic outcomes were superior or equal to comparison methods. Other outcomes also improved, including preparation, communication, interprofessional and team skills, confidence, and problem solving. While I have not conducted a formal analysis of the impact of TBL on my own teaching, I strongly believe that I have seen many of the positive cognitive and affective outcomes demonstrated in the TBL research. This conclusion is based on my own and peer observations of my TBL classes, student academic achievement, and both formal and informal, qualitative and quantitative student feedback.

First, virtually every single student has been highly engaged and on-task during all classroom tasks, especially the intra-team activities. They have consistently and frequently explained to each other how they interpreted the reading, what they thought each question was really asking, or why they believed the option they chose was correct, often spontaneously citing assigned reading in the process. I have seen and heard a great deal of active listening. Students ask for and offer clarification about contributions, again often relating back to specifics from the course readings. Several peer observers in my classroom have been struck by how on-task and actively engaged the whole group was.

Individual and team behaviors related to teamwork improved visibly, even during their first semester of TBL. This makes sense because TBL was built around accomplishing "two purposes simultaneously: deepening student learning and enhancing team development" (Fink, 2004, p. 13). This assessment is based on my classroom observations as well as student self-assessments and comments on course evaluations. One common example of the improvement that I have noticed is that, over time, very quiet students contributed more consistently, and dominant students withdrew their participation to more appropriate levels and listened more actively. This has been true during both the intra- and inter-team discussions. Furthermore, team skills have generally continued to improve more with each use of TBL: quiet students participate more consistently, and the more vocal students listen more and allow others to speak. These improvements in team skills are often spontaneously mentioned in students' written course feedback. The teams, although formed based on a desire for heterogeneous backgrounds and interests, have nearly always bonded very closely. End-of-course surveys have consistently shown that 85% to 95% of my students would prefer to stay with the same team of students in future classes if given the opportunity.

Individual student preparation has been consistently very high, which the students have consistently attributed to the reading guides provided and to the individual and team readiness assurance processes that occurred at the beginning of each module. Students knew they were going to be assessed individually and that their team would also be assessed, and those team scores would be dependent on each members' preparation. Student preparation has also been influenced by the formative peer review process, in which students have sometimes been criticized by peers for not consistently or effectively contributing. The summative peer evaluations at the end of the semester have nearly always demonstrated improvements in these problematic individuals' preparation and contributions.

Academic achievement has been consistently high as required by our curriculum's very tough admission and retention standards, but I feel that weaker students particularly benefited from the structure provided by the reading guides, as well as the ongoing self-assessment provided through readiness assurance processes and team discussions. I believe they also benefited in several ways from the close and consistent association with stronger students. The weaker students received frequent direct instruction and clarification from the stronger students, and were able to model the stronger students' ways of reasoning and explaining their thinking. It should be noted, however, that even the weaker students actively participated and made meaningful contributions to their team's decision making.

I formally solicit student feedback through both standard course evaluations as well as more specific supplemental anonymous surveys. Standard course evaluations following TBL have been consistently positive, and these improve with each of their TBL experiences. Early on, students recognize the value of the process, but a number of them comment on the effort required for class preparation and their mental fatigue at the end of class. However, by the second and especially the third time they encounter TBL with me, their perceptions have been almost universally enthusiastic. Their comments have suggested they recognized that they were learning to think like a therapist and felt they had actually understood the material. They have consistently indicated an appreciation for my role in preparing their materials carefully and in facilitating their whole class discussions in ways that deepened that understanding. These later comments occasionally mentioned their increased effort to prepare, but these comments were nearly always accompanied by the recognition of how strongly that preparation paid off during class and when preparing for the exams. One student commented anonymously following the third TBL encounter, "No other class has nailed down concepts in treatment and clinical skills as well as this class. This class makes me feel okay about the student loans I will be paying for 20 years after I graduate" (Anonymous, 2018).

The TBL Student Assessment Instrument, a valid and reliable TBL assessment tool (Mennenga, 2012), was administered anonymously to my third-year students in 2019 to get more specific student feedback. All had experienced TBL in both the first and second year of our physical therapy curriculum. Every student responded and their average total score was 127 out of a possible 165 points (77%). This indicates very favorable overall student perceptions of TBL. The average score for each of the three subscales was well above neutral. The strongest result (85% of the maximum available) was for the "Accountability" subscale, followed by the "Student Satisfaction" and "Preference for TBL" subscales: 78% and 73% of the maximum scores available, respectively (Mincer, 2019). These scores indicated that after three experiences of varying lengths, my students were very satisfied with TBL, especially regarding the level of accountability, and that they strongly preferred TBL to lecture.

Some of the most valuable student feedback has been during informal in-the-hall discussions and emails initiated by students after the course was completed and even sometimes at the end of the curriculum. A student recently stopped me to say that our sixth semester class had been the "best academic experience I've ever had, bar none" (S. Maggioni, personal communication, 2018). Months after our last class together, as students were beginning to prepare for their licensure exams, more than one student spontaneously told me that my content was much easier to recall than other curricular content and that they felt the TBL approach was the reason for the difference. One student summarized in an email how significant TBL had been for her:

> Now that I have completed the curriculum and taken the [licensure] review course, I realize how much I learned from your classes. I could quickly and easily recall the answers to questions...that related to your classes. [TBL] is also beneficial because most of the learning takes place...during discussions...very little studying was necessary before exams. Overall, ...this teaching method was the most beneficial to my education...(L. Herman, personal communication, April 29, 2018)

In a continued effort to maximize my students' chances of success, I do plan to make a change in my courses based on the results of the Swanson and colleagues (2019) meta-analysis, which found more significant improvements in academic outcomes when team size was five or less. I will reduce my usual team size from six students to five.

APPLICATION TO CROSS-DISCIPLINARY CONTEXTS

Larry Michaelsen used organizational and behavioral psychology principles to develop TBL in 1979 for his business management students (Michaelsen et al., 2003; Sweet & Michaelsen, 2012). His aim was to continue active student learning despite a sudden and dramatic increase in class sizes. Word of his success led to today's widespread international adoption of TBL in multiple educational levels and subjects. A recent reflection by faculty development personnel with very extensive TBL experience stated:

> Over the years, we have worked with hundreds of faculty to implement the original TBL model in large and small classroom settings and continue to marvel at its applicability and reliability across a wide range of teaching situations. The growing use of TBL reflects its effectiveness in creating classroom conditions that help students to develop analytical, critical-thinking, and lifelong learning skills. (Roberson & Sibley, 2019, p. 1)

These comments were not limited to health professions, but certainly the outcomes mentioned are among the most important goals of educators who are trying to develop their students' ability to reason clinically and translate a large body of disciplinary knowledge into an ever-changing clinical environment. "The entire process of dialogue and debate within teams and between teams teaches students about judgment, and…many of us would consider judgment to be the foundation of sound clinical reasoning" (Parmelee, 2007, p. 7). TBL is most appropriate when students are encountering a significant body of information and when they are learning to solve complex problems (Swanson et al., 2019). This makes TBL "ideally suited for dealing with the challenges of the professional school curriculum" (Parmelee, 2007, p. 4). It may not be surprising, then, that the health professions represent the single largest discipline group using and researching TBL. Successful application has already been widely documented in medicine, nursing, dentistry, pharmacy, and others in the United States and internationally, and the density varies from a single module or course to entire curricula. It has been most often applied in graduate programs but has also been used successfully in undergraduate programs. TBL is also being applied to interprofessional education and even for online course delivery in a variety of subject areas.

While my TBL teaching experience has been limited mostly to clinical patient care, this is a function of my particular curricular responsibilities and not because I would not or could not use it for other types of content. TBL is widely used and applicable to other kinds of content in the health professions. In fact, the inherent emphasis that TBL places on thought and decision-making processes makes it exceptionally well suited for topics that are even less black and white and more situationally influenced than patient care, including, but not limited to, health care ethics, cultural competence, and communication, as well as direction and supervision of support personnel.

One other significant positive attribute of TBL is that it is easily scalable. It can be applied successfully to very large classes with little need for additional faculty. In fact, the trigger that led Michaelsen to develop TBL was the sudden tripling of his class sizes from 40 students to 120 students (Sweet & Michaelsen, 2012). Writing specifically about professional education, Sibley and Parmelee (2011) wrote, "TBL's learner-centered perspective and tried-and-true practices can help create practitioners of tomorrow within environments of limited resources, high faculty work loads (sic), and large class settings" (p. 52). TBL is also easy to modify for fluctuating class sizes.

Academic success has been documented when TBL is applied to a single module, but most experienced TBL faculty do not recommend this. There is an organizational learning curve for implementing the multiple elements of TBL. This is not difficult and it is relatively small investment when used for a semester, but takes up a larger proportion of available time if only one module will be taught using this method. The up-front time required for student orientation and team formation generally outweighs the modestly increased academic outcomes likely to result from such limited exposure. Additionally, single modules do not allow for meaningful peer evaluation, which is an important element for improving team skills. Ideally, a whole quarter or semester should be devoted to TBL instruction. If possible, in fact, TBL is best applied to the same group of students over multiple quarters or semesters because their understanding and appreciation of the benefits seem to increase (Cheng et al., 2014; Parmelee et al., 2009; Swanson et al., 2019). This recommendation is particularly applicable in health professions programs that use a cohort model because the same student group is often encountered repeatedly over multiple years.

High-level and high-quality research has demonstrated that cognitive domain achievement has been shown to be at least as good and sometimes better than more traditional approaches to content delivery. Affective gains related to team behaviors have also been widely documented, and these are almost exclusive to this particular approach. TBL is a powerful strategy for preparing students to think and act like good clinicians in any health profession. It provides nearly continuous faculty assessment of individual and team decision making with meaningful clinical application of content. This allows the instructor to provide ongoing clarification and correction through facilitation so that course objectives are achieved. TBL also provides ongoing individual student self-assessment that allows health professions students to adjust and improve their approach to the course and the materials, which facilitates improvement of their clinical reasoning.

ADDITIONAL RESOURCES

- "Team-Based Learning: Teamwork that Works," produced by the Faculty Innovation Center at The University of Texas at Austin, provides a 12-minute video introduction to TBL, and includes the voices of students and faculty:
  - https://vimeo.com/51713733

- The Team-Based Learning Collaborative is an international nonprofit with the mission of encouraging and supporting the use of TBL. Information on additional resources, as well as introductory through advanced courses and certifications, are publicly available through the Team-Based Learning Collaborative:
  - http://www.teambasedlearning.org

- Larry Michaelson (the founder) and others provide an overview of the origins, rationale, and structure of TBL:
  - Michaelsen, L. K., Bauman Knight, A., & Fink, L. D. (Eds.). (2004). *Team-based learning: A transformative use of small groups in college teaching.* Greenwood Publishing Group.

REFERENCES

Abrami, P. C., Bernard, R. M., Borokhovski, E., Waddington, D. I., Wade, C. A., & Persson, T. (2015). Strategies for teaching students to think critically: A meta-analysis. *Review of Educational Research, 85*(2), 275-314.

Cheng, C.-Y., Liou, S.-R., Tsai, H.-M., & Chang, C.-H. (2014). The effects of team-based learning on learning behaviors in the maternal-child nursing course. *Nurse Education Today, 34*(1), 25-30. https://doi.org/10.1016/j.nedt.2013.03.013

Fink, L. D. (2004). Beyond small groups: Harnessing the extraordinary power of learning teams. In L. K. Michaelsen, A. B. Knight, & L. D. Fink (Eds.), *Team-based learning: A transformative use of small groups in college teaching.* Stylus.

Haidet, P., Kubitz, K., & McCormack, W. T. (2014). Analysis of the team-based learning literature: TBL comes of age. *Journal on Excellence in College Teaching, 25*(3), 303-333.

Haidet, P., Levine, R. E., Parmelee, D. X., Crow, S., Kennedy, F., Kelly, P. A., Perkowski, L., Michaelsen, L., & Richards, B. F. (2012). Perspective: Guidelines for reporting team-based learning activities in the medical and health sciences education literature. *Academic Medicine, 87*(3), 292-299.

Mennenga, H. A. (2012). Development and psychometric testing of the team-based learning student assessment instrument. *Nurse Educator, 37*(4), 168-172.

Michaelsen, L. K. (2004). Getting started with team-based learning. In L. K. Michaelsen, A. B. Knight, & L. D. Fink (Eds.), *Team-based learning: A transformative use of small groups in college teaching.* Stylus.

Michaelsen, L. K. (2012). *Team-based learning in the social sciences and humanities: Group work that works to generate critical thinking and engagement.* Stylus.

Michaelsen, L. K., Knight, A. B., & Fink, L. D. (Eds.). (2003). *Team-based learning: A transformative use of small groups in college teaching*. Stylus.

Mincer, A. B. (2016, October). *Optimizing clinical reasoning using team-based learning*. Presented at the Educational Session Leadership Conference, Phoenix, AZ.

Mincer, A. B. (2019). *Physical therapist student perceptions measured using the Team-Based Learning Student Assessment Instrument* [Unpublished raw data].

Parmelee, D. X., DeStephen, D., & Borges, N. J. (2009). Medical students' attitudes about team-based learning in a pre-clinical curriculum. *Medical Education Online, 14*(1), 1-7. https://doi.org/10.3885/meo.2009.Res00280

Parmelee, D. X. (2007). Team-based learning in health professions education: Why is it a good fit? In L. Michaelsen, D. Parmelee, K. K. McMahon, & R. E. Levine (Eds.), *Team-based learning for health professions education: A guide to using small groups for improving learning*. Stylus.

Reimschisel, T., Herring, A. L., Huang, J., & Minor, T. J. (2017). A systematic review of the published literature on team-based learning in health professions education. *Medical Teacher, 39*(12), 1227-1237. https://doi.org/10.1080/014215 9X.2017.1340636

Roberson, B., & Sibley, J. (2019, June 17). Team-based learning revisited. *EducauseReview*. https://er.educause.edu/blogs/2019/6/team-based-learning-revisited

Sibley, J., Ostafichuk, P., Roberson, B., Franchini, B., & Kubitz, K. (2014). *Getting started with team-based learning*. Stylus.

Sibley, J., & Parmelee, D. X. (2011). Knowledge is no longer enough: Enhancing professional education with team-based learning. In L. K. Michaelsen, M. Sweet, & D. X. Parmelee (Eds.), *Team-based learning: Small-group learning's next big step*. John Wiley & Sons, Inc.

Sibley, J., & Spiridonoff, S. (n.d.). Why TBL works. www.teambasedlearning.org

Swanson, E., McCulley, L. V., Osman, D. J., Scammacca Lewis, N., & Solis, M. (2019). The effect of team-based learning on content knowledge: A meta-analysis. *Active Learning in Higher Education, 20*(1), 39-50.

Sweet, M., & Michaelsen, L. K. (Eds.). (2012). *Team-based learning in the social sciences and humanities: Group work that works to generate critical thinking and engagement*. Stylus.

16

LESSONS LEARNED
Embedding Undergraduate Research Into Educational Practice

Joy Myers, PhD; Amanda G. Sawyer, PhD;
Maryam S. Sharifian, PhD;
and Chelsey M. Bahlmann Bollinger, PhD

DESCRIPTION OF TEACHING/LEARNING CONTEXT

In 2016, we began the journey of making undergraduate research more visible in the College of Education (COE) at our institution. Although undergraduate research was prominent in many other disciplines, such as the natural sciences, there seemed to be less focus in other areas. This is not uncommon according to Seymour and colleagues (2004), who found that there were fewer opportunities for undergraduate research in the social sciences and humanities. We suspected that some professors in the COE were conducting research with students, but there was no support system in place.

The focus of our COE is the preparation of undergraduate students to become classroom teachers in early, elementary, middle, secondary, and special education. Faculty are housed in different departments within the college, but because we share the common goal of working with undergraduate preservice teachers, we decided to join together to create the undergraduate research group (URG). For the first time, this group brought together professors from various departments in the COE who either currently conducted research with students or wanted to learn more.

One of the first steps we took as an URG was to see what our institution was doing overall to support undergraduate research. We learned that there was a yearly conference where students could present their research, and there was a publication where they could further disseminate their work. However, upon closer examination, no COE faculty or students had participated in either option since their conception. However, this was not very surprising because research suggests that although it is beneficial for teacher preparation programs to engage students in research, it is not standard practice. In fact, students majoring in education are notably underrepresented in undergraduate research (Manak & Young, 2014).

Friberg, J. C., Visconti, C. F., & Ginsberg, S. M. (Eds.). *Evidence-Based
Education in the Classroom: Examples From Clinical Disciplines* (pp. 143-150).
© 2021 Taylor & Francis Group.

This underrepresentation spurred us to investigate how other similar size institutions and, in particular, how other teacher preparation programs supported undergraduate research. Several of the exemplar institutions that fostered undergraduate research had a strong online presence on their university websites, which included how they defined undergraduate research and what opportunities they provided for students and faculty to connect. Next, our URG determined a few easy and inexpensive steps we could take to implement some of what we had learned thus far. First, each of us created information sheets that included our photo, research interests, and current projects undergraduate researchers could become involved in. We posted one copy by our office doors. We took additional copies to the "meet and greets" that brought together students and faculty. We also worked with a web designer to add an undergraduate research tab to the COE webpage. We were able to upload our information sheets to the page, and this made the work of the URG more visible to faculty as well as students.

REVIEW OF LITERATURE

Undergraduate research plays an important role in the Scholarship of Teaching and Learning. Often, those of us who work in higher education struggle to balance research and teaching, sometimes leaving these areas compartmentalized. As a result, students do not see the connections between our research and teaching, nor do they understand what we do when we are not teaching (Slobodzian, 2014). When we conduct inquiry in partnership with students, we have more opportunities to make our work public (Bonney, 2018; Franzese & Felten, 2017). Plus, students often provide a clearer perspective on our work because they may not necessarily have any background knowledge of the subject (Green & Scoles, 2016).

Engaging in undergraduate research not only benefits instructors, but it is also identified as a high-impact practice that increases students' retention and success (Kuh, 2008). Furthermore, students in all disciplinary fields can benefit (Healey & Jenkins, 2009), although specific benefits may vary from discipline to discipline (Craney et al., 2011). However, research suggests that two particular groups of students, first generation and underrepresented minority students, are less likely to participate in undergraduate research (Bhattacharyya et al., 2018). Researchers at the University of Michigan implemented a research apprenticeship program to engage these students in undergraduate research and found that providing early opportunities and financial incentives were key. Students who participated in the research apprenticeship program completed an online self-paced course called Research Methods and Ethics, which provided an overview of basic research skills that are common to most disciplines. Similar to the work of Myers and colleagues (2018), Bhattacharyya and colleagues (2018) found that novice researchers, with little disciplinary background or prior research experience, perceived that they made gains in skills and content knowledge as a result of being engaged in mentored research. Because there are so many benefits for students, interest in undergraduate research has grown all around the world in recent years (Jenkins & Healey, 2010).

Those who support undergraduate research know that it extends learning outside of the classroom and allows an instructor's passion and excitement for subjects to motivate students in their own exploration (Derounian, 2017). Multhaup and colleagues (2010) provide a framework of several different models of undergraduate research for faculty members to consider. The traditional model of undergraduate research is typically short term with the student supporting a professor's current research agenda. In the consultant model, the student takes more responsibility for the research by choosing the topic and methodology, whereas the faculty member serves as a supervisor by guiding the initial development of the study and monitoring student progress. The joint creation model combines the interests and expertise of the faculty and the student, resulting in a shared research project. Because the relationship between faculty members and undergraduate research students is an important component of the undergraduate research experience (Craney et al., 2011), Slobodzian (2014) stresses the importance of offering students opportunities to engage in all models of undergraduate research.

APPLICATION OF LITERATURE/DATA

In this section, three case studies will highlight how professors used undergraduate research to inform or change instruction, content, and/or course design in the fields of early childhood, mathematics, and literacy education.

Maryam

One of the first basic principles in the field of early childhood education is observation. Teachers, teacher assistants, student teachers, and interns always observe students for their safety, development domain progress, and lesson planning. Data from observations help adults in the classroom plan to improve students' education and well-being. As an early childhood education professor, I teach one of the fundamental courses, Introduction to Early Childhood Education. Undergraduate students take this course during their junior year. This is also when they experience being in a school 1 day a week during which they work to observe and understand children's development, and practice being a teacher in an early childhood setting. In addition to taking this course, students usually take a child development course, which requires writing a case study as the final assignment. A major goal for both courses is that students learn how to observe and collect data while interacting with students.

While undergraduate students were collecting data for their case study and lesson plan assignment, they were not making the connection between these observations/documentations and the idea of research. I noticed this gap during my first year when I invited students to join me in writing a proposal to present at the Virginia Association for Early Childhood Education Conference. Students responded that they were interested, but they were concerned because they had never done research and did not feel comfortable presenting in a professional setting.

As soon as I started as a new professor at James Madison University (Harrisonburg, Virginia), I began encouraging all undergraduate and graduate students to get involved in professional organizations and conduct research to build their professional experiences. After joining the URG, I learned about different opportunities to encourage and educate our students in research and scholarship.

One of the changes I made to the course requirements after my involvement with the URG was assigning small groups of students to pick a research topic related to the most current challenges and issues in early childhood education, interview an expert, and conduct a literature review. I wanted students to understand how they can study a topic, collect data, and present what they learned to their peers. This small group activity helped students to feel more confident about their presentation abilities and grew their interest related to research. I invited a group who researched mindfulness practices in early childhood classrooms to submit their presentation to the next Virginia Association for Early Childhood Education Conference conference. Two students accepted the invitation and met with me a few times to develop the conference proposal, which was accepted. However, when the conference presentation date came closer, both students sent me emails letting me know they were unable to present. It was an eye-opening moment for me as an educator and member of the URG. We need to continue to encourage students to become actively involved in the professional presentation of their research achievements.

Through these experiences, I have changed my methods of preparing undergraduate students through teaching the significant relationship among observation, data collection, and research during their junior year of course work. In addition, I now require my students to participate in research workshops and college symposiums that are offered every semester by the URG in order to improve their knowledge about research, as well as to create presentation opportunities. My hope is that students will continue to share their research as classroom teachers at state, national, and/or international conferences.

Amanda

I was very interested in looking at social media's influence on mathematics education, and I did not have any difficulty finding undergraduate research students who also were interested in this topic during one of the URG meet and greets. However, within the first month, one student dropped out because of time restrictions. The other undergraduate research student worked with me to begin creating a conceptual framework of how to classify quality online mathematical tasks. We decided to use Stein and Smith's (1998) framework, and she even started doing initial analysis of the quality of Pinterest pins. Difficulty arose as this project continued because the student, however motivated to do research, was also burdened with her coursework. Over time, communication became nonexistent. This experience helped me understand that there needed to be more than self-motivation to sustain research with undergraduate students.

I discussed this with a fellow mathematics education colleague at a small private liberal arts college. Although my university was a large public institution, her university offered summer grants to undergraduate research students to help professors conduct research. She also knew two students who were interested in investigating the same topic. In the end, with the help of the smaller university, we were able to find two grants that provided $3,000 to each undergraduate research student over the summer to conduct investigations into the quality of mathematical tasks on Pinterest, Teachers Pay Teachers, as well as other online resources elementary mathematics teachers use. We also offered them each first authorship on one of the publications.

The undergraduate research student provided substantial knowledge about social media use and how to approach the research in a new way. One undergraduate research student investigated how elementary teachers use social media in the classroom. She obtained 601 surveys of elementary mathematics teachers across the United States. This was mind-boggling to me because I had a very difficult time getting individuals I did not know to actually complete a survey. Using her knowledge of Facebook; Twitter; and hashtags, such as #elemmathchat, #edchat, #mathchat, #elemchat, #mtbos, #iteach, #iteachmath, and #numbersenseroutines, the undergraduate research student was able to reach a large population of elementary teachers. We would not have had the same results or data without her assistance. The second researcher was tasked to determine the quality of resources on Teachers Pay Teachers and Pinterest, using the framework we determined was appropriate from my first investigation with an undergraduate research student. She also created a codebook and analyzed more than 1,000 online resources that summer. In contrast, it took an undergraduate research student, who was unpaid during the school year, 3 months to categorize 100 online resources. This resulted in an epiphany for me! Summer work with undergraduate research students produced a larger substantial outcome, than research done during the school year. Currently, from this investigation, four papers have been published and two are under review. We also had six national presentations, with four of them conducted solely by the undergraduate research students.

Through these experiences, I learned undergraduate research students need incentives. Although some students are self-motivated, when incentives, like authorship and money, are provided, they tend to be more successful at completing tasks. I also learned that I needed to conduct research in the summer to create a stress-free environment for the student researchers. Furthermore, I learned the value of collaboration with other universities. If you are at a university that does not provide funding for undergraduate research, work with colleagues at other universities. My experience with undergraduate research has been fruitful, and I would not have had as much scholarship success without their assistance. Specific to my discipline—mathematics education—I found that many people misinterpret what undergraduate research could mean for education. Many believe that mathematics is a set of already constructed rules that does not need to be studied (Ernest, 1989); however, I love to debunk this common misconception. Anyone can do mathematics education research. Depending on the subject that is being investigated, the research group will have to come together and construct a common understanding that is not necessarily based on past knowledge or classes. If the student has a willingness and a drive to conduct this research, they can be taught the nuances necessary within the subject matter.

Chelsey

During my first year as a new faculty member, I was invited by my departmental mentor, Joy Myers, to create an information sheet that included my research interests, projects I was working on, and recent publications. This was displayed on the COE website along with other faculty who were interested in working with undergraduate research students. In addition, she invited me to attend a faculty/student meet and greet at the beginning of the year, sponsored by the URG. Like Amanda, I met several students who were interested in my research. However, I was not sure as a new faculty member that I was quite ready to work with undergraduate students on my own yet because it was my first year and I was mainly focused on acclimating to my new institution.

Joy suggested that we work together on a project since we have a shared interest in early literacy. We included two undergraduate students as coresearchers. Specifically, our research focused on writing in a play-based preschool. Joy and I handled the institutional review board (IRB), made the initial contacts with the school, conducted the first interviews, and did a couple of observations before we invited the undergraduate research students to join in. At our initial meeting with them, we provided background on what we had done so far and shared several options on how they could become involved, including observations, helping us with data analysis, co-conducting the final interviews, and/or assisting in writing a manuscript. After discussion of what all of these components would look like, both undergraduate students were interested in conducting observations and helping with data analysis. Throughout the semester we met with the undergraduate research students about once a month to discuss how the observations were going and to do some data analysis together so they understood what our process looked like. In addition, they both submitted proposals to the COE's URGs semi-annual research showcase where they highlighted the research they did with us. One of the students even received an award for her presentation.

During my second year, I decided to become a member of the URG and assisted in planning various events throughout the year. I wanted to continue working with undergraduate research students since the first year was so rewarding. Joy and I decided to continue our same line of research on early writing in play-based preschool classrooms, but this year at a different school. This time we applied for and received a grant, which provided funds to pay an undergraduate research student. I contacted previous students that I knew may be interested in this line of research and who were dependable. I had them fill out an application form, and then Joy and I decided on one undergraduate research student from the pool of applicants. Similar to the previous year, Joy and I wrote to the IRB, contacted the school, and conducted the initial interviews and observations. Then we invited the undergraduate research student in for a meeting. Because this study included a larger population of teachers than the previous study, we really needed her to assist us with all aspects of data collection. We also included her in the data analysis process and manuscript writing.

We noticed that in both of these experiences working with undergraduate research students, one where students were unpaid and the other where the student was paid, were fairly similar. The undergraduate research students who were unpaid missed a few observations, which affected our data collection; however, because they were volunteering their time and working on building their resumes and experiences with research, they chose to participate in the undergraduate research showcase. The undergraduate research student who was paid did not miss observations or many deadlines because she was being paid; however, because she saw it as a job she decided not to present at the undergraduate research showcase.

Working with undergraduate research students is important to me as an assistant professor because it helps students understand first-hand the work professors do outside of teaching. In addition, I believe that involving students in research encourages them to become more critical about their teaching. Specifically with our research, all three undergraduate research students we involved became more thoughtful about how they would teach writing with their future students.

APPLICATION TO CROSS-DISCIPLINARY CONTEXTS

We just shared three case studies, based on professors' experiences with undergraduate research at our institution. As one can see, these experiences range from supporting students' understanding of research within courses to working with undergraduate research students during the summer. Although the professors all taught within the COE, their different disciplines raised different challenges and opportunities. This suggests that even within the same field, we need to consider disciplinary differences and avoid a "one size fits all" way of linking research and teaching (Lueddeke, 2008).

The three professors, Maryam, Amanda, and Chelsey, are all pretenured faculty. Their duties include research, teaching, and service, but studies suggest that although the first priority at many institutions is research, early career faculty spend more time on teaching and service (Chen, 2015). Undergraduate research can play an essential role to junior faculty regardless of discipline in terms of supporting their research efforts. As Amanda mentioned, working with undergraduate research students increased her scholarly productivity.

You may be fortunate to be at an institution that has a lot of support for undergraduate research or perhaps there is not as much interest within your college or department. The final section of the chapter highlights lessons we have learned since establishing the URG, tips for creating cultures within institutions that value undergraduate research, ways of applying this knowledge to disciplines beyond teacher education, and resources to help you get started.

Start at the Top

The reality is that higher education is a top-down enterprise. The higher up the chain of leadership you can start, the more money and support you might be able to gain. For us, that meant initially meeting with the Associate Dean of the COE at that time, Dr. Maggie Kyger. The URG, which initially consisted of only three faculty members, scheduled a meeting so we could share ideas about incorporating undergraduate research into the COE and to get feedback from her about how to move forward. She put us in contact with several people at the university level who she thought might have funding for this type of endeavor.

Small Steps

However, since we were not able to secure funding through the university, we made a request to our dean to pay a stipend to three COE undergraduate research students and five faculty members for a summer data analysis workshop. This endeavor was funded, and we were able to focus on data that examined where preservice teachers get their ideas for lesson plans (Myers et al., 2018) We secured IRB approval, and once we began working, the undergraduate research students shared their unique "insider" perspectives on this topic. Please note that IRB may not allow undergraduate research students to work with certain data, so before beginning a project, be sure to double check with your IRB office. One important lesson we learned during this summer initiative was to divide projects into pieces and allot plenty of time for students to complete tasks. In fact, Bonney (2018) suggests allowing six times the amount of time estimated for experienced faculty members to complete the work.

Build on Success

We published two articles and presented at several conferences based on the work we did that summer with undergraduate research students, all of which we shared with our dean. We also included a detailed plan for the following year, with a budget slightly larger than what we had requested the previous summer, outlining how we would grow the URG and involve more faculty and students. Because we were able to produce tangible products, such as publications, the dean agreed.

Involve Others

By continuing to invite faculty, year after year, the URG has expanded. As more departments have gotten on board, department heads have also provided funding. With additional resources, and in an effort to increase involvement, we created an undergraduate research fall and spring research showcase where students present research they completed with faculty or research they conducted for a class in roundtable or poster sessions.

Maintain Momentum

Over time, the URG joined with the Faculty Research Group. This resulted in more faculty being involved and allowed us to look at research in the COE from multiple perspectives. In addition to the two research showcases, we continue to host meet and greets in the fall connecting faculty with students. We have also tried to bring classroom teachers to campus to speak to preservice teachers about what research looks like in their contexts.

Create a Culture

All the steps detailed previously helped create a culture of undergraduate research in our college. It is possible for others who also teach in clinical professions to find ways to connect students and faculty through research. Whether that research is faculty- or student-driven, studies suggest that offering research opportunities to undergraduate students in all disciplines yields benefits for growth and intellectual development (Craney et al., 2011; Osborn & Karukstis, 2009).

In conclusion, undergraduate research plays an important role in assisting higher education faculty to balance research and teaching. The lessons we share in this chapter highlight how we have been able to achieve that balance while developing a more nuanced understanding of the importance of undergraduate research for faculty and students. We hope the suggestions we provided help you maintain or create an environment that supports undergraduate research at your institution.

ADDITIONAL RESOURCES

There are a number of resources that helped us in our journey to embed undergraduate research into our Scholarship of Teaching and Learning. These include:

- Council on Undergraduate Research:
  - https://www.cur.org/
- *American Journal of Undergraduate Research:*
  - http://www.ajuronline.org/
- *Journal of Undergraduate Research:*
  - http://www.jurpress.org/
- National Association for Early Childhood Education:
  - https://www.naeyc.org/resources/pubs/vop/about-teacher-research
- National Head Start Association:
  - https://nhsa.org/action-research
- Perry, G., Henderson, B., & Meier, D. (2012). *Our inquiry, our practice: Undertaking, supporting, and learning from early childhood teacher research(ers)*. The National Association for the Education of Young Children.
- National Council of Teachers of Mathematics. (2014). *Principles to action: Ensuring mathematical success for all*. Author.

REFERENCES

Bhattacharyya, P., Chan, C., & Waraczynski, M. (2018). How novice researchers see themselves grow. *International Journal for the Scholarship of Teaching and Learning, 12*(2), Article 3. https://doi.org/10.20429/ijsotl.2018.120203

Bonney, K. M. (2018). Students as partners in the scholarship of teaching and learning. *International Journal for the Scholarship of Teaching and Learning, 12*(2), Article 2. https://doi.org/10.20429/ijsotl.2018.120202

Chen, C. Y. (2015). A study showing research has been valued over teaching in higher education. *Journal of the Scholarship of Teaching and Learning, 15*(3), 15-32.

Craney, C., McKay, T., Mazzeo, A., Prigodich, C., & de Groot, R. (2011). Cross-discipline perceptions of the undergraduate research experience. *The Journal of Higher Education, 82*(1), 92-113. https://doi.org/10.1080/00221546.2011.11779086

Derounian, J. G. (2017). Inspirational teaching in higher education: What does it look, sound and feel like? *International Journal for the Scholarship of Teaching and Learning, 11*(1), 1-5. https://doi.org/10.20429/ijsotl.2017.110109

Ernest, P. (1989). The impact on beliefs on the teaching of mathematics. In P. Ernest (Ed.), *Mathematics teaching: The state of the art* (pp. 249-254). Falmer Press.

Franzese, A. T., & Felten, P. (2017). Reflecting on reflecting: Scholarship of teaching and learning as a tool to evaluate contemplative pedagogies. *International Journal for the Scholarship of Teaching and Learning, 11*(1), 1-4. https://doi.org/10.20429/ijsotl.2017.110108

Green, U., & Scoles, J. (2016). Pioneering a peer review initiative: Students as colleagues in the review of teaching practices. *Teaching and Learning Together in Higher Education, 19*(1), 1-10.

Healey, M., & Jenkins, A. (2009). *Developing undergraduate research and inquiry.* The Higher Education Academy.

Jenkins, A., & Healey, M. (2010). Undergraduate research and international initiatives to link teaching and research. *Council on Undergraduate Research Quarterly, 30*(3), 36-42.

Kuh, G. D. (2008). *High-impact educational practices: What they are, who has access to them, and why they matter.* Association of American Colleges and Universities.

Lueddeke, G. (2008). Reconciling research, teaching and scholarship in higher education: An examination of disciplinary variation, the curriculum and learning. *International Journal for the Scholarship of Teaching and Learning, 2*(1), Article 18. https://doi.org/10.20429/ijsotl.2008.020118

Manak, J. A., & Young, G. (2014). Incorporating undergraduate research into teacher education: Preparing thoughtful teachers through inquiry-based learning. *Council on Undergraduate Research Quarterly, 35*(2), 35-38.

Multhaup, K., Davoli, C., Wilson, S., Geghman, K., Giles, K, Martin, J., & Salter, P. (2010). Three models for undergraduate-faculty research: Reflections by a professor and her former students. *Council on Undergraduate Research Quarterly, 31*, 21-26.

Myers, J., Sawyer, A., Dredger, K., Barnes, S., & Wilson, R. (2018). Examining perspectives of faculty and students engaging in undergraduate research. *Journal of the Scholarship of Teaching and Learning, 18*(1), 136-149. https://doi.org/10.14434/josotl.v18i1.22348

Osborn, J. M., & Karukstis, K. K. (2009). The benefits of undergraduate research, scholarship, and creative activity. In M. K. Boyd & J. L. Wesemann (Eds.), *Broadening participation in undergraduate research: Fostering excellence and enhancing the impact* (pp. 41-53). Council on Undergraduate Research.

Seymour, E., Hunter, A. B., Laursen, S. L., & DeAntoni, T. (2004). Establishing the benefits of research experiences for undergraduates in the sciences: First findings from a three-year study. *Science Education, 88*, 493-594. https://doi.org/10.1002/sce.10131

Slobodzian, J. T. (2014). Integrating undergraduate into teacher training: Supporting the transition from learner to educator. *Council on Undergraduate Research Quarterly, 34*, 43-47.

Stein, M. K., & Smith, M. S. (1998). Mathematical tasks as a framework for reflection: From research to practice. *Mathematics Teaching in the Middle School, 3*(4), 268-275.

17

MAPPING TEAMING CONCEPTS
Organizing Student Knowledge Through Active Learning

Allison Sauerwein, PhD, CCC-SLP

DESCRIPTION OF TEACHING/LEARNING CONTEXT

Augmentative and alternative communication (AAC) includes a variety of communicative systems, both high-tech (e.g., speech-generating devices) and low-tech (e.g., sign language, portable communication boards or books) that people with communication disorders use to augment or replace their verbal speech. Speech-language pathologists typically receive the most preservice preparation in this highly collaborative practice area. In our graduate program, the AAC course is a 3-credit hour, face-to-face class students take in their second year of the program. Students are expected to demonstrate knowledge of professional issues, ethical conduct, and evidence-based practices for AAC assessment and intervention for individuals with diverse communication disorders across the lifespan. Speech-language pathologists work with families and professionals, such as physical therapists, occupational therapists, and educators, to provide high-quality comprehensive services. Because effective teaming is a critical evidence-based practice for AAC assessment and intervention, it is discussed frequently throughout the course (American Speech-Language-Hearing Association, 2019; Calculator & Black, 2009).

The importance of interprofessional practice and collaboration with clients, families, and peers is not unique to speech-language pathology. Thus, students in many clinical disciplines learn early, and often in their preservice education, that teaming is vital for effective clinical practice. Teaming, however, is highly complex and varies across contexts. Who is included in the team? What skills are needed to collaborate with different team members? How might teaming with a family member differ from teaming with a professional colleague? As experts, we are likely to have ready answers to these questions. For our students, on the other hand, the answers may not be clear.

Friberg, J. C., Visconti, C. F., & Ginsberg, S. M. (Eds.). *Evidence-Based Education in the Classroom: Examples From Clinical Disciplines* (pp. 151-158). © 2021 Taylor & Francis Group.

I argue it is unrealistic to expect students to enter the workforce and engage effectively in teaming without a solid conceptual understanding of teaming to guide their efforts. In this course, I want my students to gain knowledge related to teaming. Further, it is important that they purposefully organize that knowledge, so they can apply what they know in the real world when they are completing externships or practicing as speech-language pathologists. My research on teaming has informed how I frame content, so students can unpack the nuances of collaboration and other teaming skills. Moreover, my scholarship has directed my attention to ideas and content that students might need extra support for understanding. This chapter describes how a knowledge organization framework based on data from an original Scholarship of Teaching and Learning (SoTL) study was used to inform content delivery in a graduate-level AAC course for preservice speech-language pathologists.

REVIEW OF LITERATURE

Ambrose and colleagues (2010) argue that students' organization of content knowledge plays a major role in their learning and in application of their knowledge. As experts in our clinical professions, faculty have extensive content knowledge that we connect and organize in our minds. These knowledge connections are rich and meaningful, which helps us apply what we know in clinical settings and teach what we know in the classroom. For our novice students, organizing the knowledge they obtain through coursework and clinical experiences is typically significantly more effortful.

The expert-novice gap in knowledge organization is related to the density and nature of the connections among concepts. That is, experts develop more dense knowledge organizations when compared to novices. Experts organize their knowledge hierarchically or in a cross-referenced fashion, whereas novices have sparse connections, such as simple associations between concepts (Ambrose et al., 2010). Furthermore, expert connections are meaningful and contextual based on their experiences. Because novices are not likely to have comparable experience to draw from, we would not expect our novice students to independently develop meaningful connections. Rather, they are more likely to identify superficial knowledge connections; however, in the classroom, we can model and teach students how to develop robust schemas (Ambrose et al., 2010).

Research suggests that learning is more efficient and effective when students are provided knowledge organization frameworks for consideration than when they are expected to organize their knowledge independently (Ambrose et al., 2010). Sharing our own knowledge organization frameworks not only makes the connections visible for students, but students can then use that framework to make connections of their own and deepen their understanding (Eppler, 2006; Lang, 2016). When faced with teaching students about a challenging topic or problem, one can look to literature for frameworks, flowcharts, or diagrams; however, creating a concept map based on one's personal knowledge organization may be more productive. As diagrams that represent relationships between subconcepts and a primary concept, concept maps make connections visible (Eppler, 2006). Lang (2016) recommends teachers provide students with concept maps that represent our own knowledge organizations, making clear the connections we have drawn. Then, we can facilitate students' development of their own connections. Small group work can be particularly useful in additionally shaping knowledge organizations, as students have access to multiple frameworks to draw from—the instructor's, their peers', and their own (Lang, 2016). Ultimately, students with deeper connections and more dense knowledge organizations are more likely to successfully apply what they know about teaming in practice (Ambrose et al., 2010).

Returning to AAC, researchers have begun to explore the knowledge organization experts (i.e., speech-language pathologists with AAC expertise) and novices (i.e., preservice speech-language pathologists or general practice speech-language pathologists) bring to AAC assessment. My knowledge organization framework related to teaming and AAC is constantly evolving as data from these studies are disseminated. For example, Lund and colleagues (2017) found that speech-language pathologists with AAC expertise include counseling with the family as well as goal setting with

TABLE 17-1	
Teaming Skills Codebook Definitions	
TEAMING SKILL	CODEBOOK DEFINITION
Seeking outside input	Indicating that they would seek further detail about history, skills, or preferences, or they would consult with other disciplines to get more information
Collaboration	Planning to work jointly to problem solve, set goals, or implement therapy plans from multiple perspectives relevant to the case
Educating others	Planning to teach families/professionals/peers about goals or implementation

the child and their family in their AAC assessment plans. When I conceptualize AAC assessment, these teaming skills and activities are included in my mental knowledge organization framework. However, far less data are available about the knowledge organization experts or novices bring to AAC intervention. Thus, when designing a study that explored the expert-novice gap in intervention planning for children who use AAC, I was especially interested in the data related to teaming, recognizing the potential to inform both my knowledge organization and instruction in the course.

ORIGINAL DATA

My teaming and AAC intervention knowledge organization framework was informed by an original SoTL study that explored the expert-novice gap in intervention planning for children who use AAC. Expert and novice performance on the tasks were compared to identify cognitive "bottle-necks" to student learning (Middendorf & Pace, 2004). In other words, the study aimed to reveal areas in which students' thinking was less developed or complex as compared to expert speech-language pathologists. Study methods included think-alouds for data collection and grounded theory methods for data analysis. Eight novices (i.e., preservice speech-language pathologists) and eight experts (AAC specialist speech-language pathologists) participated in the study. Novices were first-year, speech-language pathology masters-level students who had completed an introductory AAC course and/or clinical practicum with at least one client who used AAC, but had not yet begun off-campus externships. Experts held the certificate of clinical competence in speech-language pathology, had practiced as speech-language pathologists for at least 5 years, and reported supporting children who used AAC for at least 50% of their daily work activities at the time of participation.

Think-aloud tasks made participants' decision-making and generative processes observable as they planned for intervention in a private practice setting (Ericcson & Simon, 1993). Participants read two fictional case studies of children with developmental disabilities (i.e., autism and cerebral palsy) who used AAC systems and subsequently verbalized their thoughts (i.e., thought aloud) as they planned for intervention with each child. Experts and novices planned for the first therapy session as well as more long-term intervention. Think aloud recordings were transcribed and analyzed using open, axial, and selective coding (Strauss & Corbin, 1998). I developed a codebook with definitions and examples of skills observed during the think-aloud tasks. Peer debriefing, member checks, and research memos were used to authenticate the analyses and findings (Brantlinger et al., 2005; Creswell & Creswell, 2018). Intervention planning skills, clinical reasoning skills, and teaming skills emerged from the data. The teaming skills, which are the focus of this chapter, are presented and defined in Table 17-1.

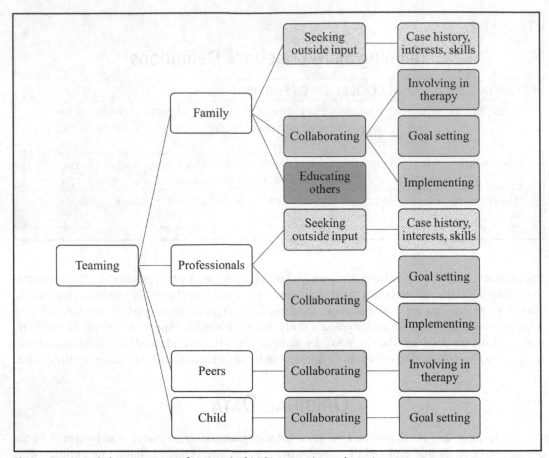

Figure 17-1. Knowledge organization framework of AAC intervention and teaming concepts.

All participants—experts and novices—planned to use three teaming skills (i.e., seeking outside input, collaboration, educating others); team with the same stakeholder groups, including family members and related professionals; and incorporate the same activities, such as collecting a case history and goal setting in their plans. Figure 17-1 presents a concept map that represents my knowledge organization framework of AAC intervention and teaming concepts. Stakeholder groups are organized top to bottom by frequency (i.e., participants most frequently mentioned team with families and least frequently mentioned team with the child). Teaming skills are presented from least complex (seeking outside input) to most complex (educating others). Color coding simply allows visual comparison of skills across stakeholders.

Overall, both expert and novice participants planned to team most frequently, using a variety of teaming approaches, with the children's family members. This is not surprising as they planned for intervention in private practice, which is typically family-centered and sometimes involves bringing family members in the room during therapy sessions. In addition, family members were the only stakeholders participants planned to educate or offer training to. Expert and novice participants planned to seek outside input from and collaborate with professionals, noting they would involve professionals in goal setting and therapy implementation across contexts. On the other hand, both experts and novices planned less intensive teaming with the children in the case studies and their peers. They planned to incorporate peers into therapy sessions with the child and collaborate with the child when setting goals for intervention.

While experts and novices approached teaming rather similarly overall, some marginal differences were noted in the details of experts' and novices' plans. For example, experts were more likely to seek information from parents about the child's interactions with their siblings. In addition, five of the experts indicated they would seek out reports, such as an AAC evaluation report or other speech and language evaluation report, whereas novices did not mention obtaining them. Novices recognized the importance of providing education or training but talked broadly about providing parent education, while experts generated specific topics for education, such as core vocabulary targets and language facilitation strategies, like modeling and providing wait time.

APPLICATION OF LITERATURE/DATA

I used data obtained in the SoTL study while designing the AAC graduate course. Application of this data was twofold. First, I proposed the concept map for students' consideration and adaptation. Second, because the study revealed expert–novice gaps, I thoroughly addressed the knowledge gaps, or areas in which novices in the study struggled, in my classroom instruction.

Concept Map

In the AAC course, we discuss communication solutions for individuals with a variety of communication disorders; however, the concept map (see Figure 17-1) aligned with the unit on developmental disabilities, such as autism, cerebral palsy, and Down syndrome. During a class period in this unit in the most recent course offering, I provided background information about the study, how data were collected, and my understanding of the concepts and connections displayed on the concept map. Then, students analyzed and evaluated the concept map. I prompted them to first review the map independently, and afterward, dedicated time for discussion in pairs or small groups. These discussions followed students' interests. For example, one group generated lists of stakeholders who might be included in each group. They listed parents, siblings, and grandparents for family members and a large number of professionals, including physical therapists, occupational therapists, general education teachers, special education teachers, audiologists, and vision specialists. Another group envisioned the teaming activities by questioning, for example, what involving family members in therapy sessions would look like and how they might initiate conversations with professional colleagues about collaborative goal setting. Flexibility during these small-group discussions allowed students the opportunity to consider, adapt, and challenge the concept map at their own pace based on their current level of understanding.

The pairs and groups adopted some of the concepts and connections in the concept map as is, but they challenged other aspects. For example, students acknowledged that collaboration was a large, overarching theme and encompassed many activities (i.e., involving the stakeholder in therapy, collaborative goal setting, coimplementation), perhaps including additional activities that the participants did not mention during the think-aloud tasks. Thus, they agreed that the major teaming skills were seeking outside input, collaborating, and educating others. On the other hand, one group discussed why participants in the study had planned to educate family members but not professionals. They concluded that some professionals with no prior AAC experience might also need training, hence developing a connection of their own in their knowledge organizations.

As a large group, we contemplated how the larger framework might be applied to other communication disorders. Another unit in the AAC class was dedicated to assessment and intervention for adults with acquired motor disorders, such as amyotrophic lateral sclerosis, multiple sclerosis, and Parkinson's disease. We talked about how some aspects of the concept map might need minor adjustments for this population. For example, in pediatric cases, parents are likely to be the primary team member from the family unit. On the other hand, spouses or adult children might be included in adult clients' teams. Family education would be important for both spouses and parents. We also discussed how adults with acquired motor needs would likely play a larger role in goal setting and providing input regarding their interests and priorities as compared to pediatric clients. Therefore, overall, we concluded that considering stakeholders, skills, and activities could be useful for organizing our knowledge about AAC intervention across diverse clinical populations.

During in-class discussions, I watched students analyze and evaluate the concept map, which are cognitive processes in Bloom's taxonomy (Bloom et al., 1956). I recognized the opportunity for students to engage in creation, a more complex process in the taxonomy. In future offerings of the course, I plan to scaffold student learning, so they can develop their own concept maps by organizing their knowledge of relevant stakeholders, skills, and activities. If students were to visualize their knowledge organizations using concept maps, they could have a visual reference of their understanding in the beginning of a unit. As they build knowledge and refine their connections and organizations, they could refine their existing concept maps or create new maps. Comparing early iterations to later versions throughout and at the end of the course would provide opportunities to students to self-monitor their learning.

Knowledge Gaps

Because the SoTL study investigated an expert-novice gap, I was also able to pinpoint areas in which students struggled compared to their expert counterparts. Recall the following examples: (1) Novices were less likely to seek information from parents about the child's interactions with their siblings, (2) novices did not plan to seek evaluation reports from other professionals, and (3) novices did not generate specific topics for parent or family education. Each of these incongruities were addressed in content delivery.

In class, we discussed using interviews with family members and consultations with professionals to seek pertinent case information needed for assessment and intervention. In relevant lectures and discussions throughout the semester, I explicitly highlighted the importance of asking parents about their child's relationship and communication with siblings at home, as well as the importance of obtaining evaluation reports from collaborating professionals, particularly if the child had a recent speech and language evaluation. Other applications of these data fostered more active learning. For example, students worked together during class time to formulate a list of potential topics for parent education. They reflected on the topics and information we had covered in the course and considered which would be most meaningful for parents and other family members to know and be able to implement at home. The students learned from each other while generating and organizing this list, and they were able to obtain my feedback on their ideas in real time. These learning opportunities directly addressed knowledge gaps I uncovered among other novices' performance in the SoTL study.

APPLICATION TO CROSS-DISCIPLINARY CONTEXTS

These principles of evidence-based education (e.g., developing knowledge organizations and addressing specific learning challenges) can be applied across clinical disciplines, as teaming is an essential component of evidence-based practice in many health professions. The knowledge organization framework for teaming and AAC service provision presented in this chapter may be useful for faculty attempting to conceptualize teaming in their own discipline or to present related content to students in coursework. In particular, considering the stakeholders, skills, and activities related to teaming may be a useful first step in creating a concept map that represents the knowledge organization framework for teaming in your discipline. Instructors can facilitate students' deep understanding of teaming concepts by developing concept maps, sharing them with students, and assisting students in connecting and organizing their own knowledge. Furthermore, faculty can pinpoint challenging aspects of teaming specific to their profession or that their students have struggled with in coursework or clinical contexts, and address those challenges head on.

While teaming is certainly a relevant topic across clinical disciplines, it may be more meaning-ful for faculty to apply the principles described in this chapter to specific bottlenecks to learning experienced by their students. Bottlenecks to students and threshold concepts learning exist in all disciplines. Teaming related to AAC service provision is a complex concept I have encountered in my scholarship, while supervising in the clinic, and while teaching in the classroom; however, for a scholar in another discipline, the troublesome bottleneck or threshold concept may be completely different. Readers of this chapter may have their own SoTL data that expose their students' bottle-necks to learning, or this chapter may have simply sparked an idea of a potential bottleneck worth exploring. SoTL scholars in a given discipline may have already identified bottlenecks unique to their students and reported them in the literature. The Decoding the Disciplines framework can be a useful guide for identifying and defining bottlenecks. A cross-disciplinary framework for improving student learning, the Decoding the Disciplines process encourages faculty to consider where students' learning breaks down (i.e., a bottleneck) and to reveal the mental tasks students need to accomplish to address the bottleneck (i.e., decoding the challenging aspects of the disci-pline; Middendorf & Pace, 2004). The decoding process may be surprisingly challenging for faculty because their knowledge organizations naturally evolve over time without major conscious effort. The outcomes of this process are important, however, for teaching our novice students.

Ultimately, after a bottleneck or threshold concept has been identified and defined and the underlying knowledge and skills have been uncovered, faculty can use the strategies described in this chapter to inspire use of their own SoTL-informed knowledge organization frameworks. The two main principles are supporting students in improving their knowledge organizations and addressing specific areas in which students have been observed to struggle. Recall that the expert-novice gap in knowledge organization can be addressed by improving the density and nature of the connections among concepts (Ambrose et al., 2010; Lang, 2016). Faculty can demonstrate how they organize knowledge using concept maps and scaffold student learning to make connections of their own. Perhaps students can represent their knowledge organizations in concept maps, or faculty can facilitate in-class opportunities for students to reflect on their knowledge organizations with their peers. Finally, this chapter provides an example for considering how SoTL data can be used to iden-tify areas in which students may need additional support and how to design instruction accordingly. Supporting our students in acquiring and organizing their knowledge is vital for preparing them to be complex thinkers in complex clinical contexts.

ADDITIONAL RESOURCES

- The Decoding the Disciplines website provides an overview of the decoding process, resources for a variety of disciplines, and a bibliography of Decoding the Disciplines works:
  - http://decodingthedisciplines.org/
- Middendorf and Shopkow (2018) offers a step-by-step guide for using Decoding the Disciplines methodology:
  - Middendorf, J., & Shopkow, L. (2018). *Overcoming student learning bottlenecks: Decode the critical thinking of your discipline*. Stylus.
- Calder (2018) and Ginsberg and colleagues (2016) describe examples of using think-alouds to make student learning and bottlenecks to learning visible:
  - Calder, L. (2018). Student-think alouds: Making thinking and learning visible. In N. Chick (Ed.), *SoTL in action: Illuminating critical moments of practice* (pp. 109-116). Stylus.
  - Ginsberg, S. M., Friberg, J. C., & Visconti, C. F. (2016). Diagnostic reasoning by experienced speech-language pathologists and student clinicians. *Contemporary Issues in Communication Science and Disorders, 43*, 87-97.

- The Center for Instructional Innovation and Assessment at Western Washington University has an online video module on using concept maps as a classroom assessment technique. The website links to a variety of resources for using concept maps in the classroom:
  ○ http://pandora.cii.wwu.edu/cii/resources/modules/concept/

- The Interprofessional Education Collaborative website houses the Interprofessional Education Collaborative Core Competencies for Interprofessional Collaborative Practice:
  ○ https://www.ipecollaborative.org

- Ogletree and colleagues (2017) illustrate the principles of interprofessional collaborative practice using a case study of a child who uses AAC:
  ○ Ogletree, B. T., Brady, N., Bruce, S., Dean, E., Romski, M., Sylvester, L., & Westling, D. (2017). Mary's case: An illustration of interprofessional collaborative practice for a child with severe disabilities. *American Journal of Speech-Language Pathology, 28*, 217-226. https://doi.org/10.1044/2017_AJSLP-15-0065

- The National Joint Committee for the Communication Needs of Persons with Severe Disabilities website provides additional teaming resources for supporting individuals with severe disabilities who are likely to benefit from AAC:
  ○ https://www.asha.org/NJC/

REFERENCES

Ambrose, S. A., Bridges, M. W., DiPietro, M., Lovett, M. C., & Norman, M. K. (2010). *How learning works: Seven research-based principles for smart teaching*. Jossey-Bass Inc.

American Speech-Language-Hearing Association. (2019). Augmentative and alternative communication. http://www.asha.org/practice-portal/professional-issues/augmentative-and-alternative-communication

Bloom, B., Englehart, M., Furst, E., Hill, W., & Krathwohl, D. (1956). *Taxonomy of educational objectives: The classification of educational goals. Handbook I: Cognitive domain*. Longmans, Green & Company LTD.

Brantlinger, E., Jimenez, R., Klinger, J., Pugach, M., & Richardson, V. (2005). Qualitative studies in special education. *Exceptional Children, 71*, 195-207. https://doi.org/10.1177/001440290507100205

Calculator, S. N., & Black, T. (2009). Validation of an inventory of best practices in the provision of augmentative and alternative communication services to students with severe disabilities in general education classrooms. *American Journal of Speech-Language Pathology, 18*, 329-342. https://doi.org/10.1044/1058-0360(2009/08-0065)

Creswell, J. W., & Creswell, J. D. (2018). *Research design: Qualitative, quantitative and mixed methods approaches* (5th ed.). SAGE Publications.

Eppler, M. J. (2006). A comparison between concept maps, mind maps, conceptual diagrams, and visual metaphors as complementary tools for knowledge construction and sharing. *Information Visualization, 5*, 202-210.

Ericcson, K. A., & Simon, H. A. (1993). *Protocol analysis: Verbal reports as data*. MIT Press.

Lang, J. M. (2016). *Small teaching: Everyday lessons from the science of learning*. Jossey-Bass Inc.

Lund, S., Quach, W., Weissling, K. S. E., McKelvey, M. L., & Dietz, A. R. (2017). Assessment with children who need augmentative and alternative communication (AAC): Clinical decisions of AAC specialists. *Language, Speech, and Hearing Services in Schools, 48*, 56-68. https://doi.org/10.1044/2016_LSHSS-15-0086

Middendorf, J., & Pace, D. (2004). Decoding the disciplines: A model for helping students learn disciplinary ways of thinking. *New Directions for Teaching and Learning, 98*, 1-11.

Strauss, A., & Corbin, J. (1998). *Basics of qualitative research: Techniques and procedures for developing grounded theory* (2nd ed.). SAGE Publications.

ENGAGING STUDENTS TO WRITE THROUGH CONFERENCES AND PEER REVIEW

Jean Sawyer, PhD, CCC-SLP

DESCRIPTION OF TEACHING/LEARNING CONTEXT

Not many Communication Sciences and Disorders (CSD) programs offer stand-alone courses in professional writing, yet writing effectively is a critical component of practice in speech-language pathology and audiology. The writing we do as speech-language pathologists and audiologists reflects our competence and our ethics (American Speech-Language-Hearing Association, 2010; Goldfarb & Serpanos, 2014). In 2011, the CSD department at Illinois State University (Normal, Illinois) decided to add a 2-credit required course in professional writing to its undergraduate program. As students would eventually be writing diagnostic reports, progress reports, individualized educational plans, and many other types of writing in their professional careers, the curriculum committee felt they should have an opportunity for instruction and practice in professional writing as undergraduates. Additionally, students may be asked to do short research papers in classes or may elect to do independent research projects as undergraduates. At the graduate level, students also elect to do theses or dissertations. Thus, the scope of the professional writing class included a review of conventional writing and practice in writing a short review of literature on a self-selected topic. The course was designed for students in their junior or senior year of study, and enrollment was capped at 25 students.

A term paper assignment in any class can encourage students to evaluate and synthesize course material. Instructors can spend class time up front to prepare students for writing and include peer editing to help the students produce a better product. After the paper is submitted, instructors spend time evaluating the papers and may write comments justifying a grade. This type of evaluation is largely summative. After receiving their papers, students may not even look at the comments, and

Friberg, J. C., Visconti, C. F., & Ginsberg, S. M. (Eds.). *Evidence–Based Education in the Classroom: Examples From Clinical Disciplines* (pp. 159-166).

thus miss an opportunity to learn about writing in the discipline or learn how to improve their written work (Sommers, 1982; White, 1984). There is little, if any, research on writing in the discipline of CSD at the undergraduate level. Instructors who assign a paper may give students opportunity for peer review, but due to time constraints both in the course and on the instructor, there may be no more opportunities for rewriting once the paper is submitted.

In teaching the professional writing class at Illinois State University, the instructor wanted to give the students a different writing experience by teaching writing as a process. Whether they were writing clinical reports or a literature review, students completed multiple drafts of their work before the final submission. Responding effectively to that work should, in theory, help students learn about writing and make them better writers (Sommers, 2006). This chapter describes two types of reviews of writing used in the professional writing course, which were taken from the field of teaching writing and composition. The first review was an individual meeting with the instructor to discuss a draft of clinical writing: a diagnostic report or progress report. The second was a group peer review of a literature review. This chapter reviews the effectiveness of these two types of reviews from the viewpoint of the students.

REVIEW OF LITERATURE

A traditional and typical way to respond to students' writing is through written comments. The motivation for instructors to write comments on drafts of student papers includes the hope of helping their students become better writers (Sommers, 1982, 2006, 2012). One university-wide study on writing showed that in actual practice, however, not much specific feedback was given to help students with writing (Sommers, 2006). The Harvard Study of Undergraduate Writing examined college writing assignments for 400 students over 4 years (Sommers, 2006). Students rarely received specific writing instruction in their courses and were not asked to revise. Comments on the final papers served for most students as the only instruction they received about how to write.

Making Written Comments to Provide Writing Feedback

Whereas teachers in general courses may not give much feedback on written drafts, for teachers of writing composition, having students write drafts and commenting on them is a way to teach writing as a process. Writing comments is time consuming, and not only teachers but also students may feel overwhelmed by writing and receiving comments on written work (Sommers, 2012). Comments can actually take the students away from their own purpose in writing, and students might put their revision focus on pleasing the instructor or trying to discern what the teacher's purpose in commenting was (Sommers, 1982). Instructors may be directing comments more to the paper than to the student (Sommers, 2012). Students may also have difficulty prioritizing what is important, as comments can focus on the mechanics of writing as well as organization and content. In her study of comments of 35 teachers of writing at two universities, Sommers (1982) indicated that students may use comments to see first drafts as finished drafts, and believe if they simply respond to the comments, their paper will be complete.

Scholars agree that not much is known about what students take away from the comments teachers make (Ferris, 2014; Rutz, 2006; Sommers, 2006). The Harvard Study of Undergraduate Writing revealed that comments were often not read, and students often viewed them as judgmental (Sommers, 2006). Students found some comments difficult to understand and wished instructors would have given specific feedback and commented more frequently. Students who felt they had grown as writers paid attention to the comments and felt they had received constructive criticism of their writing.

The nature of comments differs according to individual instructors. Rutz (2006) conducted interviews of teachers in a first-year writing classroom and found inconsistencies in approaches to comments, with some instructors writing comments line by line, some who never made comments on writing errors, and some choosing to meet with their students in conferences rather than provide written comments. An alternative to writing comments is to hold conferences with the students to talk about their papers. Personal conferences may provide focused guidance to students.

Ferris (2014) found similar variability in instructors' responses to student writing after surveying and interviewing first-year writing instructors in eight different institutions in northern California. Some instructor feedback included checklists and some instructors made marginal comments and/or a summary paragraph at the end of a paper. The length of comments varied, as did the type, with instructors using questions, statements, and imperatives. As with the Rutz study (2006), Fitzgerald (1987) found many instructors made use of writing conferences.

Best practices for responding to student writing include providing feedback on all drafts, having students receive feedback from both instructors and peers, and giving feedback in one-on-one conferences (Ferris, 2014). If feedback is given in the form of a conference, instructors should discuss the goals and format of the conference and encourage students to take notes. If students feel intimidated by coming in for a conference, instructors may wish to conduct conferences with students in pairs.

Using Peer Review to Give Writing Feedback

Peer review is another effective way to help students improve their writing. Research has shown that comments made by peers and instructors are not meaningfully different (Falchikov & Goldfinch, 2000; Marcoulides & Simkin, 1991, 1995). Peer review is part of a formative evaluation and usually involves students working in pairs to read and provide input to the writer on ways to revise the paper, without assigning a grade. The peer review may take place over a class period, or students may do the peer review on their own time, outside of class (Haswell, 1983; Sommers, 2012; White, 1984).

Rieber (2006) examined grades on papers of 57 students in his business communications class. Papers that were peer reviewed received grades that were significantly higher than those that were not. Rieber felt that peer review forced students to be more organized, as they had to finish their drafts before the actual due date. Another advantage of peer review was that it forced his students to look at the assignment a second time. Additionally, students may see peer comments as less evaluative than those of instructors. Students may also be encouraged to re-assess their own papers after having examined another student's paper. Peer review may be done in pairs or in small groups. If done in groups, students can benefit from other perspectives, but it does take more time than when done in pairs (Rieber, 2006). Peer review does take class time, and weaker students may not be able to help stronger stundents. Ferris (2014) recommends providing training to students if using peer review. Instructors should assign the groups thoughtfully and require accountability, which may be in the form of a reflection of the process.

ORIGINAL DATA

Project 1: Engaging Students by Evaluating Writing Through Conferences

While there is ample evidence about providing students with feedback on writing through written comments, less is known about the effects of providing feedback via conferences. The evidence for holding individual conferences with students in the professional writing course about their clinical papers came from previous research done by the instructor in a different undergraduate class. The goal of the research was to determine the effectiveness of conducting individual writing conferences. The class was an introduction to stuttering, and students were to write a three- to four-page paper to a specific audience explaining what causes stuttering. Students taking this 3-credit course were juniors and seniors. The purpose of the conference was to provide formative feedback to students as to how they could strengthen their papers. Eighty students in two classes over two semesters participated in the study, which was approved by the institutional review board at Illinois State University.

Students were to write their papers in the American Psychological Association style. The paper was worth 35 points, broken into 3 points for peer editing with another student, 17 points for a rewrite of the peer-evaluated paper, and 5 points for attending the conference with the instructor. The final draft was worth 10 points. Prior to the conference, the instructor evaluated the paper holistically by assessing it on a score of 17 points and highlighted areas to discuss in the conference. The students were given the highlighted paper and instructed to think about changes they might want to make before coming to the conference. Students signed up for a 15-minute conference. It took approximately 1 week to meet with all the students, and students were given 2 weeks to revise their papers and resubmit them. After the conference, students could elect to complete an anonymous questionnaire about the process.

The questionnaire had one question asking about previous experiences with writing feedback. There were four Likert-type questions about students' experiences with the conference, with 1 being "strongly disagree" and 5 being "strongly agree." There were also three open-ended questions about the students' experiences with the conferences.

All students had feedback on drafts of papers prior to taking the current class. Ten percent of students had just one experience, while 37% of students had two to three experiences. Twenty-four percent had feedback three to four times. Beyond that, 10% had feedback five to six times, and 14% had feedback on their drafts seven or more times.

Students were largely positive about getting feedback through a conference. The mean response to the question of "verbal comments made it easy to determine how I could strengthen my paper" was 4.39 on a 5-point scale (SD = 0.57). Almost all students agreed or strongly agreed with the statement, with one student marking disagree. On the question of, "I would prefer written over verbal feedback about my paper," most students (38) marked disagree, and some (17) marked strongly disagree. The mean response to that question was 2.52 (SD = 0.91). Most students (65) agreed or strongly agreed with the statement, "I learned more about writing from the conference than I would have learned from written comments." The mean for that question was 3.94 (SD = 0.81).

Even though students overwhelmingly felt the conference format was helpful, it was still intimidating for some to attend. The question "I felt intimidated about coming in for feedback about my paper" had a mean response of 2.56 (SD = 1.24). Thirty-eight percent of respondents agreed with the statement, with 35% disagreeing, 25% strongly disagreeing, and 2.9% had no opinion.

Students were asked to list some of the advantages of a writing conference. Several felt they could easily ask questions (14) and learn the strengths and weaknesses of their paper (12). Many (17) felt they could more easily learn how to change their papers through conferences. A few students (5) felt they could use the conference to strengthen their papers in other courses and also appreciated the opportunity to meet with the instructor.

When asked about the disadvantages of the conference, 30 students wrote that there were none. Scheduling was a problem for 10 students, and 10 students felt it was "intimidating to hear what I had to work on." One student said she wrote notes on a piece of paper and admitted it would have been easier to take the notes on the actual term paper. Six students took minimal notes and could not remember how to revise their paper.

Most students (52) indicated they would like to take another course that offered conferences about written drafts. One student felt the conference "pushed me to do better." Five students were more ambivalent, with one student writing, "It doesn't make a difference either way," and another writing, "It's not my favorite thing, but it wasn't all that bad."

From the instructor's viewpoint, even though the conferences took time, it was a good use of time, and she felt it was productive in helping students learn about writing. The time spent on getting the drafts ready for the conferences was minimal in comparison to using written comments to guide students. The final drafts were of high quality, and the instructor spent less time evaluating them than if she had not met with students individually. It was enjoyable to meet with students and talking to them was easier than writing comments to help them guide their revisions. Additionally, conferences made it easier to let students know what they had done well.

Based on the positive feedback about the writing conferences used in the undergraduate stuttering course, the instructor decided to use conferences in the professional writing courses for two assignments: the diagnostic report and the progress report. One advantage of the conference format was that it was similar to the way students are likely to get feedback in their graduate clinical experiences; they will be meeting clinical supervisors regularly for feedback on both treatment and clinical reporting. Both the diagnostic report and progress report were done in pairs, and students were asked to come to the conference together, which may serve to minimize any feelings of intimidation during the conferences. The format of the conferences in the professional writing class was similar to that done with the stuttering class. The instructor marked areas of the report to discuss and asked the students to think about those areas and the report in general before meeting with the instructor. The conference meeting represented approximately 10% of the grade for the paper. Clinical papers were also peer-reviewed before the conference, so students had several opportunities to work with their papers. No formal assessment of the efficacy of individual conferences for the professional writing class was conducted, but students have commented that they found the conferences helpful to their development as clinical writers.

Project 2: Developing Critical Thinking in Student Writers Through Group Peer Review

Peer review is another way of providing feedback to students about their writing. Instructors may typically elect to have students read papers in pairs. The instructor of the professional writing class wanted to investigate the efficacy of a group peer review. The goal of the peer review was to expose students to multiple examples of written work and give them more experience evaluating writing, with a focus on increasing their confidence and skills to improve their own writing.

Twenty-one students taking the professional writing course participated in the study, which was approved by the institutional review board at Illinois State University. The assignment was to write a six- to eight-page literature review on a topic of interest, using American Psychological Association style. The paper was worth 75 points, broken into 10 points for preliminary work (topic selection, library visit, and outline), 30 points for peer review, and 35 points for the final draft.

For the peer review, the class was divided into two groups of 11 and 12 students. Individual students printed copies of their papers for each member of the group. Students were instructed to mark the papers with editing comments and to write a letter to the author giving suggestions as to how to improve the paper. The 50-minute class period was spent on reviewing three students' papers at a time, one group at a time, and the students in the group came to class with the papers and discussed them as a group. The student writer began the discussion, stating the purpose of the paper and giving a short summary. Students received points for commenting on the paper, and at the end of the discussion, gave the student the letter summarizing the suggested changes and the draft copies. The instructor also participated and gave the students comments and wrote them letters. Students then rewrote their papers and submitted them at the end of the semester.

Twenty-one of 23 students agreed to participate in the research by answering a survey at the end of the peer review period. The survey consisted of two questions that asked about students' experiences with peer review, eight Likert-type questions on their opinions and preferences regarding the peer review, and three open-ended questions. The Likert-type questions ranged from 1 (strongly agree) to 5 (strongly disagree).

Three students had never had experience with peer review in a one-on-one basis. Two students had experienced this type of peer review once. Six students had two to three prior experiences with one-on-one peer review. The other respondents had more experience, with six responding they had done this four to five times, and four having done it six or more times.

The students had not had as much experience with group review. Fifteen students had never reviewed papers in groups, three students had done it once, two students had done group review two to three times, and one student had significant experience with group peer review, having done it four to five times.

The overall opinion of doing peer review in groups was mixed. More than half the class indicated one-on-one peer review was preferential to group peer review. Nearly 48% agreed with the statement "I prefer one-on-one peer review to group peer review" and 4.8% strongly agreed. Almost 43% disagreed, and 4.8% had no opinion. Another version of the question was asked later in the survey, focusing on the feedback students received: "I prefer group feedback to one-on-one feedback." One-third of the participants disagreed with the statement, 42.8% had no opinion, and 23.8% agreed.

Although students were evaluating 10 or 11 papers over the semester, most did not find it time-consuming. For the statement, "The group peer review was too time consuming," 38% of students agreed and 62% of students disagreed.

The group format meant students received many comments on their papers, but they largely felt that they could understand their peers' comments. Seventy-one percent disagreed with the statement, "The comments I received were difficult to understand because they were coming from so many different people." In fact, students seemed to regard multiple viewpoints positively, as 76.2% marked the statement, "Getting the perspective of more than one person in a group peer review made my paper stronger," either "agree" or "strongly agree."

Reading more papers seemed to help students learn about their writing, as 76.2% agreed or strongly agreed with the statement, "I learned more about writing using group peer review than I do in on-on-one review because I read so many papers." Additionally, most students felt their writing improved after the peer review. Sixty-seven percent agreed or strongly agreed with the statement, "My writing has improved as a direct result of participating in the group peer review process."

If it is uncomfortable for students to get feedback from instructors, it might be uncomfortable for students to get feedback from several peers. Participants' responses to the statement, "I felt uncomfortable hearing others make remarks about my paper," indicated that most (67%) disagreed or strongly disagreed.

Students were asked to provide written comments addressing the strengths and weaknesses of group peer review. For the strengths, seven students mentioned they got to see multiple perspectives on their writing. Six felt the review helped them not overlook their mistakes. Five felt the comments helped them become better writers, and two enjoyed having written copies of the suggestions. One student mentioned "the environment was welcoming," and another wrote that she "felt much more confident in my writing."

Students pointed out weaknesses as well. Five felt the groups were too large, and five felt there were too many comments, making it difficult to know which to focus on in the revision. Five students wrote that the peer review was "time consuming and tedious." Four students did not like the timing of the draft due dates and felt they were due too early.

The final open-ended question asked students if they would want to take another class that implemented group peer review feedback. Sixteen students said they would like to do so, and indicated the feedback was beneficial (five students) and they had become more confident in their writing (eight students). Two students said "no," that group peer review was too time-consuming, one student said "maybe," and two did not respond to this question.

The instructor enjoyed having joint responsibility for giving feedback, and found student comments to be insightful. She found students were able to make comments on areas that she had overlooked. It was also a positive experience to be able to explain what students had done well. The instructor found students to be respectful and interested in what each other had to say about the papers.

APPLICATION TO CROSS-DISCIPLINARY CONTEXTS

Writing is a complex skill, and meeting students individually or in small groups to discuss what they have written helps students understand and think about how they might improve their papers. Additionally, group peer reviews give student writers more opinions about their writing and expose the students to other styles of writing. These two methods of review have enhanced the undergraduate courses described in this chapter. The instructor plans to continue soliciting feedback to make these experiences effective.

Any discipline that asks professionals to produce written documents could benefit from asking students to attend writing conferences and participate in group peer reviews of writing. Other health professions, such as occupational therapy or physical therapy, may require their students to write treatment plans or other professional reports, and students may benefit from receiving feedback in the ways outlined in the chapter.

Group peer review and writing conferences could be beneficial outside the classroom as well. Students who are working on independent study projects, theses, or dissertations may find it helpful to share written drafts in small groups and meet to talk about what the writers have done well or ways they could improve their drafts. Course instructors who require writing assignments in a particular department could collaborate and have small groups of students from each class read drafts of papers and meet to comment on them.

As instructors, we want to help our students learn to write effectively, and that means giving them feedback on what they are doing and providing a course structure that enables several drafts, treating writing as a process. Getting feedback in conferences and giving feedback to peers are two ways to effectively facilitate writing as a process.

ADDITIONAL RESOURCES

- Elbow, P. (1999). Options for responding to student writing. In R. Staub (Ed.), *A sourcebook for responding to student writing* (pp. 197-202). Hampton Press.
- Fitzgerald, J. (1987). Research on revision in writing. *Review of Educational Research, 57*(4), 481-506.
- The Harvard Study of Undergraduate Writing. (2014). Study of undergraduate writing. *Harvard University.* https://writing.gse.harvard.edu/
- Marcoulides, G. A., & Simkin, M. G. (1995). Evaluating student papers: The consistency of peer review in student writing projects. *Journal of Education for Business, 70*(4), 220-224.
- Straub, R. (1999). *A sourcebook for responding to student writing.* Hampton Press.
- Topping, K. J. (2003). Self and peer assessment in school and university: Reliability, validity and utility. In M. S. R. Segers, F. J. R. C. Dochy, & E. C. Cascallar (Eds.), *Optimizing new modes assessment: In search of qualities and standards.* Kluwer Academic Publishers.

REFERENCES

American Speech-Language-Hearing Association. (2010). Code of ethics. http//www.asha.org/policy

Falchikov., N., & Goldfinch, J. (2000). Student peer assessment in higher education: A meta-analysis comparing peer and teacher marks. *Review of Educational Research, 70*, 287-322.

Ferris, D. R. (2014). Responding to student writing: Teachers' philosophies and practices. *Assessing Writing, 19*, 6-23.

Fitzgerald, J. (1987). Research on revision in writing. *Review of Educational Research, 57*(4), 481-506.

Goldfarb, R., & Serpanos, Y. C. (2014). *Professional writing in speech-language pathology and audiology* (2nd ed.). Plural.

Haswell, R. H. (1983). Minimal marking. *College English, 45*(6), 600-604.

Marcoulides, G. A., & Simkin, M. G. (1991). Evaluating student papers: The case for peer review. *Journal of Education for Business, 67*(2), 80-86.

Marcoulides, G. A., & Simkin, M. G. (1995). The consistency of peer review in student writing projects. *Journal of Education for Business, 70*(4), 220-223. https://doi.org/10.1080/08832323.1995.10117753

Rieber, L. J. (2006). Using peer review to improve student writing in business courses. *Journal of Education for Business, 81*(6), 322-326.

Rutz, C. (2006). Recovering the conversation: A response to "responding to student writing" via "across the drafts." *College Composition and Communication, 58*(2), 257-262.

Sommers, N. (1982). Responding to student writing. *College Composition and Communication, 33*(2), 148-156.

Sommers, N. (2006). Across the drafts. *College Composition and Communication, 58*(2), 248-257.

Sommers, N. (2012). *Responding to student writers.* St. Martin's.

White, E. M. (1984). *Teaching and assessing writing: Recent advances in understanding, evaluating, and improving student performance* (2nd ed.). Jossey-Bass Inc.

CURRICULAR INTEGRATION IN CLINICALLY BASED FIELDS
A Case Study From Speech-Language Pathology

Lisa A. Vinney, PhD, CCC-SLP
and Jennine M. Harvey-Northrop, PhD, CCC-SLP

DESCRIPTION OF TEACHING/LEARNING CONTEXT

Like other allied health professionals, speech-language pathologists are trained to address a wide variety of disorders. Thus, graduate-level speech-language pathology curriculum is often siloed into courses focused on these disorders (e.g., one course in aphasia, another in motor speech disorders) based on the nine broad areas required for graduate speech-language pathology programs. On the other hand, basic courses that discuss the foundations of speech, language, and swallowing (e.g., speech science, neuroanatomy, neurophysiology) are traditionally the focus of undergraduate study. Given that most professors who teach undergraduate and graduate speech-language pathology courses are specialists in one or two disorder-based areas and their foundations, the segmentation of the field into silos has been a logical and traditional feature of graduate-level speech-language pathology programs. Unfortunately, students educated within this model may struggle to see the interrelatedness of clinical presentations and etiologies and apply foundational knowledge/basic science across those presentations (Friberg & Harbers, 2016; Harvey & Vinney, 2019; Vinney & Harvey, 2017). Specific to our experience, we noticed that students struggled to integrate foundational knowledge common to motor speech disorders (MSDs) with similar foundations in the aphasias. Furthermore, students had difficulty applying these foundations to the assessment and treatment practices for co-occurring presentations of these disorders. Students' exposure to foundational neuroanatomy and neurophysiology also often occurred 2 or more years prior to their graduate study. Because students had difficulty recalling much of this foundational information, we both implemented a time-intensive review of basic neuroanatomy and neurophysiology. This review significantly delayed discussion of the applied content representing "the meat" of our courses.

Friberg, J. C., Visconti, C. F., & Ginsberg, S. M. (Eds.). *Evidence-Based Education in the Classroom: Examples From Clinical Disciplines* (pp. 167-174).
© 2021 Taylor & Francis Group.

Figure 19-1. Vertical and horizontal integration of course content.

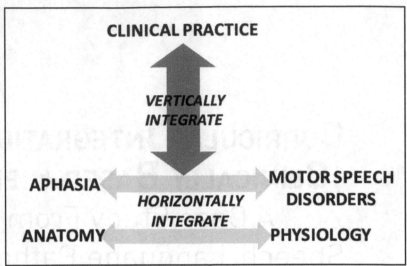

Thus, in Spring 2016, we were motivated to integrate aspects of our MSDs and aphasia courses to foster horizontal and vertical integration (Snyman & Kroon, 2005). Horizontal integration addresses the links between basic sciences/foundational knowledge (i.e., anatomy and physiology and basic knowledge of aphasia and MSDs) and vertical integration addresses the links between the basic sciences/foundational knowledge and clinical practice (i.e., assessment and treatment of MSDs and aphasia within one client). For a visual of vertical and horizontal integration relevant to our learning context, please see Figure 19-1.

The current chapter describes integrating intradisciplinary curriculum in the classroom by describing the following: (1) considerations and frameworks for curricular integration based on the literature, (2) our research into the implementation and study of integrated curricular features across courses in graduate-level MSDs and aphasias, and (3) how integration may be applied in other disciplinary contexts.

REVIEW OF LITERATURE

Integrated instruction is a new area of scholarship of teaching and learning in speech-language pathology, but concerns over curricular silos have been discussed and studied for decades in many health science fields (Cohn et al., 2014; Elangovan et al., 2016; Harden et al., 1984; Howard et al., 2009; Husband et al., 2014; Malik & Malik, 2011; Pfeifer, 2018). We believe that the discussion of integrated curricula has relevance to all clinical professions, given their common challenges. Thus, we detail four major ideas in the following sections regarding the impetus, potential design, and pros/cons of curricular integration.

Idea 1: Integrating the Basic and Clinical Sciences Is a Potential Opportunity

Many clinical degree programs' curricula include basic sciences/foundational information courses, like anatomy and physiology, followed by clinical sciences (i.e., courses focused on assessment and treatment of specific health conditions). This traditional structure may date back to the Flexner Report of 1910, which called for a new 4-year standard medical curricula that exposed students to 2 years of basic science education followed by 2 years of clinical science education (Bolender et al., 2013; Elangoven et al., 2016; Flexner, 1910). Recently, many scholars have expressed concerns over a lack of opportunities for medical and dental students to horizontally and, in particular, vertically integrate information (Howard et al., 2009; Pfeifer, 2018). Thus, although the Flexner Report is credited with spurring tremendous scientific advancement and improving medical practice, it has led to modern concerns about the curricular organization facilitating professional training in clinical fields. Indeed, in a follow-up report that came out 100 years since the Flexner Report, the authors call for more explicitly uniting the basic sciences with clinical practice in medical education (Cooke et al., 2010; Irby et al., 2010).

Idea 2: Problem- and Case-Based Learning May Act as Vehicles for Integration

Clinical and basic information have frequently been integrated by case-based learning and problem-based learning (PBL) practices. When students are provided with real-world clinical cases or problems that they must assess or solve, they are more likely to connect basic information to clinical contexts and become critical thinkers (AlSaggaf et al., 2010; Harman et al., 2015). Research documents how a case-based approach to learning has aided in facilitating transfer, over and above lecture and discussion (Harman et al., 2015; Loghmani et al., 2011; Yoo & Park, 2015).

Instruction that is case-based has reportedly facilitated gains in clinical skill development and the critical analysis and evaluation of problem scenarios in fields such as medicine, dentistry, and other health care disciplines, including dietetics, nursing, physical therapy, and speech-language pathology (Harden, 2000; Harman et al., 2015; Hassan, 2013; Howard et al., 2009; Kantar & Massouh, 2015; Loghmani et al., 2011; Malik & Malik, 2011; Meilijson & Katzenberger, 2015; Yoo & Park, 2015). Further, activities that involve the evaluation of cases via students from many disciplines have led to horizontal integration of foundational knowledge that is both intradisciplinary and interdisciplinary in nature (Trommelen et al., 2014).

Idea 3: Integration Occurs Along a Continuum

Besides specific pedagogies like case-based learning and PBL, educators in clinically based fields should make their goals for implementing integrated instruction explicit in order to determine the level of integration required to meet those goals and the policies and procedures needed to support such integration (Fogarty, 1991; Harden, 2000). Harden (2000) models these levels as rungs of an integration ladder (Table 19-1).

Starting at level 8, courses are unlikely to be segmented by subject boundaries. Thus, curricular integration at levels 8 through 11 may require extensive revisions of traditional clinical training programs such that several courses are subsumed into one block (Brauer & Ferguson, 2015; Elangoven et al., 2016; Kitzes et al., 2007; Malik & Malik, 2011; Pfeifer, 2018). These blocks may be directed by a single instructor, multiple instructors within the health science discipline's degree program, or include instructors from other disciplines. For example, a new speech-language pathology program at McMaster University has semester-long units based around a core theme (Hamilton et al., 2019). While specific diseases and disorders are covered throughout the semester, the core principles and knowledge and skills inherent to clinical practice in speech-language pathology are emphasized and addressed via a PBL approach. Thus, learning is focused on clinical problem solving, specific clinical tasks related to solving each clinical problem, and the foundational and clinical knowledge inherent to them with the preservation of core subject areas (e.g., aphasia, MSDs, articulation) discussed in reference to these principles. This program is shaped by the McMaster University's approach to medical education developed in the 1970s and 1980s and subsequently adapted by the university's occupational and physical therapy programs (Brauer & Ferguson, 2015; Hamilton et al., 2019; Neufeld & Barrows, 1974).

TABLE 19-1

Levels Along the Integration Continuum

INTEGRATION LEVEL	NAME	DESCRIPTION
1	Isolation	Specialists in an academic area prepare their courses and teach them without regard for other courses in the curriculum.
2	Awareness	Instructors teach their own subject area but communicate with other teachers about the elements of their courses. The connection between other topics or courses in the curriculum is not explicitly discussed with students in class.
3	Harmonization	Instructors explicitly discuss the connection between other topics or courses in the curriculum during their specific class.
4	Nesting	Instructors teach their own subjects, but integrate specific concepts or skills (e.g., counseling, applying the scientific method to clinical cases) across courses.
5	Temporal coordination	Instructors teach their own subjects, but related topics are taught at the same time within each course. Explicit links between these subjects are not made, but because the timing of their delivery is coordinated, students may be able to better conceptualize their relationship.
6	Sharing	Two or more instructors from different fields or subfields work together to teach a course on a topic that relates to each (e.g., a course on counseling run by a number of allied health departments like occupational therapy and physical therapy).
7	Correlation	Instructors primarily teach their own subjects, but they include some courses/class periods and assignments that are integrated.
8	Complementary	Instructors are unlikely to teach their own subject in a silo. Instead, many courses or class periods are based around core themes to which multiple disciplines or subdisciplines may contribute.
9	Multidisciplinary	All class periods integrate a number of subjects with the focus of learning on ideas or themes. Individual subjects still retain their identity, but instruction encompassing many subjects is developed and delivered together.

(continued)

TABLE 19-1 (CONTINUED)		
Levels Along the Integration Continuum		
INTEGRATION LEVEL	NAME	DESCRIPTION
10	Interdisciplinary	All class periods integrate a number of subjects. Individual disciplines may not be acknowledged as separate and distinct at this level. In this model, interdisciplinary does not necessarily imply that two different areas of study (e.g., physical therapy and occupational therapy) must come together to produce curricula as is the common understanding of this word.
11	Transdisciplinary	Instruction occurs through clinical immersion experiences (e.g., clinical practice experiences that expose students to multiple disciplines, settings, clients, specialty areas).

Idea 4: Curricular Integration Challenges Traditional University Structures

Faculty time and resources are typically related to semester credit hours based on a siloed system of coursework. Higher levels of integration introduce significant challenges to calculating faculty workloads. For example, if a theme subsumes silo-based courses and leads to a rearrangement of the curriculum, one instructor may not be responsible for an individual course or courses. The effects of this rearrangement on each faculty person's course load and promotion and tenure must be determined early on. Furthermore, if such a rearrangement is a hindrance to professional advancement or not supported by the department or institution, motivation to integrate is unlikely to be sustained (Brueckner & Gould, 2006; Elangoven et al., 2016). Higher levels of curricular integration may also result in the loss of valuable discipline-based perspectives and potential "turf-wars" between experts (Brueckner & Gould, 2006; Ferguson & Wilson, 2011). Finally, the need to collaborate and co-teach with one's colleagues should not be taken lightly, given that communication and relationship building is an endeavor requiring time, dedication, and a shared vision (Bacharach et al., 2008; Brueckner & Gould, 2006; Ferguson & Wilson, 2011; Morelock et al., 2017). The considerations noted earlier have been reflected in the research. Specifically, when 44 basic and clinical scientists were surveyed about the possibility of an integrated health science curriculum at their institution, they showed a high degree of interest but cited similar barriers to implementation (Brueckner & Gould, 2006).

APPLICATION OF LITERATURE/DATA

Given the literature, we believed that we had an opportunity to design our separate aphasia and MSD classes with integrated components. We discussed our core learning objectives for integration which were to help students (1) integrate foundational knowledge related to both aphasias and MSD and (2) use that knowledge to make sense of clinical presentations including both classes of disorders. In clinical practice, aphasias and MSDs are diagnosed separately and typically require distinct assessment and treatment practices. Thus, we wanted our classes to maintain their own identities. Logistically, we also hoped to decrease curricular redundancy and increase efficiency across both our courses. We reasoned that our goals and objectives aligned best with correlation (level 7), so we would remain responsible for our own subjects but together would implement integrated class periods, exams, and assignments. This level of integration was also most appropriate given the arrangement of our curriculum (aphasia and MSDs were offered to the same cohort at the same point in their plan of study).

Thus, we integrated components of aphasia (Harvey was instructor of record) and MSD (Vinney was instructor of record) for a cohort of 38 master's-level speech-language pathology students in Spring 2016. In particular, we developed and co-taught an introductory foundational review of neuroanatomy and physiology that included modules consisting of narrated lectures for each of the five different neurological systems (e.g., brainstem) and associated case questions illustrating how potential speech and language deficits might be linked to neurological damage. Students reviewed each module prior to the beginning of the semester. During the first week of the semester, students attended MSD and aphasia class periods led by both instructors. During this class time, students asked questions about the integrated content, and engaged in small- and large-group discussions about their case question responses. Following the out-of-class modules and in-class augmentation, students took an exam, which included multiple choice and short answer case-based questions, on the integrated foundational content.

After the foundational integrated review, the core foundations and assessment practices for aphasia and MSDs were reviewed separately. However, to show students how assessment practices for aphasia and MSDs might appear together, we designed a lab requiring pairs of students to assess cranial nerve, cognition, and language function in partner-assigned specific neurological deficits. The student giving the exam gained experience administering the clinical procedure, while observing the acted out or described partner's deficits. Conversely, the student acting out or describing the deficits had to think through how a person with their assigned area of damage might present given each of the exam tasks. We once again engaged in distinct classroom teaching following this lab to go over the classification schemes for the aphasias and MSDs, respectively, but the last segment of our course included a case-based integrated final. Students worked with another peer to write up a full diagnostic report based on an assigned clinical case in which a fictional patient demonstrated both an aphasia and MSD. Students were required to integrate background and assessment information to differentially diagnose both the specific aphasia and MSD, as well as provide treatment and referral recommendations. Each of the three cross-course components were created and scored by both Vinney and Harvey.

Original Data

After the conclusion of the semester, we used a rubric to address whether and at what level students' case responses demonstrated content knowledge and its application. Case responses were scored anywhere from 0 (content knowledge or application was not demonstrated overall) to 16 (content knowledge or application was demonstrated overall). Every student received an average content knowledge and clinical application rubric score for the foundational exam case questions (beginning of both courses) and clinical application final (end of both courses). We reasoned that growth from the beginning to the end of the semester might suggest the accomplishment of our core learning objectives for integration.

Based on our analysis using a repeated measures analysis of variance, students' average rubric scores for both content knowledge and application improved significantly for both application and content knowledge from the beginning to the end of the semester (for detailed results, see Harvey and Vinney [2019]). Average scores for demonstrated content knowledge increased from 4.4 (foundational case questions) to 14.7 (final case questions), whereas average content application scores increased from 7.9 (foundational case questions) to 13.2 (final case questions). While it is impossible to tease out whether these results were simply a result of overall learning across the semester and unrelated to our integrated pedagogies, our findings certainly do not contraindicate integration and suggest such components may support the application and recall of integrated speech pathology content (Harvey & Vinney, 2019; Vinney & Harvey, 2017).

APPLICATION TO CROSS-DISCIPLINARY CONTEXTS

Integration within any health science field may (1) expose students to overlapping content without redundancy, (2) facilitate connections between basic and clinical knowledge, and (3) illustrate the interrelatedness of subareas within a discipline. Curricular integration may vary substantially depending on the objectives of integration and the unique features of a discipline. Thus, the learning objectives that may be accomplished by integration should be identified before making any curricular changes. Next, the integration level (Harden, 2000) that would address those objectives and is also logistically possible within one's university structure will guide the specific design of the integrated curricular components. We contend that the earlier mentioned items two and three are often, at least, partially addressed by embedding clinical cases into integrated components. The following are two potential examples for implementing integration and how it might vary by levels in the integration ladder:

1. If faculty of a physical therapy program had the objective of students applying anatomy and physiology to functional movement, they might transition from integration at level 1 (isolation) to level 5 (temporal coordination). Thus, instead of one course addressing physiology and another addressing anatomy being taught and prepared totally separately, these two courses might be delivered at the same time in the students plan of study. Alternatively, faculty might determine that creating a course that included both anatomy and physiology (level 9 of the integration ladder) may more directly address this objective.

2. If faculty of a nurse practitioner program had the objective of students planning and implementing patient care in the context of an interdisciplinary team, they might transition from having a course on evidence-based practice with one instructor (level 1, isolation) to having multiple instructors share how evidence-based practice is applied in their subdiscipline (level 6, sharing). Then, they can hierarchically build on these skills in an applied skills lab in which students engage in a simulated team approach to assessment and treatment (level 9, multidisciplinary) of disease, and finally expand to the highest level of complex integration through clinical immersion during clinical externships (level 11, transdisciplinary).

ADDITIONAL RESOURCE

- Example of integration across a plan of study from McMaster University's speech-language pathology master's program:
  - https://srs-mcmaster.ca/slp-program-information/#1491929439427-cc0a7c2c-c84c\

REFERENCES

AlSaggaf, S., Ali, S. S., Ayuob, N. N., Eldeek, B. S., & El-Haggagy, A. (2010). A model of horizontal and vertical integration of teaching on the cadaveric heart. *Annals of Anatomy, 192*(6), 373-377.

Bacharach, N., Heck, T. W., & Dahlberg, K. (2008). Co-teaching in higher education. *Journal of College Teaching and Learning, 5*(3), 9-16.

Bolender, D. L., Ettarh, R., Jerrett, D. P., & Laherty, R. F. (2013). Curriculum integration = course disintegration: What does this mean for anatomy? *Anatomical Sciences Education, 6*(3), 205-208.

Brauer, D. G., & Ferguson, K. J. (2015). The integrated curriculum in medical education: AMEE Guide No. 96. *Medical Teacher, 37*(4), 312-322.

Brueckner, J., & Gould, D. (2006). Health science faculty members' perceptions of curricular integration: Insights and obstacles. *Journal of International Association of Medical Science Education, 16*(1), 31-34.

Cohn, E. S., Coster, W. J., & Kramer, J. M. (2014). Facilitated learning model to teach habits of evidence-based reasoning across an integrated Master of Science in Occupational Therapy curriculum. *American Journal of Occupational Therapy, 68*, S73-S82.

Cooke, M., Irby, D. M., & O' Brien, B. C. (2010). *Educating physicians: A call for reform of medical school and residency.* Jossey-Bass Inc.

Elangovan, S., Venugopalan, S. R., Srinivasan, S., Karimbux, N. Y., Weistroffer, P., & Allareddy, V. (2016). Integration of basic clinical sciences, PBL, CBL, and IPE in U.S. dental schools' curricula and a proposed integrated curriculum model for the future. *Journal of Dental Education, 80*(3), 281-290.

Ferguson, J., & Wilson, J. C. (2011). The co-teaching professorship: Power and expertise in the co-taught higher education classroom. *Scholar-Practitioner Quarterly, 5*(1), 52-68.

Flexner, A. (1910). *Medical education in the United States and Canada.* Carnegie Foundation for the Advancement of Teaching.

Fogarty, R. (1991). Ten ways to integrate curriculum. *Educational Leadership, 49*(2), 61-65.

Friberg, J. C., & Harbers, H. (2016). Encouraging cross-curricular integration in communication sciences and disorders. *The Journal of Research and Practice in College Teaching, 1*(1), 1-14.

Hamilton, J., Phoenix, M., Campbell, W., & Turkstra, L. (2019, June). Problem-based learning in speech-language pathology graduate education. *AHSA Journals: Academy.* https://academy.pubs.asha.org/2019/06/problem-based-learning-in-speech-language-pathology-graduate-education/

Harden, R. M. (2000). The integration ladder: A tool for curriculum planning and evaluation. *Medical Education, 34*(7), 551-557.

Harden, R. M., Sowden, S., & Dunn, W. R. (1984). Educational strategies in curriculum development: The SPICES model. *Medical Education, 18*(4), 284-297.

Harman, T., Bertrand, B., Greer, A., Pettus, A., Jennings, J., Wall-Bassett, E., & Babatunde, O. T. (2015). Case-based learning facilitates critical thinking in undergraduate nutrition education. *Journal of the Academy of Nutrition and Dietetics, 115*(3), 378-388.

Harvey, J. M. T., & Vinney, L. A (2019). Bridging the gap: An approach to facilitating integrated application of neuroanatomy and neurophysiology in graduate-level speech-language pathology across the semester. *Teaching and Learning in Communication Sciences & Disorders, 3*(2), Article 6.

Hassan, S. (2013). Concepts of vertical and horizontal integration as an approach to integrated curriculum. *Education in Medicine Journal, 5*(4), e1-e5.

Howard, K. M., Stewart, T., Woodall, W., Kingsley, K., & Ditmyer, M. (2009). An integrated curriculum: Evolution, evaluation, and future direction. *Journal of Dental Education, 73*(8), 962-971.

Husband, A. K., Todd, A., & Fulton, J. (2014). Integrating science and practice in pharmacy curricula. *American Journal of Pharmaceutical Education, 78*(3), 63.

Irby, D. M., Cooke, M., & O'Brien, B. C. (2010). Calls for reform of medical education by the teaching: 1910 and 2010. *Academic Medicine, 85*(2), 220-227.

Kantar, L. D., & Massouh, A. (2015). Case-based learning: What traditional curricula fail to teach. *Nurse Education Today, 35*(8), e8-e14.

Kitzes, J. A., Savich, R. D., Kalishman, S., Sander, J. C., Prasad, A., Morris, C. R., & Timm, C. (2007). Fitting it all in: Integration of 12 cross-cutting themes into a school of medicine curriculum. *Medical Teacher, 29*(5), 437-442.

Loghmani, M. T., Bayliss, A. J., Strunk, V., & Altenburger, P. (2011). An integrative, longitudinal case-based learning model as a curriculum strategy to enhance teaching and learning. *Journal of Physical Therapy Education, 25*(2), 42-50.

Malik, A. S., & Malik, R. H. (2011). Twelve tips for developing an integrated curriculum. *Medical Teacher, 33*(2), 99-104.

Meilijson, S., & Katzenberger, I. (2015). A clinical education program for speech-language pathologists applying reflective practice, evidence-based practice and case-based learning. *Folia Phoniatrica Et Logopaedica, 66*(4), 158-163.

Morelock, J. R., Lester, M. M. G., Klopfer, M. D., Jardon, A. M., Mullins, R. D., Nicholas, E. L., & Alfaydi, A. S. (2017). Power, perceptions, and relationships: A model of co-teaching in higher education. *College Teaching, 65*(4), 182-191

Neufeld, V. R., & Barrows, H. S. (1974). The "McMaster philosophy": An approach to medical education. *Journal of Medical Education, 49,* 1040-1050.

Pfeifer, C. M. (2018). A progressive three-phase innovation to medical education in the United States. *Medical Education Online, 23*(1), 1427988.

Snyman, W. D., & Kroon, J. (2005). Vertical and horizontal integration of knowledge and skills: A working model. *European Journal of Dental Education, 9*(1), 26-31.

Trommelen, R. D., Hebert, L., & Nelson, T. K. (2014). Impact on physical therapy and audiology students of an interprofessional case-based learning experience in education of vestibular disorders. *Journal of Allied Health, 43*(4), 194-200.

Vinney, L. A., & Harvey, J. M. T. (2017). Bridging the gap: An integrated approach to facilitating foundational learning of neuroanatomy and neurophysiology in graduate-levels speech-language pathology coursework. *Teaching and Learning in Communication Sciences & Disorders, 1*(2), Article 1.

Yoo, M., & Park, J. (2015). Effect of case-based learning on the development of graduate nurses' problem-solving ability. *Nurse Education Today, 34*(1), 47-51.

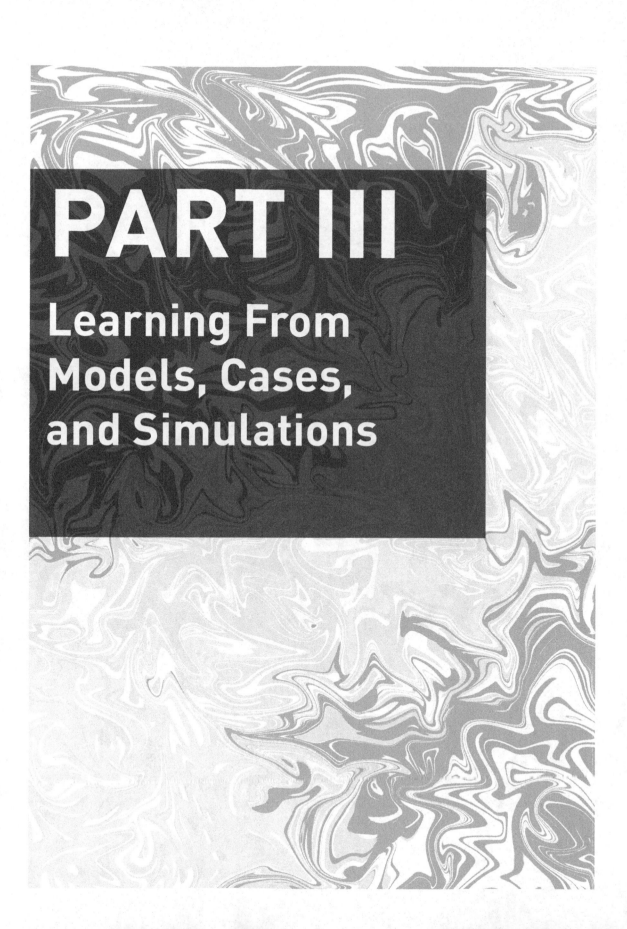

PART III

Learning From Models, Cases, and Simulations

20

UNFOLDING CASE STUDIES
A New Active Learning Pedagogy

Hilary Applequist, DNP, APRN-NP, ACHPN;
Marla Kniewel, EdD, MSN, RN;
Krystina Eymann, MSN, RN; and Eric Kyle, PhD

DESCRIPTION OF TEACHING/LEARNING CONTEXT

Undergraduate and graduate nursing student education requires a variety of teaching methods to facilitate learning of the complex health care needs in society. An unfolding case study is one teaching method that is effective in connecting theory to practice through the analysis of real-world situations. This modality is not equivalent to a traditional case study (Phillips, 2016). A case study is a descriptive and exploratory analysis of a patient situation, but it is static and does not allow for assessment of the student decision-making process. In comparison, an unfolding case study provides patient data that evolves in an unpredictable manner over time, requiring students to evaluate and re-evaluate a situation. An unfolding case study is also known as an evolving or scaffolding case study and starts with a brief scenario, with or without the addition of virtual reality, followed by challenge questions for the students to answer. Additional information is added to the scenario intermittently, with each addition followed by student challenge questions.

Several semesters ago, unfolding case studies were developed as a teaching modality for courses for baccalaureate nursing students and Doctor of Nursing Practice students at our small, private Midwestern health sciences college. Undergraduate students typically live locally and attend traditional classrooms. The graduate students are from across the United States and the program is online. Unfolding case studies were developed in a paper and pencil format for the traditional undergraduate nursing classroom and in an online format for the graduate nursing course. The use of unfolding case studies has demonstrated broadened critical thinking, use of the nursing process, and/or diagnostic reasoning.

Friberg, J. C., Visconti, C. F., & Ginsberg, S. M. (Eds.). *Evidence-Based Education in the Classroom: Examples From Clinical Disciplines* (pp. 177-184).

REVIEW OF LITERATURE

A review of the literature on unfolding case studies provided guidance on the development and implementation of the teaching methodology. Research on the effectiveness of unfolding case studies is limited but showed positive results. The literature provided information on the use of unfolding case studies in a variety of settings, disciplines, and academic levels of students. Unfolding case studies were being used in the classroom and online courses, the nursing laboratory, or in simulation (Pilcher, 2018).

One focus in the literature was on the development and use of unfolding case studies in nursing education. Kaylor and Strickland (2015) described the use of an unfolding case study on cardiovascular alterations for junior nursing students to connect pathophysiology with clinical manifestations as well as describe lifespan, legal, ethical, psychosocial, spiritual, and cultural considerations. Unfolding case studies used in a nursing labratory facilitated learning of psychomotor skills and enhanced student understanding of the decision-making processes in skill performance (Meiers & Russell, 2019). This approach encouraged students to link relevant assessment findings necessary with the performance of skills. Contextual psychomotor skill development was learned within the context of a patient's story over several labratory sessions.

With limited clinical sites, Bowman (2017) showed how an online unfolding case study can be used as an alternative learning experience with undergraduate students. The four-part unfolding case study used a simulated patient with multiple comorbidities and a change in status. Students reported feeling challenged in a safe environment while increasing self-confidence in clinical decision making. Additional research on unfolding case studies with undergraduate nursing students has shown positive results in learning, confidence, and clinical reasoning. Studies have shown statistically significant results on critical thinking disposition when compared to the teaching methodologies of traditional lecture and single-episode case-based learning (Dehghanzadeh & Jafaraghaee, 2018; Hong & Yu, 2017).

Student and faculty perceptions on the impact of unfolding case studies on learning were also studied (Meiers & Russell, 2019). Themes derived from students centered on knowledge synthesis, holistic patient care, and transferability to practice. Knowledge synthesis was the most affected with the use of unfolding case studies, as students were able to make sense of the experience and build upon previous knowledge from pathophysiology and nursing fundamentals. Themes derived from faculty on the impact of the unfolding case study on student learning were transferability to practice and increased clinical competence.

The literature on graduate nursing student learning has shown unfolding case studies as an effective teaching methodology. Positive feedback on the benefits in preparing graduate students for new roles was evident in the literature (Peery, 2015). Vogt and Schaffner (2016) found that the majority of nurse practitioner students were satisfied with the use of technology-enhanced unfolding case studies as part of the course work. Other findings demonstrated increased clinical reasoning skills in graduate nursing students (Granger et al., 2018; O'Rourke & Zerwic, 2016).

Another option discussed for an online format was the use of a branching unfolding case study in which decisions can lead students down a different path, changing the outcome of the patient (Snegirev, 2016). The branching case study focused on the real-world application of the content, in terms of the level of detail needed, in the decisions made by the student, and in the evolving outcome. A branching unfolding case study begins with a brief scenario requiring a student response. Due to varied responses, students may branch down different routes in the scenario. There are multiple decision points as the scenario progresses, leading to different patient outcomes, depending on the student's response. Branching scenarios can be developed with software programs, like Adobe Captivate, Lectora (eLearning Brothers, LLC), and Articulate Storyline (Articulate Global Inc), and are invaluable in assessing student clinical reasoning skills, as learning occurs through trial and error.

APPLICATION OF LITERATURE/DATA

Unfolding case studies were shown to facilitate the development of critical thinking, decision making, and self-confidence in nursing students in the classroom and in online environments (Bowman, 2017; Dehghanzadeh & Jafaraghaee, 2018; Hong & Yu, 2017; Meiers & Russell, 2019). Nurses and nurse practitioners use a wide array of skills in practice, to provide safe and effective care for patients.

Undergraduate Context

In a senior undergraduate nursing classroom, unfolding case studies were used as the teaching modality for a concept-based lesson on inflammation and immunity. In preparation for a lesson, students were provided assigned reading related to specific conditions of Guillain-Barré syndrome, multiple sclerosis, rheumatoid arthritis, scleroderma, and systemic lupus erythematosus. Students were introduced to the unfolding case study process at the beginning of class, then assigned to groups of six to seven students. Each group of students was provided an introduction to one of five patient scenarios. Students then periodically checked in with faculty as the case study unfolded. Students were expected to determine the appropriate nursing care for the patient in the assigned scenario by the end of the lesson. Each patient scenario unfolded into five parts with the patient introduction, physical examination, labs and diagnostics, medications and treatments, and putting it all together.

Part 1: Patient Introduction

The patient introduction section started with a brief history of the present illness. Students listed potential conditions the patient may be experiencing and were asked the following question: What further information and assessment data is needed to help differentiate between the potential conditions? Students then obtained physical assessment findings from the faculty before moving forward in the case study. Faculty checked-in with each student group to ensure the correct patient condition was identified. If a student group was on an incorrect path, students were encouraged to review additional information. The faculty also questioned students on further assessment data needed from the patient or the patient's chart.

Part 2: Physical Examination

In the second step, students were to determine anticipated labs, diagnostics, and consultations prior to calling the health care provider for orders. Challenge questions that students were to answer included: (1) What are the labs, diagnostics, and/or consults expected to be ordered by the health care provider? and (2) Knowing the patient's history, what contributing factors/risk factors do they have? The faculty discussed with each student group the anticipated labs, diagnostics, and consultations. The student group utilized SBAR (situation, background, assessment, and recommendation) communication and requested orders from the health care provider, a role played by the faculty member. During the recommendation stage, the faculty and student group discussed rationale for orders that may or may not have been provided. This helped to ensure the student group stayed on the correct path to meet the final objectives of the activity.

Part 3: Labs and Diagnostics

Students reviewed the orders from Part 2 and were provided the results of tests. Students were asked to determine the patient's condition based on the collected assessment data. Challenge questions asked in this part to promote critical thinking included the following: (1) What other manifestations/complications are you monitoring for? and (2) What medications and/or consults do you anticipate the health care provider ordering? Again, the students called the health care provider with the test results and orders were received from the health care provider (played by the faculty). During the recommendation stage, the faculty and student group discussed the rationale for the anticipated orders.

Part 4: Medications and Treatments

Students reviewed medications and treatments ordered by the health care provider. Challenge questions in this part asked students to (1) explain the rationale for each medication to the patient, (2) teach important side effects, and (3) list interventions and education to be provided to the newly diagnosed patient.

Part 5: Putting It All Together

The final question of the unfolding case study asked the students to discuss how the patient's condition related to the assigned concept(s). Each group then presented the patient and findings to the entire class. Through this process students were able to learn about the assigned conditions and compared and contrasted the conditions. At the end of the activity, faculty collected the unfolding case studies from the student groups and posted them within the learning management system (LMS) for students to access and utilize as a study guide.

Graduate Context

An online graduate advanced pathophysiology course used an unfolding case study approach via the LMS related to the weekly topic. It was utilized to facilitate diagnostic reasoning with first semester students, as research suggests unfolding case studies are important in developing clinical reasoning skills (Kantar & Massouh, 2015; Lawson, 2018; Pilcher, 2018). Additionally, students applied growing knowledge and understanding of pathophysiology in a creative assessment modality. Cases developed via a patient introduction section (chief complaint, history of present illness), followed by a patient interview (review of systems), and then a physical examination, concluding with diagnostic and laboratory data. Each section contained critical thinking questions to guide students, ultimately, to provide a diagnosis with rationale. Students worked individually through each section of the case study and were required to discuss other students' responses to a part or parts of the case study via the discussion board. Reading other students' work prompted some students to rethink the approach and/or answers previously provided. Faculty provided feedback to individual students after the assignment was complete. A case study review video was posted for students by faculty after the case study was complete to share the answers to each section with rationales.

Part 1: Patient Introduction

This section began with a brief history of present illness similar to what a provider would learn about a patient prior to a visit. Students were asked to provide a list of three differential diagnoses with rationale based on course learning materials. The following sections of the case study opened on a set date and time after the patient introduction responses were due. Each of those sections, as described later, provided the student with more data to analyze and synthesize into a final diagnosis. Ideally, the subsequent sections would open once the student turns in the previous section; however, that is precluded by limitations in the LMS.

Part 2: Patient Interview

More medical history and history of present illness information was shared in Part 2, including social and family history as well as medications and allergies. Patient questions that the student "provider" must answer were included in some case studies. Challenge questions for this section included the following: (1) How does this history help you rule a differential diagnosis in or out?, (2) What other questions do you have for the patient?, (3) What is important about the question(s) included for the patient?, and (4) What are your responses to questions the patient/family have for you?

Part 3: Physical Examination

Students were provided a focused physical examination based on patient symptoms including vital signs. To continue to build upon previous sections of the case study, the challenge questions for this section were the following: (1) What do these data suggest may be going on with the patient?, (2) What differential diagnoses can you discard and why?, (3) Hypothesize which differential diagnosis is the correct diagnosis, (4) What lab test/diagnostic test may be ordered and why?, and (5) What do you predict results will show based on the hypothesized diagnosis?

Part 4: Diagnosis/Solution

The final section provided students with results of any lab tests and other diagnostic studies performed on the case study patient. Final challenge questions ask the students to make a diagnosis based on all components of the case study and included the following prompts: (1) What diagnosis do you make?, and (2) Provide rationale based on course learning materials and explain the pathophysiology causing the disease/illness/syndrome.

Students shared in end-of-course evaluations how much benefit and enjoyment were gleaned from the unfolding case studies. One student commented, "I like how faculty incorporated case studies in this course and clarified it with a sample case study without leaving us wondering what to do. It created a confidence that would enable me to practice." Another student reported:

> Overall, I liked how the case study was set up. It made me use critical-thinking skills and the skills to research things to try to find the correct diagnosis and all the rationales that led to the diagnosis. Through this process of researching, gathering information, and critical thinking, I feel like I was able to grasp the knowledge about disease processes.

These comments demonstrated outcomes of the unfolding case study process highlighted in the literature review earlier.

APPLICATION TO CROSS-DISCIPLINARY CONTEXTS

The use of unfolding case studies in other education and health care fields has been widely documented. Meta-analyses of educational studies on real-world teaching strategies showed a significant effect on student learning (Hattie, 2009). Overall, these studies have found that real-world activities are very effective for lower achieving students and helped students build upon previously obtained knowledge. Similarly, a health care education literature review found these pedagogical methods were common in fields such as occupational therapy, allied health, child development, and dentistry (McLean, 2016). These studies involved both undergraduate and graduate students and unfolding case studies used in on-ground and online environments. Overall, these studies confirm the effectiveness of these types of teaching strategies across disciplines.

Furthermore, when integrated with clinical simulations, unfolding case studies have been effectively used to foster interprofessional competencies across health care disciplines (New et al., 2015; Zook et al., 2018). In these studies, students from different health care disciplines, such as nursing, medicine, psychology, speech-language pathology, and pharmacy, worked together on various unfolding case studies. Here, the focus was not just on developing health care–specific knowledge and skills, but also interprofessional teamwork skills. Other case study–based strategies that have been found to be effective in nursing and other health care disciplines include the use of simulated patients, simulation-based learning environments, and large-scale simulations (Gude et al., 2015; Jorm et al., 2016; Makransky et al., 2016; Rue & Doolen, 2015; Zimmerman et al., 2015). Each of these approaches can have a significant impact on student learning, attitudes, and interprofessional skills. As a result, we assert that this chapter's exploration of unfolding case studies in nursing will be applicable to health care educators in other fields.

ADDITIONAL RESOURCES

- The National League for Nursing (2019) provides several unfolding case studies on their website in the Advancing Care Excellence series. The Advancing Care Excellence series provides teacher-ready curricula focusing on the vulnerable populations of seniors, Alzheimer's patients and their caregivers, pediatrics, veterans, caregivers, and persons with disabilities:
  - http://www.nln.org/professional-development-programs/advancing-care-excellence-series
- The Quality and Safety Education for Nurses (2019) website provides several case studies for nurse educators to utilize as a teaching strategy in the classroom and simulation for undergraduate nursing students:
  - http://qsen.org/tag/case-studies

Example of Graduate Nursing Unfolding Case Study

- Part 1—Introduction
  - G. A. is a 59-year-old Black man who presents to the clinic with a 3-month history of progressive dyspnea, cough, and increasing amounts of mucus production, especially in the morning. He remembers having similar symptoms last winter that seemed to improve somewhat as the weather got warmer. However, the cough has not totally gone away.
  - Challenge Question:
    - List three differential diagnoses for the case described. Provide rationale based on course learning materials.
- Part 2—Patient Interview
  - G. A. reports that he usually coughs up minimal clear sputum during the day after fairly intense coughing with more mucus production after arising in the morning. He denies fever, chills, night sweats, weakness, muscle or joint aches, or bloody sputum. He does express increased fatigue and poor exercise tolerance. Walking upstairs to the second floor of his home leaves him out of breath. He denies tuberculosis, asbestos exposure, occupational exposure, heart disease, morning headaches, sleeping difficulty, or asthma; also denies dysphagia or throat pain. G. A. reports unintentional 25 lb weight loss over the last 5 years.
  - Past Medical/Surgical History: H/O depression w/ one suicide attempt at 22 years old, HTN x 15 years, L lateral malleolus fracture 2015 (s/p surgical repair), acute bronchitis x 3 since December 2018, mild CVA 5 months ago with no residual deficits
  - Family History:
    - Mom: alive, 87 years old, COPD and on oxygen; Dad: deceased 50 years old, lung cancer; one sister, age 62 years old with HTN, bronchiectasis, three children without chronic medical issues
  - Social History: two ppd Camel cigarettes, H/O excessive ETOH, currently social use of ETOH, denies illicit drugs, works at beef packing plant, divorced, lives with mom
  - Medications: HCTZ 25 mg PO daily, amlodipine 5 mg PO daily, aspirin 325 mg PO daily, clopidogrel (Plavix) 75 mg PO daily
  - Allergies: NKDA
  - Challenge Questions:
    - How does this history help you rule a differential diagnosis in or out?
    - What other questions do you have for the patient? What is important about the question(s) included for the patient?
    - What are your responses to questions the patient and family have for you?

- Part 3—Physical Examination
  - Vital Signs: BP 166/95, HR 110, RR 26, T 97.5°F, weight 141 lbs, height 5'11"
  - Constitutional: Thin, appears older than stated age, ill appearing. Skin: Cold and dry, poor turgor noted, no cyanosis, nodules, masses, rashes, or jaundice. HEENT: PERRLA, anicteric; tympanic membrane intact, pearly gray bilaterally with cone of light at 5 o'clock position (R) and 7 o'clock position (L); mucous membranes dry and intact; palate intact; pharynx without exudate or erythema; (+) pursed lip breathing; poor dentition. Neck: Supple without masses, thyroid without masses or edema, complete range of motion, no carotid bruits noted bilaterally, nonpalpable lymph nodes, mild JVD bilaterally. Lungs: Use of accessory muscles at rest, barrel chest appearance, poor diaphragmatic excursion bilaterally, hyper resonant to percussion, diminished lung sounds throughout, prolonged exhalation with occasional wheeze, no rhonchi/crackles noted bilaterally, (-) axillary/supraclavicular lymphadenopathy. CV: Tachycardic and regular rate, no murmur/gallops/rubs, prominent S3, radial and dorsalis pedis pulses 2+ bilaterally, capillary refill less than 2 seconds. GI: Soft, nondistended, normoactive bowel sounds in all 4 quadrants, negative hepatosplenomegaly. Neuro: Alert and oriented x4, no focal deficits, CN II-XII intact, sensation intact UE/LE bilaterally, steady gait. Extremities: 1+ LE edema bilaterally, cyanotic nail beds UE/LE, mild clubbing UE/LE. MSK: Full ROM in all joints, no crepitus/edema/erythema/pain in any joints.
  - Challenge Questions:
    - What do these data suggest may be going on with the patient?
    - What differential diagnoses can you discard and why? Hypothesize which differential diagnosis is the correct diagnosis.
    - What lab test/diagnostic test may be ordered and why?
    - What do you predict results will show based on hypothesized diagnosis?
- Part 4—Diagnosis/Solution. The following diagnostic tests were performed:
  - CMP: Na 146 mEq/L, K 4.3 mEq/L, Cl 113 mEq/L, Ca2+ 8.9 mg/dL, Bicarbonate 25 meq/L, Blood Urea Nitrogen 29 mg/dL, Creatinine 1.2 mg/dL, Glucose (fasting) 89 mg/dL, PO4 3.5 mg/dL, Mg 2.5 mg/dL. CBC: WBC 9,200/mm^3, PMNeutros 65%, Lymphs 28%, Monos 6%, Basos 1%, Eos 3%, Hct 56%, Hgb 19.1 g/dL, Plt 176,000/mm^3. LFTs: Aspartate aminotransferase 14 IU/L, Alanine aminotransferase 36 IU/L, Total Bilirubin 0.2 mg/dL, Albumin 3.9 g/dL, Protein, total 6.6 g/dL, Alk phos 78 IU/L, Alpha1-antitrypsin 137 mg/dL. ABG: pH 7.32, PaO$_2$ 65 mmHg, PaCO$_2$ 54 mmHg, SaO$_2$ 90%.
  - Pulmonary Function Tests: FEV1=1.67 L (45% of expected), FVC=4.20 L (85% of expected), FEV1/FVC=0.41 (expected 0.77)
  - Chest X-Ray: Impression: Hyperinflation with flattened diaphragm; large anteroposterior diameter, diffuse scarring and bullae in all lung fields, especially prominent in bilateral lower lobes; no effusions or infiltrates; large pulmonary vasculature
  - Challenge Questions:
    - What diagnosis do you make? Provide rationale based on course learning materials.
    - Explain the pathophysiology causing the disease/illness/syndrome.

REFERENCES

Bowman, K. (2017). Use of online unfolding case studies to foster critical thinking. *Journal of Nursing Education, 56*(11), 701-702. https://doi.org/10.3928/01484834-20171020-13

Dehghanzadeh, S., & Jafaraghaee, F. (2018). Comparing the effects of traditional lecture and flipped classroom on nursing students' critical thinking disposition: A quasi-experimental study. *Nurse Education Today, 71*, 151-156. https://doi.org/10.1016/j.nedt.2018.09.027

Granger, T., Zappas, M., Walton-Moss, B., & O'Neill, S. P. (2018). A patient panel of case studies to teach across the family nurse practitioner curriculum. *Journal of Nursing Education. 57*(8), 512. https://doi.org/10.3928/01484834-20180720-14

Gude, T., Grimstad, H., Holen, A., Anvik, T., Baerheim, A., Fasmer, O. B., Hjortdahl, P., & Vaglumet, P. (2015). Can we rely on simulated patients' satisfaction with their consultation for assessing medical students' communication skills? A cross-sectional study. *BMC Medical Education, 15*, 225. https://doi.org/10.1186/s12909-015-0508-x

Hattie, J. (2009). *Visible learning: A synthesis of over 800 meta-analyses relating to achievement* (pp. 230-231). Routledge.

Hong, S., & Yu, P. (2017). Comparison of the effectiveness of two styles of case-based learning implemented in lectures for developing nursing students' critical thinking ability: A randomized controlled trial. *International Journal of Nursing Studies, 68*, 16-24. http://dx.doi.org/doi:10.1016/j.ijnurstu.2016.12.008

Jorm, C., Lim, R., Roper, J., Skinner, C., Robertson, J., Gentilcore, S., & Osomanski, A. (2016). A large-scale mass casualty simulation to develop the non-technical skills medical students require for collaborative teamwork. *BMC Medical Education, 16*(1), 1-10. https://doi.org/10.1186/s12909-016-0588-2

Kantar, L. D., & Massouh, A. (2015). Case-based learning: What traditional curricula fail to teach. *Nurse Education Today, 35*(8), e8-e14.

Kaylor, S. K., & Strickland, H. P. (2015). Unfolding case studies as a formative teaching methodology for novice nursing students. *Journal of Nursing Education, 54*(2), 106-110.

Lawson, T. N. (2018). Diagnostic reasoning and cognitive biases of nurse practitioners. *Journal of Nursing Education, 57*(4), 203-208. https://doi.org/10.3928/01484834-20180322-03

Makransky, G., Bonde, M. T., Wulff, J., Wandall, J., Hood, M., Creed, P. A., Bache, I., Silahtaroglu, A., & Nørremølle, A. (2016). Simulation based virtual learning environment in medical genetics counseling: An example of bridging the gap between theory and practice in medical education. *BMC Medical Education, 16*, 2-9.

McLean, S. F. (2016). Case-based learning and its application in medical and health-care fields: A review of worldwide literature. *Journal of Medical Education and Curricular Development, 3*, 39-49. https://doi.org/10.4137/JMECD.S20377

Meiers, J., & Russell, M. J. (2019). An unfolding case study: Supporting contextual psychomotor skill development in novice nursing students. *International Journal of Nursing Education Scholarship, 16*(1), 1-9. https://doi.org/10.1515/ijnes-2018-0013

National League for Nursing (2019). Advancing Care Excellence series. http://www.nln.org/professional-development-programs/advancing-care-excellence-series

New, S. N., Huff, D. C., Hutchison, L. C., Bilbruck, T. J., Ragsdale, P. S., Jennings, J. E., & Greenfield, T. M. (2015). Integrating collaborative interprofessional simulation into pre-licensure health care programs. *Nursing Education Perspectives, 36*(6), 396-397.

O'Rourke, J., & Zerwic, J. (2016). Measure of clinical decision-making abilities of nurse practitioner students. *Journal of Nursing Education, 55*(1), 18-23. https://doi.org/10.3928/01484834-20151214-06

Peery, A. I. (2015). Use of the unfolding case study in teaching nurse educator master of science in nursing students. *Journal of Nursing Education, 54*(3), 180.

Phillips, J. M. (2016). Strategies to promote student engagement and active learning. In D. Billings & J. Halstead (Eds.), *Teaching in nursing: A guide for faculty* (5th ed., pp. 255-256). Elsevier.

Pilcher, J. (2018). Promoting learning using case-based strategies in nursing professional development. *Journal for Nurses in Professional Development, 34*(4), 199-205.

Quality and Safety Education for Nurses. (2019). Tag: Case studies. http://qsen.org/tag/case-studies/

Rue, S., & Doolen, J. (2015). Pseudostandardized patients in undergraduate nursing health assessment. *Journal of Nursing Education, 54*(11) 663-664. https://doi.org/10.3928/01484834-20151016-11

Snegirev, S. (2016, October 31). Branching scenarios: What you need to know. *eLearning Industry.* https://elearningindustry.com/branching-scenarios-need-know

Vogt, M. A., & Schaffner, B. H. (2016). Evaluating interactive technology for evolving case study on learning and satisfaction of graduate nursing students. *Nurse Education in Practice, 19*, 79-83.

Zimmermann, K., Bachmann Holzinger, I., Ganassi, L., Esslinger, P., Pilgrim, S., Allen, M., Burmester, M., & Stocker, M. (2015). Inter-professional in-situ simulated team and resuscitation training for patient safety: Description and impact of a programmatic approach. *BMC Medical Education, 15*, 189. https://doi.org/10.1186/s12909-015-0472-5

Zook, S. S., Hulton, L. J., Dudding, C. C., Stewart, A. L., & Graham, A. C. (2018). Scaffolding interprofessional education. *Nurse Educator, 43*(2), 87-91. https://doi.org/10.1097/NNE.0000000000000430

21

A LITTLE BIT OF SUGAR
Creating Powerful Learning Experiences by Integrating Unfolding Cases and Zull's Neuroscience

Carole Bennett, PhD, PMHCS-BC

DESCRIPTION OF TEACHING/LEARNING CONTEXT

Several years ago, in a new job, I was asked to design a course for family nurse practitioner students, which would prepare them for treating common psychiatric symptoms of depression, anxiety, insomnia, and stress in primary care. Uncomplicated mental health care had shifted to primary care and most people without serious mental illness, such as schizophrenia or bipolar disorder, were relying on their primary care provider to treat mild to moderate cases of anxiety and depression. In addition, people with serious mental illness were now receiving health care from primary care providers who had little instruction regarding mental illness and health concerns that may be related (Druss et al., 2010).

At the same time, as a gift in that new job, the dean of my college gave me a copy of James E. Zull's (2002) *The Art of Changing the Brain: Enriching the Practice of Teaching by Exploring the Biology of Learning*. It was this coincidence that created an opportunity for me to apply Zull's ideas about stimulating different parts of the brain during learning, in essence, changing the brain as a teaching/learning tool. As a neuroscientist, he had developed a teaching strategy that, by assigning different types of learning tasks to the students, would engage multiple parts of the brain sequentially. Using this process, the students link multiple small brain networks together into large, complex networks, which would allow them to respond effectively to complex situations in this teaching/learning process that is then transferable to clinical practice (Perry, 2015).

Friberg, J. C., Visconti, C. F., & Ginsberg, S. M. (Eds.). *Evidence-Based Education in the Classroom: Examples From Clinical Disciplines* (pp. 185-192).

Based on years of advanced clinical practice in psychiatric nursing, I recognized that most patients present with what the casual observer could assume to be a simple complaint, such as "I am tired all the time," but, which after a thorough investigation, is recognized to be a very complicated often contentious situation that the patent is hoping you will recognize and lead them through to a healthy resolution. First of all, I wanted my students to experience the practice of supporting a patient through a guided process of treatment and education toward health and improved quality of life. I also wanted them to develop a systematic approach to this process, as Tanner described in her editorial, *The Case for Cases: A Pedagogy for Developing Habits of Thought* (Tanner, 2009), which I believed would translate to their clinical practice and encourage them to become excellent nurse practitioners. To this end, I thought that using unfolding case studies as a deliberative, engaged process while applying Zull's learning strategies would challenge my students to develop critical-thinking skills (Bowman, 2017) applicable to any clinical setting. To describe the implementation of this practice, this chapter describes a course that integrates these two teaching strategies of using unfolding case studies with brain-based types of learning (i.e., watching, listening, recalling, describing, investigating, integrating, testing hypotheses), which alternately uses cognitive and emotional centers of the brain to stimulate complex learning with significant retention over time.

REVIEW OF LITERATURE

Unfolding Case Studies

In today's health care environment, nurse practitioners must be prepared to diagnose and treat people with complex comorbid illnesses; one of these illnesses is, all too often, addiction. Unfolding case studies can prepare students for that challenge. Unfortunately, most texts explore individual classes of diagnoses separately and fail to adequately prepare students for the diversity and complexity of real-world cases in clinical practice (Granger et al., 2018). Case studies have been used successfully in health care education to integrate multiple learning objectives in a single case, which is carefully designed and authentically presented. Beers and Bowden (2005), in comparing a traditional lecture format and a case-based learning format for teaching endocrine disorders, found that immediately following the learning experience, students tested similarly on the content. However, when retesting the students a year following the learning experiences, the students who had learned from a case-based method scored significantly higher than the students who had received the traditional lecture; perhaps because case studies engage students both cognitively and emotionally, making the experience meaningful to them and, therefore, more memorable. Bowe and colleagues (2009) found that multiple clinical problems could be successfully introduced to medical students within one case, and that this type of instruction led to an engaged discussion relating biological processes to clinical presentation.

Anderson and Bradshaw (2016) describe a face-to-face classroom experience teaching human development to graduate students using an interrupted case study method. Over an 8-week period using a documentary film that followed several individuals from 7 years old to 54 years old, while using previous knowledge of developmental theorists, students hypothesized, made predictions, and then discovered the pattern of development of these individuals was revealed. Over the course of the experience, students showed an increase in complex levels of clinical thinking, which demonstrated the method's effectiveness. These authors also described their views that students' ongoing curiosity related to these cases stimulated students forward to pursue clinical knowledge and understanding.

Personally and anecdotally, I have found the unfolding case study method to be very adaptable. It allows for information to be provided over time to students to consider and reconsider when engaged in clinical thinking. Additionally, an entire case can be changed suddenly by posting a phone message from a patient requesting a prescription for opiates, a report of a visit to an emergency room where the patient reported suicidal thoughts, or news of an unexpected discovery of stimulants in a drug screen. The use of unexpected findings requires that patient priorities suddenly shift forcing the student's thinking process to expand.

Brain-Based Model of Adult Learning

The idea that the brain can change its own structure and function through thought and activity is, I believe, the most important alteration in our view of the brain since we first sketched out its basic anatomy and the workings of its basic component, the neuron. (Doidge, 2007, p. xix)

Zull (2004), in applying this idea of changing the brain as a learning tool, interweaves the ideas of neuroscience with learning. He points out that all nervous systems have three basic elements: sensory elements that respond to outside stimuli, motor elements that generate action, and association elements that link sensory and motor. It is the strategic use of these elements that change the brain while learning. His ideas are based on scientific research conducted on learning to juggle. In this research, magnetic resonance imaging was done before and after the subjects were taught to juggle. It was discovered that learning to juggle produced more density of brain cells in specific regions of the brain and convinced Zull that learning actually changes the brain (Draganski et al., 2004). Based on this work, he developed a model of teaching in which regions of the brain are repeatedly stimulated changing neuronal cell density and extending neuronal networks.

He explains that the neocortex, the large forebrain that differentiates humans, is organized into two large areas for cognitive association, which is essential for understanding. Insight into unsolved problems, which occurs in the back half of the neocortex, comes slowly and needs time for associations to become apparent. However, the frontal neocortex is heavily engaged in conscious associations by sorting and organizing memories and information necessary for recall and application to problem solving and creativity. The frontal neocortical region sends signals to the motor regions for control of movement. There are neurons that modify the signaling through the production and distribution of neurotransmitters associated with emotional responses. Zull (2004) wrote that learning is most powerful and long-lasting when multiple neocortical regions are engaged. Thus, the more regions of the cortex that are used, the more neurological change will occur, creating a more potent learning experience (Table 21-1, Steps 1 through 8).

APPLICATION OF LITERATURE/DATA

Course Planning

My colleagues and I decided that in a class of 13 weeks, we would develop four cases for use, each lasting for 3 weeks. We wanted the students to work with cases that would help them to develop habits of effective clinical thinking but still provide enough time that the unsolved problems could "gestate" creating deeper understanding and insights for the students.

Each unfolding case study was developed by taping four large pieces of paper on the wall, following a process outlined by Bennett and colleagues (2011). Each piece of paper represented one case study. Patient descriptions, including age, race, and gender, were created for each case and recorded on the hanging paper. My colleagues and I discussed the psychiatric disorders and addictions that students would explore and learn about in the course and selected four to focus on, one for each case. Each of these was added to the four papers. Following the same process, we considered various personality disorders that we thought students would encounter, as well as clinical emergencies and challenges that patients with such conditions often present. Four were selected for our cases and recorded. After outlining the demographic information, psychiatric disorders, and other conditions germane to our course on the four papers, we had established a framework for our four cases.

Following this, I wrote a brief script to accompany each case, found friend actors (faculty members and family), and began videotaping the cases for use in my course. To create dramatic effect and to challenge our students' observation skills, eyeshadow was used to make bruise marks on one young woman patient's upper arms to look as though she had been grabbed and shaken. An eyeliner

TABLE 21-1

Zull's Brain-Based Learning Model

STEPS IN PROCESS	BRAIN ENGAGEMENT
Step 1: Watch online video of patient	Sensory organs: Vision area in very back of neocortex/hearing area close to ears/amygdala to determine emotional response. Integrative cortex to give cognitive meaning through release of neurotransmitters.
Step 2: Post online regarding previous knowledge	Locate in brain previous experience and knowledge. Zull believes building on existing knowledge and neuronal networks is critical, encourages unity and efficiency.
Step 3: History, physical, and family genogram revealed	Sensory organs and integrative cortex in back of neocortex: Integrative cortex with previous neuronal network building larger networks (let tangles lie). Zull believes that it is best to leave misinformation alone and do not attend to it. He finds that if not attended to, the new information will take over and misinformation will be forgotten.
Step 4: Find screening tools, order labs	Associations formed in front and rear of neocortex. Students struggle to find solutions to new and untried challenges/reflections/ideas are bounced around brain literally looking for connections.
Step 5: As a group, generate eight clinical problems	Integrate experiences, working memory, in back neocortex, send to front neocortex to add information, make executive decisions, sort and organize knowledge, emotional responses to inequities, victimization, stress. These are abstract ideas and therefore risky. A search of the literature and assigned readings gives students the confidence to accept the ideas.
Step 6: Develop differential diagnoses	Visual/sensory stimulation integrates associations: Act with investment. Generates emotional response produces acetylcholine, whose job it is to cause chemicals to be released, which make synapses more responsive. When synapses get repeated signaling, it forms stronger and stronger bonds, which causes the brain to be changed and synapses to grow in responsiveness.
Step 7: Search literature	Connect visual integrative and back integrative cortex, to front neocortex to add information and to integrate finding, creating unity.
Step 8: Synthesis and final treatment plan	Action from discussion and focused writing/data flow into motor cortex.

pencil was used to make multiple superficial scars across the wrist of a teenager. Then "patients" delivered their lines, one phrase at a time while I videotaped them using my iPhone (Apple) in our simulation center examining room. The video was easily edited on my computer (see Additional Resources) and uploaded into the course management system for the course. We completed histories, physicals, and genograms for each case and uploaded those into the software, too.

Then, guided by Zull's brain-based model, the following process for unfolding each case was created (Table 21-2):

1. Students watched the initial video of the patient with their presenting complaint and posted in the discussion board, comparing the case to a similar case or experience that they had previously encountered.

2. The case unfolds further when the history, physical, and family genogram are made available. Students are organized into groups of four to discuss the case and order labs appropriate for the case. They research to find out which screening tools they think are appropriate for this patient and request that the patient complete the selected tool.

3. Lab results are posted, and screening tools are filled out by faculty (acting as the patient depicted in the case) and posted. Students must score the screens and interpret findings. Through this process, students were required to locate information on their own, using their own ingenuity to identify resources and supports for their work, as though they were in the clinic searching for information as the need arises.

4. Based on their review of each case to this point, each group must identify eight possible clinical problems for the patient depicted in the case. These are shared with and approved by the course instructor. Cases are deliberately designed with rich texture so that eight (or more) clinical problems and their appropriate psychiatric diagnoses might be identified. These are hinted at in the genogram or history (i.e., a patient's older parent with dementia who lives in an apartment in the backyard; a sister with a live-in boyfriend who drinks too much and neglects her children; a husband who is a police officer and faces danger daily, who is also depressed and has multiple firearms in the house).

5. Each group member researches two of the possible clinical problems and diagnoses using a rubric that guides them to relevant research (e.g., data on health inequities) and to specific websites with treatment guidelines, etc. They then post their research findings on an open discussion board and are encouraged to read each other's posts.

6. From here, each group develops a differential diagnosis, a final diagnosis, and a comprehensive, evidence-based treatment plan based on their discussion postings. Treatment plans are graded and various groups are asked to present sections of their plans and discuss their decision-making process during an online class.

During this complete process, online classrooms are provided for groups to meet in, and a template is provided in a care plan format to provide easy access for sharing information while completing work.

As the case unfolds and students identify their clinical problems, they learn wide-ranging but relevant information that must be considered in treating psychiatric diagnoses and related problems that they will face within primary care practice. They learn the process of noticing, questioning, gathering, researching, integrating, and ultimately, managing complex health problems and finding appropriate treatment guidelines and recommendations. Then, they must prioritize those treatment options and present a coherent plan to the patient without overwhelming the patient. It is a complex, nuanced learning experience, which they work through over a 3-week time frame as the case slowly unfolds and they engage many areas of the brain to gain insight and respond.

TABLE 21-2

Interactive Process With Unfolding Case

STEPS IN PROCESS	STUDENT LEARNING BEHAVIORS
Step 1: Watch brief case video of patient with presenting complaint	Observe verbal and nonverbal expressions of concerns. Listen for emotional expression of distress and any unusual physical presentations.
Step 2: Recall previous relevant knowledge and experience of similar patient	Post in online discussion board.
Step 3: Review history and physical, family genogram opens	After reading the history and physical, family genogram, and key, have online discussion with group to discuss which lab tests are most important and consider genetics. Email orders to instructor.
Step 4: Find screening tools, which can help to rule certain illnesses in or out	Make requests to instructor for screens to be completed by patient.
Step 5: Identify eight clinical problems as a group	Consider physical, emotional, family, interpersonal, environmental, cultural, work-related, age-related, race-related, previous trauma–related factors. Make a list for approval by instructor (hypothesis testing, metacognitive process, from individual patients to identify risk factors and vulnerabilities of groups). Get list approved.
Step 6: Review lab results and interpret screens	Synthesize with previous history and physical, and develop differential diagnoses. Score and interpret, and extend differential diagnoses.
Step 7: Explore literature for evidence-based treatment and synthesize	Post in online discussion board two clinical problems per student using rubric. Online group discussion as a treatment team to make treatment decisions.
Step 8: Write final treatment plan	Work in doc.x to present integrated treatment plan using the rubric. Sections of treatment plans and discussion boards are presented in an online class to finalize treatment plan and explore multiple learning process objectives with this case.

Exemplar Case Study

Case Unfolds on Video

A 24-year-old woman presents, and when asked, "What can I do for you today," she states, "I don't know what is wrong with me. I am tired, crying all the time. I don't understand what has happened. My boyfriend gets angry with me when I act like this. I want to stop, but I can't. Something is wrong, but I don't know what it is." She starts to cry. Viewers learn that she works as an x-ray technician at a local hospital and lives with her boyfriend who is a lawyer. She says he is stressed constantly over his work. Although the patient does not mention it, you can see that she has bilateral bruises on her upper arms.

Student Action

Students immediately respond about similar patients, friends, and family members they have known with similar concerns; women they have seen in the emergency department or roommates they have had in the past. They reference bits of previously acquired information that is relevant and start to speculate about diagnoses. They gather in their group to decide on lab tests and screening tools, emailing those requests to the instructor, and while waiting for results, begin to work on listing eight clinical problems. They often get focused on obscure problems or minute irregularities and need guidance to consider the large metacognitive issues that are illustrated by this case. Tables 21-1 and 21-2 provide further information about this process.

Case Unfolds (Posted in Course Management Software)

The patient's lab tests reveal that she is pregnant and has opiate and benzodiazepine metabolites in her urine drug screen. Screening tools reveal that she has depression (which is severe), somatic symptom disorder, and addiction to pain medication in addition to her unplanned pregnancy. She admits to her boyfriend's abuse on a domestic violence screening.

Student Action

Students begin to discuss as a group, asking questions such as the following: What are the options for this patient? What are the health effects of unplanned pregnancies? Will she opt to terminate the pregnancy? What are the current laws in this state? How will her boyfriend respond to this news? Is she a safety risk? Where is there a women's shelter locally? How do I approach her about this issue? What are my responsibilities? Is she injecting opiates? Has she shared needles? Does she have hepatitis C? What is recommended for treatment of opiate addiction during pregnancy? What risks are involved with benzodiazepine exposure in utero? How is withdrawal from benzodiazepines managed pharmacologically? Because she is an x-ray technician, has the baby had radiation exposure? How do you treat depression during pregnancy? What are treatment guidelines during pregnancy and breastfeeding? Is intrauterine exposure a concern with antidepressants? What social support does she have? Could her boyfriend be encouraging her drug misuse? Is she diverting narcotics from her hospital job? What is the impact of narcotic diversion by health care providers? Can she lose her license and job if this is exposed? What decisions and plans need to be made before she leaves your office? Might she become suicidal? These are just a few of the concerns that students will research and consider while planning care for this woman.

Once the case has unfolded, the students must integrate their researched information, identify realistic priorities, develop a coherent plan, and decide how the plan will be presented to the patient. They must decide on a sequence of events that the patient will be guided through, using conjoint decision making. They must consider prevention as well as intervention strategies. The students together practice making discrete clinical judgments about this patient's future care and identify contingency plans depending on the patient's decisions. They also must consider the unborn child and the potential impact on that child's future health and the baby's father and how he will be integrated into this process if that is his and the patient's wishes. These real-life scenarios engage the students in an effective simulation for the comprehensive, moment-to-moment thinking process of a clinical problem for a nurse practitioner. The more textured the clinical problem is, the more effective the learning process becomes, engaging multiple areas of the brain; this is Zull's learning through brain change.

APPLICATION TO CROSS-DISCIPLINARY CONTEXTS

Case-based learning is currently utilized in many disciplines, including medical education and nursing education, with all levels of students. As availability for specific clinical experiences become more competitive and simulation becomes increasingly important, this method of extending brief patient descriptions to create complex cases that unfold over time is a viable option for teaching in all clinical disciplines, particularly in preparation of clinicians who treat patients over time with multiple chronic illnesses and vulnerabilities. Using an iPhone and easily available computer software for video editing, faculty members can create unfolding cases to teach and challenge students in any clinical discipline. While the quality of the video is not highly professional, with the proliferation of YouTube and self-documenting on social media, students are unfazed by this aspect of the experience and respond enthusiastically to the challenge.

ADDITIONAL RESOURCES

- Zull, J. E. (2002). *The art of changing the brain: Enriching the practice of teaching by exploring the biology of learning.* Stylus.
- An interview with James E. Zull:
  - https://sharpbrains.com/blog/2006/10/12/an-ape-can-do-this-can-we-not/
- *The Brain That Changes Itself: A Documentary:*
  - https://www.youtube.com/watch?v=bFCOm1P_cQQ
- *TED Talk: The Woman Who Changed her Brain:*
  - https://www.youtube.com/watch?v=o0td5aw1KXA
- iMovie Basics: Video editing tutorial for beginners:
  - https://www.youtube.com/watch?v=VF2mUJ0P3xU
- iPhone movies:
  - https://www.youtube.com/watch?v=g8a4F6mVX64

REFERENCES

Anderson, J. W., & Bradshaw, S. (2016). Using interrupted video case studies to teach developmental theory: A pilot study. *Gauisus, 4,* 1-11.

Bennett, C., Kennedy, S., & Donato, A. (2011). Preparing NPs for primary care: Unraveling complexity with unfolding cases. *Journal of Nursing Education, 50*(6), 328-331.

Beers, G., & Bowden, S. (2005). The effect of teaching method on long term knowledge retention. *Journal of Nursing Education, 44,* 511-514.

Bowe, C., Voss, J., & Aretz, T. (2009). Case method teaching: An effective approach to integrate the basic and clinical sciences in the preclinical medical curriculum. *Medical Teacher, 31,* 834-841.

Bowman, K. (2017). Use of on-line unfolding case studies to foster critical thinking. *Journal of Nursing Education, 56*(11), 701-702.

Doidge, N. (2007). *The brain that changes itself: Stories of personal triumph from the frontiers of brain science.* Penguin Group.

Draganski, B., Gaser, C., Busch, V., Schulerer, G., Bogdahan, U., & May, A. (2004). Neuroplasticity: Changes in grey matter induced by training. *Nature, 427,* 311-312.

Druss, B., Mays, R., Edwards, V., & Chapman, D. (2010). Primary care, public health, and mental health. *Preventing Chronic Disease, 7*(1), 1-2.

Granger, T., Zappas, M., Walton-Moss, B., & O'Niell, S. P. (2018). A patient panel of case studies to teach across the Family Nurse Practitioner curriculum. *Journal of Nursing Education, 57*(8), 512.

Perry, A. I. (2015). Use of unfolding case study in teaching nurse educator master of science in nursing students. *Journal of Nursing Education, 54*(3), 180.

Tanner, C. (2009). The case for cases: A pedagogy for developing habits of thought. *Journal of Nursing Education, 48*(6), 299-230.

Zull, J. E. (2002). *The art of changing the brain: Enriching the practice of teaching by exploring the biology of learning.* Stylus.

Zull, J. E. (2004). Key aspects of how the brain learns. *New Directions for Adult and Continuing Education, 110,* 3-9.

CASE-BASED PERSPECTIVE TAKING
A New Active Learning Pedagogy

Jennifer C. Friberg, EdD, CCC-SLP, F-ASHA
and Lisa A. Vinney, PhD, CCC-SLP

DESCRIPTION OF TEACHING/LEARNING CONTEXT

Several semesters ago, we developed an independent study experience for our undergraduate speech-language pathology students focused on the interprofessional management of laryngeal cancer. Our intention in planning this independent study experience was that students would complete topical readings each week, then meet in a group of 10 to 12 students to engage in a fruitful discussion related to fictional patient cases. We hoped by arranging the independent study in this way, students would better understand the patients and families experience at specific time frames: before, during, and after a diagnosis of laryngeal cancer.

This chapter describes the combination of two evidence-based pedagogies for use with students enrolled in our independent study. A high-level summary of analyses undertaken to assess the effectiveness of the new pedagogy is presented, as well. That we do not provide in-depth data on the impact of our new pedagogy in this chapter is intentional, as we felt there was value in exploring the processes undertaken to develop what we have termed *case-based perspective taking*. Thus, this chapter serves as an example of application of extant research on teaching and learning to optimize student outcomes in the learning experience we subsequently describe.

Friberg, J. C., Visconti, C. F., & Ginsberg, S. M. (Eds.). *Evidence-Based Education in the Classroom: Examples From Clinical Disciplines* (pp. 193-197).

REVIEW OF LITERATURE

Based in large part on the clinical nature of our independent study subject matter, we both felt that a case-based learning approach would be ideal for our students. However, we also hoped to encourage our students to develop a deeper understanding of health care professionals' roles in the assessment and treatment of laryngeal cancer. We were not certain that case-based learning alone would facilitate this objective. Thus, we investigated case-based learning more deeply and found an additional pedagogy—*perspective taking*—that we felt could be used in conjunction with case-based learning as part of our independent study planning. Both case-based learning and perspective taking are described in the following sections.

Case-Based Learning

Case-based learning is an active learning pedagogy that requires students to analyze realistic case scenarios collaboratively and cooperatively. For students representing clinical disciplines (e.g., nursing, dietetics, physical/occupational/speech therapy), case-based learning engages students in clinical reasoning that requires deep (higher level) versus surface processing of information (Biggs, 2003). In particular, students are tasked with applying their current knowledge and understanding of a topic based on a specific clinical case scenario in order to analyze case features and synthesize potential management strategies (Trommelen et al., 2017). The implementation of case-based learning has been tied to significantly better test performance from pre to posttest when compared to lecture alone (Datta & Ray, 2016). Furthermore, discussions surrounding cases afford the opportunity to engage in cooperative learning and may enhance emotional engagement with content to foster learning outcomes and improve student interactions (Foran, 2002; Nkhoma et al., 2017).

Perspective Taking

de Bono's "six thinking hats" (1985) is a strategic pedagogy that can be used to facilitate metacognitive awareness via a framework for students to engage in six different thinking processes, represented by different colored hats students could wear when applying each process and when examining cases, questions, or problems such as the following:

1. Reporting factual evidence
2. Questioning assumptions and/or working with peers to think about topics differently
3. Advocating for alternative ideas to be developed and shared
4. Challenging problematic aspects of a topic or potential solution
5. Using emotion to engage with the topic
6. Self-regulating and reflecting upon discussion to make decisions regarding a topical problem

In particular, applying these thinking strategies in parallel as a topic is discussed may promote metacognitive knowledge and practice of metacognitive regulation.

APPLICATION OF LITERATURE/DATA

Given our review of these two approaches, the combination of case-based learning and perspective taking to create a case-based perspective taking (CBPT) pedagogy seemed advantageous. We viewed CBPT as a vehicle to engage our students in discussions about specific patient cases while integrating the six hats strategy implicitly, asking students to think as if they were a doctor, nurse, speech-language pathologist, spouse, dietitian, employer, child, psychologist, etc. Thus, rather than assigning a thinking process to each student, we assigned a perspective to be represented so students could more fully understand what it was like to think like each stakeholder. We hypothesized CBPT would lead to students' integration of a number of different perspectives into a final solution for each case.

What impacts could we expect based on research on the separate case-based learning and perspective-taking pedagogies? There is evidence that case-based learning may allow students to expand content knowledge and practice effective communication in scenarios that may be put into practice during students' future work (Nkhoma et al., 2017). Research on perspective taking supports its effectiveness in facilitating empathy in a number of situations, which, in turn, may improve professional practice (Blatt et al., 2010; Galinsky & Ku, 2004; Vescio et al., 2003). What is unknown is the efficacy of case-based learning and perspective taking when combined. Thus, CBPT was studied across two independent study cohorts.

Original Data

Over the course of two semesters, 19 students met with one or more facilitators for weekly 1-hour discussion sessions. Students prepared for each independent study session by completing preselected readings from an assigned text (Friberg & Vinney, 2017). During independent study meetings, facilitators introduced a series of CBPT activities related to the content of their assigned readings. These activities required that students represent the perspective of various stakeholders important to the management of laryngeal cancer (e.g., patient, family, doctor, psychologist, employer) in specific clinical cases to discuss various topics. See the Additional Resources section later in this chapter for an exemplar CBPT activity.

Measuring Case-Based Perspective Taking

The implementation of CBPT was studied systematically across independent study students to determine the efficacy of this pedagogy (for detailed results, see Vinney et al., 2019). Data analyzed suggest that CBPT is a pedagogy that may increase both metacognition and higher-level cognitive processing. Summarized weekly reflections from students involved in the independent study cohorts as well as pre and postindependent study experience scores on the Metacognitive Awareness Inventory (MAI; Schraw & Dennison, 1994) were analyzed to determine the effect of CBPT. The MAI measures metacognitive awareness across eight domains related to two foci:

1. Knowledge of one's own cognition, which corresponds to what students know about themselves, thinking/learning strategies, and the utility of these strategies

2. Regulation of one's own cognition, which relates to knowledge about how students plan, monitor, and evaluate their learning

Analysis of MAI data indicated statistically significant increases in students' metacognitive abilities from preindependent study to postindependent study time frames, particularly in the areas of planning and evaluating learning. These areas of growth are consistent with students' independent study experiences where they routinely evaluated their own learning and planned for next steps to add to their content knowledge specific to laryngeal cancer.

Additionally, a sentence-by-sentence analysis of student reflection data from weeks 1, 4, and 8 of the independent study experience was completed using Bloom's taxonomy to examine changes in students' thinking relative to independent study content (Bloom et al., 1956). Analyses were conducted by a trained graduate student. Data indicated changes in the complexity of students' cognitive processing over time. More reflection statements indicating low-level cognitive processing (e.g., comprehension) were noted early in the independent study experience. In later weeks, there was a shift toward higher-level processing of core material evidenced by a greater number of evaluation and synthesis statements.

In addition to these findings, students provided feedback to instructors about the CBPT framework as part of a required postindependent study reflection. Overwhelmingly, students reported their experiences with CBPT as impactful, helping to support learning and further their understanding of complex academic content. The following are excerpts from these reflections:

It's easy to look at each case through the lens of a speech-language pathologist. When given the opportunity to take on different roles of professionals within a case, we were better able to understand the importance of multidisciplinary teams.

We found [perspective taking] extremely useful in our learning, as we could get a better picture of how much laryngeal cancer transforms not only the patient's life, but also the lives of those around them.

Application to Cross-Disciplinary Contexts

Based on the measured impact of CBPT as well as informal feedback from independent study students, we intend to use CBPT again in similar teaching situations in the future. While CBPT was developed for use with speech-language pathology students, we see obvious applications to any discipline where taking on various perspectives in the context of case-based learning might be impactful. Essentially, any situation where a case-based approach can be merged with the need to understand the perspective of different stakeholders in a given context would be appropriate. For instance:

- A course instructor for a physical therapy course might use CBPT to simulate a meeting to establish a private practice. Students could take on the roles of investor, employee, owner, customer, human relations manager, etc., to explore a case focused on opening a stand-alone physical therapy clinic.
- In a course focused on dietetics, an instructor could use CBPT to facilitate exploration of the roles of teachers, parents, students, teacher aids, administrators, etc., through discussion of a school-based evaluation and treatment planning case study.

Additional Resources

- Description of de Bono's six thinking hats:
  - de Bono, E. (1985). *Six thinking hats: An essential approach to business management*. Little, Brown, & Company.
- Metacognitive Awareness Inventory:
  - https://services.viu.ca/sites/default/files/metacognitive-awareness-inventory.pdf

Exemplar Case-Based Perspective Taking Activity

Students were presented with the following case. Facilitators randomly assigned roles for each student, such as patient, spouse, surgeon, employer, best friend, child, or speech-language pathologist. Students wore nametags identifying their role for others in the discussion group. The facilitator led a discussion where each student was encouraged to respond professionally and/or emotionally to the following prompt by adopting the perspective/persona of their assigned role. Debriefing afterward helped students think about how different individuals might view cases differently based on the perspectives they represent.

Based on the perspective of your assigned role, what might you consider regarding Rose's assessment and management?

Rose, a 64-year-old long-term smoker, experienced a gradual onset of suspicious symptoms over the course of several months. Initially, Rose began to notice that her voice was raspy and hoarse. She and her primary care doctor attributed this status change to continued issues with gastroesophageal reflux disease. Her medicine was changed, yet her voice did not improve in intensity or quality. Around this same time, Rose began to notice difficulty swallowing foods that had never been problematic in the past (e.g., crackers, toast, apples). In response to this difficulty, she started eating softer foods and eventually found that even those were difficult to eat. These dysphagia symptoms led to a referral from her primary care doctor to an otolaryngologist (ENT). After completing a basic examination of Rose and considering her long history of smoking and current symptom profile, the ENT was interested in determining whether a tumor in her larynx may have been compromising her ability to eat and communicate effectively. The ENT immediately referred Rose for magnetic resonance imaging to establish the presence or absence of laryngeal cancer. After her magnetic resonance imaging was completed, Rose was diagnosed with a late-stage tumor of the larynx and subsequently consulted with a new cancer care team consisting of an ENT, a medical oncologist, and a radiation oncologist, as well as a social worker to assist Rose in managing her medical care, a speech-language pathologist to address concerns about feeding and communication, and a palliative care physician to begin conversations about pain management and living a functional life with laryngeal cancer. During this consultation, discussion focused on all the possible options for treating Rose's cancer.

REFERENCES

Biggs, J. B. (2003). *Teaching for quality learning at university: What the student does* (2nd ed.). Society for Research into Higher Education, Open University Press.

Blatt, B., LeLacheur, S. F., Galinsky, A. D., Simmens, S. J., & Greenberg, L. (2010). Perspective-taking: Increasing satisfaction in medical encounters. *Academic Medicine, 85*(9), 1445-1452.

Bloom, B., Englehart, M., Furst, E., Hill, W., & Krathwohl, D. (1956). *Taxonomy of educational objectives: The classification of educational goals, Handbook I: Cognitive domain.* Longmans, Green.

Datta, A., & Ray, J. (2016). Case based learning in undergraduate pathology: A study to assess its efficacy and acceptability as teaching-learning tool. *International Archives of Integrated Medicine, 3*(6), 93-100.

de Bono, E. (1985). *Six thinking hats: An essential approach to business management.* Little, Brown, & Company.

Foran, J. (2002). The case method and the interactive classroom. *The NEA Higher Education Journal, 17*(1), 41-50.

Friberg, J. C., & Vinney, L. A. (Eds.). (2017). *Laryngeal cancer: An interdisciplinary resource for practitioners.* SLACK Incorporated.

Galinsky, A. D., & Ku, G. (2004). The effects of perspective taking on prejudice: The moderating role of self-evaluation. *Personal Social Psychology Bulletin, 30*(5), 594-604.

Nkhoma, M., Sriratanaviriyakul, N., & Le Quang, H. (2017). Using case method to enrich students' learning outcomes. *Active Learning in Higher Education, 18*(1), 37-50.

Schraw, G., & Dennison, R. S. (1994). Assessing metacognitive awareness. *Contemporary Educational Psychology, 19,* 460-475. https://doi.org/10.1006/ceps.1994.1033

Trommelen, R. D., Karpinski, A., & Chauvin, S. (2017). Impact of case-based learning and reflection on clinical reasoning and reflection abilities in physical therapist students. *Journal of Physical Therapy Education, 31*(1), 21-30.

Vescio, T. K., Sechrist, G. P., & Paolucci, M. P. (2003). Perspective taking and prejudice reduction: The meditational role of empathy arousal and situational attributions. *European Journal of Social Psychology, 33*(4), 455-472.

Vinney, L. A., Friberg, J. C., & Smyers, M. M. (2019). Perspective-taking as a mechanism to improve metacognition and higher-level thinking in undergraduate speech-language pathology students. *Journal of the Scholarship of Teaching and Learning, 19*(3), 91-104.

23

A Competency-Based Clinical Simulation to Facilitate Fieldwork Readiness

Andrea Coppola, OTD, OTR/L; Carey Leckie, OT, OTD, OTR, CHT; and Jean McCaffery, OT, EdD, OTR

Description of Teaching/Learning Context

Occupational therapy education must prepare students to meet the demands of the current health care environment and identify best practices to bridge the gap from classroom to clinical practice. This chapter outlines a competency-based, clinical simulation experience developed by one Master of Science Occupational Therapy program that utilizes hands-on learning experiences. The intent of these experiences is to maximize student learning in preparation for the required intensive, clinical rotations that occur at the end of the didactic portion of the program, termed Level II fieldwork (Accreditation Council for Occupational Therapy Education [ACOTE], 2018).

Clinical simulation is a 20-minute, client-centered, student-led assessment and intervention session with a standardized patient in a controlled, low-risk context that incorporates objective assessment of student development of cognitive, affective, and psychomotor skills (Jensen et al., 2013). Throughout the 2-year didactic portion of the graduate occupational therapy program, students participate in a progressive sequence of hands-on learning opportunities leading up to the final competency-based clinical simulation learning experience. This midfidelity simulation involves the use of standardized patients, or trained individuals who portray persons with a specific condition, family members, or other health care professionals, in a manner that is realistic, standardized, and reproducible (Bennett et al., 2017; Bethea et al., 2014; Lopreiato et al., 2016). This learning activity requires students to prepare clinical sessions for five different standardized patients in which they must accurately and effectively administer clinical assessments, provide skilled education and training, and interpret and document clinical findings. Students receive both immediate individualized feedback and the opportunity to participate in a group debriefing session to maximize the learning experience.

Friberg, J. C., Visconti, C. F., & Ginsberg, S. M. (Eds.). *Evidence-Based Education in the Classroom: Examples From Clinical Disciplines* (pp. 199-210).

REVIEW OF LITERATURE

Faculty called upon current literature regarding various forms of experiential learning including clinical simulation, case studies, and the use of standardized patients when devising this educational experience. Practical, hands-on experiences embedded within the curriculum and learning through lived experience has been the subject of research for decades. Experiential learning theory as defined by Kolb (1984) is "knowledge [that] results from the transaction between these objective and subjective experiences in a process called learning" (p. 37). In this theoretical framework, the hands-on, practical experience that occurs within a "real" context is the key to individualized learning.

Recent studies have explored the perceived impact of experiential learning on participants within health care education, and have demonstrated consistent support for its use and effectiveness (Bell et al., 2015; Kruger et al., 2015; Tovin et al., 2017; Walls et al., 2019; Yu et al., 2017). Findings have indicated students perceive an expressed impact on practical knowledge, skill development, clinical reasoning, and increased confidence in the ability to interact within an interprofessional health care environment (Knecht-Sabres, 2013; Tovin et al., 2017; Yu et al., 2017). Within occupational therapy education, the use of experiential learning is frequently applied as a means of preparing students for clinical practice (Knecht-Sabres, 2013; Precin et al., 2018; Ryan et al., 2018; Walls et al., 2019; Yu et al., 2017). Bennett and colleagues (2017) summarize several methods of experiential learning with an emphasis on simulation. These include the use of written or video-based case studies, role plays, computer-based simulation experiences, and the use of high-fidelity simulation mannequins.

Simulation is defined as "a technique that creates a situation or environment to allow persons to experience a representation of a real event for the purpose of practice, learning, evaluation, testing, or to gain understanding of systems or human actions" (Lopreiato et al., 2016). Simulation has gained widespread popularity among occupational therapy educators for its potential as a teaching pedagogy and means for objectively assessing students' professional behaviors and overall performance (Bennett et al., 2017; Bethea et al., 2014; Gibbs et al., 2017; Giles et al., 2014). Proponents of simulation claim its capacity to foster development of core clinical competencies, clinical reasoning, critical thinking, and decision-making skills, as well as increase students' overall comfort, self-confidence and readiness for practice (Bennett et al., 2017; Bethea et al., 2014; Gibbs et al., 2017; Giles et al., 2014).

Faculty within health care educational programs can integrate clinical simulation within the curriculum through various means and can create simulated environments that can be characterized as having low, medium, or high fidelity. Fidelity within the simulated environment refers to the extent to which the clinical simulation reproduces the physical, psychological, and environmental elements of the actual event or clinical setting (Lopreiato et al., 2016). Clinical simulation has been found to be especially effective when it maximizes the authenticity of the learning environment and incorporates well-developed learning objectives and clinical scenarios, strong student engagement, and an opportunity for students to reflect on the experience through facilitated debriefing (Bennett et al., 2017; Shea, 2015).

Clinical simulation-based education, which incorporates the use of standardized patients who simulate specific conditions in a realistic manner (Lopreiato et al., 2016), affords students valuable opportunities for experiential learning with immediate and meaningful feedback and critical reflection (Giles et al., 2014). Simulated patient encounters "enrich the learner experience" (Yeung et al., 2013, p. 234) and augment traditional curriculum by promoting the core values of the rehabilitation professions, facilitating development of communication skills, interpersonal skills, interviewing skills, and competence in the administration of clinical evaluations (Armstrong & Jarriel, 2015; Kaplonyi et al., 2017; Yeung et al., 2013). Ultimately, standardized patient encounters during the prelicensure period provide students with opportunities to apply and transfer their learning beyond lectures and textbook readings, to interact with real persons and to help develop readiness, confidence, and preparedness for clinical fieldwork and practice (Gibbs et al., 2017; Giesbrecht et al., 2014).

Although perceived as challenging, students frequently identify encounters with standardized patients to be useful, meaningful, and more authentic, when compared to other traditional teaching and learning activities (Bennett et al., 2017; Giesbrecht et al., 2014; Pritchard et al., 2016; Walls et al., 2019). In particular, participation in simulated clinical encounters with standardized patients at the end of a professional occupational therapy program can act as a "springboard for transitioning from formal didactic work to integrated clinical work" (Giles et al., 2014, p. S64). This learning opportunity encourages students to review and synthesize content from previous coursework and apply that knowledge to complex patient scenarios situated within an authentic context.

APPLICATION OF LITERATURE/DATA

Clinical simulation applies a developmental learning sequence by building on foundational skills incorporated throughout the occupational therapy graduate program toward a higher-level application of knowledge within an experiential learning context (Cecilio-Fernandes et al., 2018; Verenna et al., 2018). Throughout the 2 years of the didactic portion of the occupational therapy graduate program, and prior to this competency-based, clinical simulation experience, students participate in a series of practical, hands-on learning experiences pertaining to the management of individuals with physical dysfunction. Bloom's taxonomy is a hierarchical structure in which foundations of knowledge and comprehension are necessary to progress to the higher levels of application, analysis, synthesis, and evaluation that are critical to the development of clinical reasoning (Cecilio-Fernandes et al., 2018; Verenna et al., 2018). This understanding of the taxonomy is applied in the progressive sequence of clinical simulation experiences incorporated throughout the occupational therapy program. Early clinical simulation experiences emphasize concrete and discrete skills to demonstrate knowledge and comprehension and lay the foundation for advanced reasoning and analysis.

Experiential Learning That Precedes Clinical Simulation

Students face increasing challenges throughout their academic sequence by completing clinical simulation activities that require higher-level cognitive processing. By the end of their academic sequence, students rely on basic comprehension skills for application of appropriate tests and measures and analysis of those results to inform their ability to synthesize information to complete a clinical evaluation and create a treatment plan for their simulated client. Relevance, knowledge application, and active engagement in the learning process facilitate knowledge acquisition at a deeper level using the higher Bloom's taxonomy levels, which are most appropriate for patient care (McLean, 2016; Trommelen et al., 2014). Table 23-1 displays the progressive sequence of clinical simulation experiences in the program.

The Clinical Simulation Experience

All of these preceding learning experiences build upon component knowledge and skill acquisition toward the final integration of these components into clinical simulation. This learning experience facilitates students' hands-on skill development, professional client-to-therapist communication and interactions, the application of clinical reasoning within a simulated, low-risk environment, and the ability to accurately record and reflect the session experience.

Clinical simulation occurs in the final semester of the master of science occupational therapy graduate program at this institution. Effective clinical simulation delivery relies on active participant engagement. In these learning experiences, students control "the direction and course of action in response to the clinical scenario" (Shea, 2015, p. 4), thereby maximizing student engagement during the clinical simulation. To ensure students' understanding of roles and responsibilities and to increase comfort and minimize student anxiety (noted to be prevalent in clinical simulation; Bradley

Table 23-1

Progressive Sequence of Clinical Simulation Experiences

TIMELINE	CLINICAL SKILLS COVERED	BRIEF DESCRIPTION OF CLINICAL SIMULATION EXPERIENCE
PY1 Fall	• Coordination • Visual perceptual motor skills	• Students assess an individual's coordination and visual perceptual motor skills (e.g., rapid alternating arm movements, finger to nose, finger to thumb touching, visual scanning, saccades, convergence/divergence).
PY1 Spring	• Sensation • Balance • Vital signs • Grip/pinch strength	• Students perform three separate clinical assessments on a standardized patient. • Assessments could include sensation (e.g., light touch, sharp/dull, proprioception, temperature, vibration), balance (e.g., Functional Reach, TUG, 30-second sit to stand), vital signs (e.g., manual pulse, BP, RR, oxygen saturation), and/or grip/pinch strength using a dynamometer or pinchmeter. • Students document clinical findings on varying recording forms.
PY1 Spring	• Assessment and management of client within acute care setting	• HFS lab with mannequin. • In groups, students perform a brief assessment on a standardized patient following a fall at home and with a diagnosis of AMS and UTI.
PY1 Summer	• Functional mobility	• Students are evaluated on their ability to assist a client with bed mobility, gait belt application, sit to stand, and functional ambulation using an AD.
PY1 Summer	• Intervention planning and implementation for group of community participants with CVA	• Students plan, organize, and implement an activity group for community participants that is age and skill-level appropriate. • Students are evaluated on their ability to maintain participants' safety, grade and adapt activities, and document clinical observations.
PY2 Fall	• ROM • MMT	• Students interview and practice ROM screenings on residents within an ALF. • Students are evaluated on their ability to perform UE ROM and MMT assessments on a peer. • Students document clinical findings on standard recording forms.

(continued)

TABLE 23-1 (CONTINUED)

Progressive Sequence of Clinical Simulation Experiences

TIMELINE	CLINICAL SKILLS COVERED	BRIEF DESCRIPTION OF CLINICAL SIMULATION EXPERIENCE
PY2 Fall	• Functional mobility	• Students are evaluated on their ability to perform two basic functional transfers with a peer (stand pivot, squat pivot, or slideboard).
PY2 Fall	• Assessment and management of medically complex client within the ICU	• HFS lab with mannequin. • In groups, students perform a brief assessment on a standardized patient diagnosed with acute respiratory failure and pneumonia.
PY2 Spring	• Functional mobility: complex transfers	• Students are provided with two clinical scenarios involving standardized patients with varying clinical conditions, precautions, and/ or activity restrictions. • Students are evaluated on their ability to transfer each standardized patient using a particular transfer technique.

AD = assistive device; ALF = assisted living facility; AMS = altered mental status; BP = blood pressure; CVA = cerebrovascular accident; HFS = high-fidelity simulation; ICU = intensive care unit; MMT = manual muscle testing; PY1 = professional year 1; PY2 = professional year 2; ROM = range of motion; RR = respiratory rate; TUG = Timed Up and Go; UE = upper extremity; UTI = urinary tract infection.

et al., 2013; Ohtake et al., 2013; Wu & Shea, 2009), students are oriented to the clinical simulation process, policies, and expectations several weeks prior to the day of the actual clinical simulation experience. Two weeks prior to the scheduled event, students are given brief written descriptions of five different clinical cases. Each case description includes an overview of a simulated client's primary diagnosis, history of present illness, reason for referral to occupational therapy services, activity orders and restrictions, and information surrounding each client's prior level of function and home setup. Students are provided a list of clinically appropriate assessments for each client scenario, which they may choose to conduct during their time with their standardized patient. Table 23-2 illustrates examples of clinical case scenarios utilized for the learning experience.

Students are allotted 2 weeks to develop a plan and prepare for an initial assessment with each of the five patients. Over this time frame, students are permitted and encouraged to create one "cheat sheet" that they can refer to while evaluating their standardized patient on the day of the clinical simulation. Several open lab sessions are offered within the 2-week time frame; the first of which includes representation from clinical faculty to answer questions and provide guidance as students prepare. Students use all of these sessions to practice assessments, hands-on interventions, and provision of skilled education and training as they pertain to each clinical scenario.

On the day of the clinical simulation, students arrive 15 minutes prior to their assigned testing time, at which point they receive a folder with one randomly assigned case from the initial set of five scenarios. Students are provided with a blank sheet of paper to record notes and a recording form to document findings that is completed at the end of the session. Students are allotted 20 minutes to evaluate and complete the session with the standardized patient. Occupational therapy practitioners

TABLE 23-2

Clinical Simulation Case Scenarios

CASE	DIAGNOSIS	SETTING	ACTIVITY RESTRICTIONS	CLIENT'S DEFICITS/ CONCERNS
1	Hodgkin's lymphoma	Outpatient	Activity as tolerated	• RUE edema, pain, numbness/tingling, and decreased strength and coordination • Decreased independence with daily tasks
2	Humerus fracture	Acute care	NWB LUE; sling on at all times except for exercises, bathing/dressing; permitted to engage in LUE pendulums and elbow/forearm/wrist/hand AROM	• Pain • Decreased ROM and strength • Decreased independence with ADLs
3	Rheumatoid arthritis	Outpatient	No strenuous activity; no resistive exercise or activity; avoidance of fatigue	• Weakness and pain in bilateral hands • Increasing difficulty with ADLs/IADLs/leisure participation
4	Total hip replacement	Subacute rehabilitation facility	WBAT; posterior hip precautions	• Decreased recall of precautions • Decreased independence with self-care and functional mobility • Presence of pain
5	Chronic obstructive pulmonary disease	Subacute rehabilitation facility	Maintain $SpO_2 \geq 95\%$	• Generalized weakness and debility • Shortness of breath, tachycardia, and oxygen desaturations • Decreased independence with self-care and functional mobility

ADLs = activities of daily living; AROM = active range of motion; IADLs = instrumental activities of daily living; LUE = left upper extremity; NWB = nonweightbearing; ROM = range of motion; RUE = right upper extremity; SpO_2 = oxygen saturation; WBAT = weightbearing as tolerated.

from the community serve as the standardized patients, as they are knowledgeable of the ways in which patients with varying physical conditions present. Prior to this clinical simulation experience, standardized patients are given a description of the clinical scenario that includes the patient's concerns, physical limitations and abilities, and examples of verbiage and behaviors that they must display in a standardized fashion during each student evaluation.

To ensure fidelity, faculty arrange clinical simulation testing rooms to mock a clinical setting as much as feasible. Standardized patients who are simulating inpatient clinical scenarios are dressed in hospital attire and positioned in hospital beds or wheelchairs. Relevant clinical assessment instruments and medical or therapy equipment is readily available for students, including but not limited to, oxygen tanks, sphygmomanometers, pulse oximeters, adaptive equipment for dressing, clothing, slings, assistive devices for mobility, gait belts, therapeutic exercise equipment, fine motor manipulatives, goniometers, dynamometers, pinchmeters, volumeters, tape measures, sensory evaluation kits, and some standardized testing materials. Students are instructed to wear professional attire and identification badges, which emphasizes the need to act professionally, thereby contributing to greater psychological fidelity and authenticity of the clinical simulation experience (Bradley et al., 2013).

Once students have finished their evaluations, they return to a proctored environment to document clinical findings on an evaluation recording form. Students are encouraged to complete their documentation within 30 to 45 minutes to replicate real-world time constraints and work demands typically encountered by occupational therapists working in fast-paced physical rehabilitation settings.

Faculty observe and evaluate each student's standardized patient encounter. Students are rated on their ability to provide an introduction and explanation of their role, perform three biomechanical or functional assessments, inquire about pain, and provide some relevant skilled education and training. Faculty refer to an objective grading rubric (see Additional Resources section) to assess student performance and provide feedback for an integrated set of clinical skills that incorporate components of psychomotor, affective, and cognitive learning domains. These skill areas emphasize professional communication and client-centered approaches, appropriate selection and administration of assessments and interventions, environmental awareness, time management, and the ability to ensure patient safety throughout the clinical simulation experience. Students are also rated on their ability to accurately document their clinical observations and interpretations.

Finally, recognizing the known value of debriefing (Bradley et al., 2013; Gibbs et al., 2017; Ohtake et al., 2013; Shea, 2015; Wu & Shea, 2009), a class-wide debriefing session with all involved faculty evaluators is held once all grades are calculated and individualized feedback has been provided. The purpose of this debriefing is to discuss overall themes pertaining to faculty observations, areas of strength, areas for improvement; to answer student questions; and to receive student feedback regarding their overall experience. Similar to Shea's reports (2015), faculty at this educational institution have also recognized how debriefing discussions allow students to reflect upon and gain awareness of their thought processes as related to the clinical simulation encounter, problem solve more ideal actions or responses if indicated, and consider how their clinical simulation experiences apply to future clinical experiences. In reviewing the events that occurred and the students' rationales behind their actions and behaviors, faculty also often come to appreciate "knowledge gaps among the students" (Shea, 2015, p. 5). This proves valuable and assists faculty in planning future learning activities and individualized student remediation plans toward the goal of facilitating readiness for the transition to intensive Level II fieldwork.

APPLICATION TO CROSS-DISCIPLINARY CONTEXTS

This learning experience was created with an intentional developmental sequence specific to the curricular design within the context of one occupational therapy program, and therefore, in consideration of its use within other contexts, "generalizability is not the goal, but rather transferability" (Bloomberg & Volpe, 2016, p. 47). Many elements of the design and implementation leading up to and including the clinical simulation experiential learning opportunity are applicable and could be adapted for use within other educational contexts in keeping with current evidence in support of experiential learning opportunities within health care education programs (Bell et al., 2015; Knecht-Sabres, 2013; Kruger et al., 2015; Tovin et al., 2017; Yu et al., 2017). When devising clinical simulation experiences, faculty should consider the unique curricular design and expectations of students within each program.

Specific to occupational therapy education, impending changes in accreditation standards include the use of clinical simulation environments and standardized patients as potential options to meet Level I fieldwork objectives (ACOTE, 2018). The clinical simulation scenarios and grading rubric used during this experience may be adapted and applied to create learning opportunities that contribute to enhancing classroom learning experiences, and have the potential to contribute to the development of occupational therapy Level I fieldwork experiences.

Relative to other health care professions, these cases, rubrics, and the structure of these learning experiences have the potential to be modified to address skill areas necessary to prepare students for practice within other health care professions. Additionally, accreditation standards for occupational therapy programs (ACOTE, 2018), as well as the majority of other health care education programs, require interprofessional education embedded within the curriculum. This clinical simulation experience has the potential for future development and application within other disciplines and through collaborative interprofessional learning opportunities.

ADDITIONAL RESOURCES

The following resources and texts contributed to the development of clinical learning experiences within the curriculum and toward the development of the Clinical Simulation Grading Rubric. Additional resources are also found within the reference list.

- Halloran, P., & Lowenstein, N. (Eds.). (2015). *Case studies through the health care continuum: A workbook for the occupational therapy student* (2nd ed.). SLACK Incorporated.
- Jensen, G. M., Mostrom, E., & Shepard, K. F. (2013). From curricular goals to instruction: Preparing to teach. In G. M. Jensen & E. Mostrom (Eds.), *Handbook of teaching and learning for physical therapists* (3rd ed., pp. 19-35). Elsevier.

Clinical Simulation Grading Rubric

	YES *(Meets criteria)* *1 point*	NEEDS IMPROVEMENT *(Meets partial criteria)* *0.5 points*	NO *(Does not meet criteria)* *0 points*	COMMENTS
Introduction/Interactions/ Professional Demeanor Introduced self Concisely and accurately described role of occupational therapy for setting/diagnosis Exhibited professional manner Provided information and patient instructions clearly Used appropriate terminology when conversing with patient Interacted and responded appropriately to patient questions/comments				
Assessed Pain During Evaluation (Pre/post)				
Assessment 1 Chose appropriate assessment/functional task for patient condition/setting and performed accurately				
Assessment 2 Chose appropriate assessment/functional task for patient condition/setting and performed accurately				
Assessment 3 Chose appropriate assessment/functional task for patient condition/setting and performed accurately				
Education Provided skilled education clearly and appropriately for patient condition				

(continued)

(CONTINUED)

Clinical Simulation Grading Rubric

	YES (Meets criteria) 1 point	NEEDS IMPROVEMENT (Meets partial criteria) 0.5 points	NO (Does not meet criteria) 0 points	COMMENTS
Safety Ensured patient understanding and adherence to any relevant precautions/activity restrictions throughout evaluation				
Evaluation Management Demonstrated ability to transition from one clinical/ functional test to the next; completed evaluation within allotted time frame				
Total Score (max 10): _____				

© 2021 SLACK Incorporated. Friberg, J. C., Visconti, C. F., & Ginsberg, S. M. (2021). *Evidence-based education in the classroom: Examples from clinical disciplines.* SLACK Incorporated.

Rubric for Evaluation Recording Form

	MAX SCORE	STUDENT SCORE
All fields completed thoroughly, objectively, and accurately using clinical terminology. Demonstrates skilled occupational therapy evaluation/services.		
Beginning questions (page 1) • Patient demographics • History of present illness • Activity restrictions/precautions • Prior level of function • Patient goals/concerns	0.25	
Clinical/functional assessments	1.0	
Education	0.25	
Intervention plan	0.5	
Additional Points From Evaluation Recording Form (max 2): _____		
Total Score (max 10): _____		

© 2021 SLACK Incorporated. Friberg, J. C., Visconti, C. F., & Ginsberg, S. M. (2021). *Evidence-based education in the classroom: Examples from clinical disciplines.* SLACK Incorporated.

REFERENCES

Accreditation Council for Occupational Therapy Education. (2018). *2018 Accreditation Council for Occupational Therapy Education (ACOTE) standards and interpretive guide: Effective July 31, 2020*. https://acoteonline.org/wp-content/uploads/2020/10/2018-ACOTE-Standards.pdf

Armstrong, K. J., & Jarriel, A. J. (2015). Standardized patient encounters improved athletic training students' confidence in clinical evaluations. *Athletic Training Education Journal, 10*(2), 113-121. https://doi.org/10.4085/1002113

Bell, K., Tanner, J., Rutty, J., Astley-Pepper, M., & Hall, R. (2015). Successful partnerships with third sector organisations to enhance the healthcare student experience: A partnership evaluation. *Nurse Education Today, 35*(3), 530-534. https://doi.org/10.1016/j.nedt.2014.12.013

Bennett, S., Rodger, S., Fitzgerald, C., & Gibson, L. (2017). Simulation in occupational therapy curricula: A literature review. *Australian Occupational Therapy Journal, 64*(4), 314-327. https://doi.org/10.1111/1440-1630.12372

Bethea, D. P., Castillo, D. C., & Harvison, N. (2014). Use of simulation in occupational therapy education: Way of the future? *American Journal of Occupational Therapy, 68*, S32-S39. http://dx.doi.org/10.5014/ajot.2014.012716

Bloomberg, L. D., & Volpe, M. (2016). *Completing your qualitative dissertations: A road map from beginning to end* (3rd ed.). SAGE Publications.

Bradley, G., Whittington, S., & Mottram, P. (2013). Enhancing occupational therapy education through simulation. *British Journal of Occupational Therapy, 76*(1), 43-46. https://doi.org/10.4276/030802213X13576469254775

Cecilio-Fernandes, D., Kerdijk, W., Bremers, A. J., Aalders, W., & Tio, R. A. (2018). Comparison of the level of cognitive processing between case-based items and non-case-based items on the Interuniversity Progress Test of Medicine in the Netherlands. *Journal of Educational Evaluation for Health Professions, 15*(28), 1-5. https://doi.org/10.3352/jeehp.2018.15.28

Giesbrecht, E. M., Wener, P. F., & Pereira, G. M. (2014). A mixed methods study of student perceptions of using standardized patients for learning and evaluation. *Advances in Medical Education and Practice, 5*, 241-255. https://doi.org/10.2147/AMEP.S62446

Gibbs, D. M., Dietrich, M., & Dagnan, E. (2017). Using high fidelity simulation to impact occupational therapy student knowledge, comfort, and confidence in acute care. *The Open Journal of Occupational Therapy, 5*(10), Article 10. http://dx.doi.org/10.15453/2168-6408.1225

Giles, A. K., Carson, N. E., Coker-Bolt, P., & Bowman, P. J. (2014). Conference proceedings: Use of simulated patients and reflective video analysis to assess occupational therapy students' preparedness for fieldwork. *American Journal of Occupational Therapy, 68*, S57-S66.

Jensen, G. M., Mostrom, E., & Shepard, K. F. (2013). From curricular goals to instruction: Preparing to teach. In G. M. Jensen & E. Mostrom (Eds.), *Handbook of teaching and learning for physical therapists* (3rd ed., pp. 19-35). Elsevier.

Kaplonyi, J., Bowles, K. A., Nestel, D., Kiegaldi, D., Maloney, S., Haines, T., & Williams, C. (2017). Understanding the impact of simulated patients on health care learners' communication skills: A systematic review. *Medical Education, 51*, 1209-1219. https://doi.org/10.1111/medu.13387

Knecht-Sabres, L. (2013). Experiential learning in occupational therapy: Can it enhance readiness for clinical practice? *The Journal of Experiential Education, 36*(1), 22-36.

Kolb, D. A. (1984). *The process of experiential learning. Experiential learning: Experience as the source of learning and development* (pp. 20-38). Prentice-Hall.

Kruger, J. S., Kruger, D. J., & Suzuki, R. (2015). Assessing the effectiveness of experiential learning in a student-run free clinic. *Pedagogy in Health Promotion, 1*(2), 91-94. https://doi.org/10.1177/2373379915575530

Lopreiato, J. O., Downing, D., Gammon, W., Lioce, L., Sittner, B., Slot, V., Spain, A. E. Terminology & Concepts Working Group. (2016). Healthcare simulation dictionary. http://www.ssih.org/dictionary

McLean, S. (2016). Case-based learning and its application in medical and health-care fields: A review of worldwide literature. *Journal of Medical Education and Curricular Development, 3*, 39-49. https://doi.org/10.4137/JMECD.S20377

Ohtake, P. J., Lazarus, M., Schillo, R., & Rosen, M. (2013). Simulation experience enhances physical therapist student confidence in managing a patient in the critical care environment. *Physical Therapy, 93*(2), 216-228. https://doi.org/10.2522/ptj.20110463

Precin, P., Koenig, V., Chiariello, E., Masotti, G. K., Diamond, B. N., Lashinsky, D. B., & Tierno, D. (2018). Spots: A model for the creation of sustainable, population-based, occupational therapy fieldwork sites. *Occupational Therapy in Health Care, 32*(1), 44-58. https://doi.org/10.1080/07380577.2017.1402228

Pritchard, S. A., Blackstock, F. A., Nestel, D., & Keating, J. L. (2016). Simulated patients in physical therapy education: Systematic review and meta-analysis. *Physical Therapy, 96*(9), 1342-1353. https://doi.org/10.2522/ptj.20150500

Ryan, K., Beck, M., Ungaretta, L., Rooney, M., Dalomba, E., & Kahanov, L. (2018). Pennsylvania occupational therapy fieldwork educator practices and preferences in clinical education. *The Open Journal of Occupational Therapy, 6*(1). https://doi.org/10.15453/2168-6408.1362

Shea, C.-K. (2015). High-fidelity simulation: A tool for occupational therapy education. *The Open Journal of Occupational Therapy, 3*(4), Article 8.

Tovin, M. M., Fernandez-Fernandez, A., & Smith, K. (2017). Pediatric integrated clinical experiences: Enhancing learning through a series of clinical exposures. *Journal of Physical Therapy Education, 31*(2), 137. https://doi.org/10.1097/00001416-201731020-00016

Trommelen, R. D., Hebert, L., & Nelson, T. K. (2014). Impact on physical therapy and audiology students of an interprofessional case-based learning experience in education of vestibular disorders. *Journal of Allied Health, 43*(4), 194-200.

Verenna, A., Noble, K., Pearson, H., & Miller, S. (2018). Role of comprehension on performance at higher levels of Bloom's taxonomy: Findings from assessments of healthcare professional students. *Anatomical Sciences Education, 11*(5), 433-444. https://doi.org/10.1002/ase.1768

Walls, D. J., Fletcher, T. S., & Brown, D. P. (2019). Occupational therapy students' perceived value of simulated learning experiences. *Journal of Allied Health, 48*(1), e21-e25.

Wu, R., & Shea, C.-K. (2009). Using high-fidelity simulations to prepare occupational therapy students for intensive care unit practice. *Education Special Interest Section Quarterly, 19*(4), 1-4.

Yu, M.-L., Brown, T., & Etherington, J. (2017). Students' experiences of attending an innovative occupational therapy professional practice placement in a childcare setting. *Journal of Occupational Therapy, Schools, & Early Intervention, 11*(1). https://doi-org.une.idm.oclc.org/10.1080/19411243.2017.1408443

Yeung, E., Dubrowski, A., & Carnahan, H. (2013). Simulation-augmented education in the rehabilitation professions: A scoping review. *International Journal of Therapy and Rehabilitation, 20*(5), 228-236. https://doi.org/10.12968/ijtr.2013.20.5.228

24

SIMULATION-BASED EDUCATION IN HEALTH CARE

Amber Herrick, MS, PA-C
and Sarah Bolander, DMSc, PA-C, DFAAPA

DESCRIPTION OF TEACHING/LEARNING CONTEXT

Simulation-based education in health care is an impactful teaching method to integrate medical knowledge with the psychosocial complexities of clinical practice. A dedicated course in simulation was developed for physician assistant students following the didactic phase of the curriculum, prior to transitioning to clinical rotations. This 6-week course includes a simulation encounter each week. The goal of this course, titled Clinical Simulation, is to provide students with frequent opportunities to apply medical knowledge collaboratively in a team-based approach to address health care disparities and challenging patient scenarios. The course coordinators have created novel, thought-provoking standardized patient encounters that are administered in a safe environment to foster the application of learning. This form of education requires significant advanced planning and components of prebrief, self-reflection, and debrief to be effective (Table 24-1).

This chapter introduces one physician assistant program's approach to simulation-based education utilizing standardized patients to address the psychosocial aspects of patient care. The course coordinators will emphasize the components of effective simulation and outline ways simulation can be used in health care education. Although programs may utilize various forms of simulation, the focus of this chapter will be on standardized patients, as this may be more feasible and effective in bridging the transition between didactic and clinical education. "The question is no longer *if* we should use simulation, but *how*" (Kneebone et al., 2017, p. 92).

Friberg, J. C., Visconti, C. F., & Ginsberg, S. M. (Eds.). *Evidence-Based Education in the Classroom: Examples From Clinical Disciplines* (pp. 211-220).

TABLE 24-1

Components of Simulation

COMPONENT	PURPOSE
Prebrief	• Orients students • Establishes objectives and goals • Introduces settings, materials, and available resources • Sets clear expectations • Creates a safe environment
Simulation events	• Meaningful and relevant experiences related to students' profession(s) • Appropriately designed based on predetermined objectives and goals • Formative and/or summative assessment • Creating authentic cases to enhance student buy-in
Self-reflection	• Allows for a higher level of understanding by increasing student awareness of one's own responses to the simulation event • Identifies areas of strength, needs for individualized improvement, and informs for potential change • Influences students' perceptions, attitudes, and behaviors
Debrief	• Timely feedback • Allows for analysis of the encounter and application of acquired knowledge and skills • Facilitates transfer of students' experiences to a health care practice environment

REVIEW OF LITERATURE

Simulation-based education is a teaching method used to improve real patient experiences with scenarios designed to emulate patient encounters using high-fidelity mannequins, task trainers, virtual reality, or standardized patients. Well-defined learning outcomes are required prior to planning and implementing simulation into the curriculum effectively. Simulation is more beneficial when integrated into an established curriculum instead of adding supplementary content (McGaghie et al., 2010; Motola et al., 2013). Once the goals and outcomes are determined, each component of a simulation must be considered to enable a cohesive design. Components of simulation include a prebrief, the simulation event, self-reflection, and debrief. Each element is critical in the successful implementation of simulation events (Gardner, 2013; Vandyk et al., 2018).

Prebrief

The prebrief commonly orients students to simulation and sets the tone for the event. The content often includes identifying the setting, time allotment, potential materials being used, and other expectations for the patient scenario (Stephenson & Poore, 2016). Clearly defined goals and objectives for the simulated clinical encounter should be provided and discussed with students. Student transparency allows for appropriate preparation and focus on learning outcomes (Stephenson & Poore, 2016). Simulation also requires establishment of a safe environment for students to learn. This decreases student anxiety and encourages participation without the fear of failure or academic consequences (McGaghie et al., 2010; Stephenson & Poore, 2016; Vandyk et al., 2018). It is important for team-based encounters to define role expectations and communicate how the team will be assessed. Students may be provided with resources on teamwork or communication to assist with their preparation.

Prebriefs can be delivered through modules, videos, reading assignments, small group discussions, and/or live lectures. Prebrief guides the simulation, facilitates goal achievement, and improves student satisfaction (Stephenson & Poore, 2016).

Simulation Events

Simulation events require appropriate design based on predetermined goals, implementation, and structured evaluation methods (Motola et al., 2013; Vandyk et al., 2018). The outcome goals of simulation vary amongst institutions and should direct the focus of the encounter and the assessment measures. Medical knowledge assessment is the most widely accepted use for simulation (Coerver et al., 2017; Huang et al., 2012). There is value in moving beyond using simulation to solely evaluate cognitive abilities. Additional uses of simulation include motivational interviewing, communication skills, interpersonal skills, team training, error disclosure, patient safety, delivering bad news, empathetic behavior, and interprofessional education (IPE; Floyd et al., 2015; Guinane & Molloy, 2013; McGaghie et al., 2010; Motola et al., 2013).

A challenge with simulation is achieving student buy-in. There are numerous ways to enhance the realism of simulation to better represent clinical scenarios. Increasing student buy-in will not only improve the overall experience but will lead to more authentic responses from the students (Gormley et al., 2012; Stokes-Parish et al., 2017). Although actual patients may be able to portray the desired positive findings needed for a simulation, these patients may be difficult to locate, or the findings may not be conducive to repeat exams. For example, recruiting a patient for a specific heart murmur may not be feasible, or a patient with a sprained ankle may not tolerate repeat exams by students. Therefore, standardized patients are commonly used. To enhance the realism of the encounter, adjunct elements can be incorporated, such as task trainers, props, or moulage. A task trainer, such as an electronic audio pad or specialized stethoscope, can be programmed to provide the exact murmur needed. A prop, such as crutches and the use of moulage to mimic the appearance of bruising, can enhance the patient presentation of a sprained ankle. Moulage is the art of creating lifelike physical examination findings or mock injuries using makeup, prosthetics, or theater elements and is an effective tool in simulation (Gormley et al., 2012; Zorn et al., 2018). Simple additions made to a case, as in these examples, can significantly improve the overall student experience.

Hybrid simulation can also be used to allow students to develop procedural skills (Gormley et al., 2012). The integration of mannequins or task trainers into the simulation event with a standardized patient maintains much of the realism while allowing students to practice skills, such as inserting an intravenous needle, injecting a medication, or suturing a wound. Standardized patients are still able to display feelings of pain, worry, aggravation, irritation, etc.

Another component to set the stage for these events is to replicate the atmosphere. The environment should simulate the typical clinical setting (Gormley et al., 2012). This may depict an operating room, emergency department, intensive care unit, office exam room, etc. Successful incorporation of auditory, olfactory, and/or visual senses can provide additional layers enhancing the authenticity of the case and ultimately leading to student buy-in. The auditory conditions may also be considered, such as the sounds of monitors, overhead announcements, or urgent phone calls. Smells such as alcohol or a fruity odor may complement the scenario. Additional visual cues, such as droplets applied with a spray bottle, could be used to portray diaphoresis or the application of foam or gel pads to the ankles could signify lower extremity edema.

Once goals are established, planning requires consideration of location, delivery mode, time frame, faculty support, and feedback/evaluation tools (Motola et al., 2013). Evaluation measures should not only assess students' abilities, but also the quality of the encounter. Simulation encounters often require revision based on a continuous evaluation process. This may lead to altering content, additional training for standardized patients or faculty facilitators, adjustments to the evaluation tools, or adjusting some of the logistics to improve successful implementation (McGaghie et al., 2010; Motola et al., 2013).

Self-Reflection

Reflection provides a higher level of understanding by bringing conscious awareness to the responses evoked by the encounter (Paterson & Chapman, 2013). Beyond the goal of learning from the experience, students can identify individual areas in need of improvement. Kolb's experiential learning cycle requires reflective observation followed by abstract conceptualization in order to change the approach to a similar scenario in the future (Kolb, 1984).

Self-reflection and clinical reasoning can be incorporated successfully with video reviews of the simulated encounter, medical knowledge checklists, and/or guided open-ended questions. Self-reflection provides students with dedicated time to critically think about the encounter, analyze the experience, and reflect on their responses to the challenging scenario. If the event occurs in teams, often peer-evaluations are incorporated. Simulation has the potential to influence students' perceptions, attitudes, and behaviors facilitated by self-reflection (Gardner, 2013).

Debrief

Students require immediate feedback for a simulation event to be effective. Feedback may occur simultaneously as part of the activity or directly following the event and should be specific to the individual's or teams' learning needs (Motola et al., 2013). Feedback is the most critical component of simulation-based education and initial feedback may be provided by the standardized patient, peers, or facilitators (Cleland et al., 2009; Issenberg et al., 2005). Debriefing sessions to review the overall encounter are typically facilitator- or student-led and delivered to an individual or a group. Debrief should allow for analysis of the experience and provide ways to integrate the activity into clinical practice (Gardner, 2013). The key to debrief is empowering the student to transfer the simulated encounter directly to a health care practice environment (Rudolph et al., 2008). This application creates relevance for the activity and improves student perceptions. Students must receive feedback in a nonjudgmental and confidential environment (Fanning & Gaba, 2007; Rudolph, et al., 2008). Facilitators should remain supportive and encourage various learning styles tailored to the student and specific to the encounter.

The controlled environments of simulation foster deliberate practice and quality assessment opportunities (Motola et al., 2013). Deliberate practice is commonly used to facilitate repetitive task training with continuous feedback. Corrective feedback ultimately will allow the opportunity for mastery (Gaba, 2004; Guinane & Molloy, 2013). On-demand training allows for convenience and flexibility with learning. Because simulation allows for deliberate practice, simulation-based education has become an important tool in interprofessional training and development of health care teams (Coerver et al., 2017).

APPLICATION OF LITERATURE/DATA

There is evidence to suggest that adult learners benefit the most when they are actively engaged and can apply what they have learned to their own experiences (Fanning & Gaba, 2007; Gardner, 2013). In Kolb's experiential learning cycle, adults learn through experience, and the more relevant the experience is, the more meaningful the activity is (Gardner, 2013; Kolb, 1984). As a learning strategy, simulation is valuable in creating authentic clinical scenarios that simulate real patient encounters, applicable to the student's own profession, while in a controlled and supervised environment. Current literature supports the effectiveness of simulation in health care education and has shown to increase knowledge, develop student confidence, and improve clinical judgment (Spies et al., 2015; Vandyk et al., 2018).

Our Clinical Simulation course is intentionally placed in the pre-clinical quarter to complement where students are at as learners. The pre-clinical quarter immediately follows the completion of the didactic phase of the curriculum and precedes the clinical phase as physician assistant students start clinical rotations. The sequencing of the curriculum allows for enrichment of pedagogy and application of acquired knowledge and skills. The overall course structure is designed using evidence-based practices previously discussed, including components of prebrief, the simulation event, self-reflection, and debrief. The objective of this course is to provide students with simulated clinical scenarios that not only incorporate medical knowledge but are compounded by the complex psychosocial elements that influence patient care. The purpose of the simulated clinical encounters with standardized patients is to provide students with an educational experience that fosters critical thinking, effective communication, strengthens teamwork, and encourages self-reflection as they prepare for the transition to clinical rotations and real patients.

Prebrief

It is generally agreed upon by educators that there should be some form of a prebrief to prepare students for a simulated event (Motola et al., 2013; Vandyk et al., 2018). On the first day of the course, prior to students' first standardized patient event, we review the course objectives, discuss expectations, and highlight the evidence behind simulation and debrief. Additionally, we stress that the simulation events are safe places to make mistakes and to learn from them. This process in the literature is referred to as *normalizing* (Gardner, 2013).

Simulation Event

Students are placed in pairs for standardized patient encounters. Each pair of students is provided a chief complaint and vital signs prior to entering the examination room. For one of the cases, the patient that awaits them is in obvious distress, guarding their face, and has a disheveled appearance (Figures 24-1 and 24-2). The standardized patient complains of severe facial pain and a possible sunburn. Students are expected to collect a problem-focused history, complete a physical examination, and make a diagnosis of herpes zoster ophthalmicus. As this condition is sight-threatening, the patient requires immediate treatment; however, added layers of complexity intentionally interfere with students' available options for management. The goal is for students to discover that the patient is homeless and without health insurance or transportation. This challenges students to act in an empathetic manner while considering additional resources and maintaining the standard of care. Although the patient has moulage applied to replicate the herpes zoster virus manifestation and the overall unkempt appearance is consistent with poor hygiene and lack of shelter, the simulation still creates a wide variety of responses from the students with varying approaches to patient care.

Self-Reflection

Immediately following the standardized patient encounter, each student reviews their own video and completes a guided self-reflection. The purpose of the self-reflection is to focus on improvement rather than judgment. The student is asked to reflect on their experience and critique themselves and their partner, recognize gaps in knowledge, and identify areas where they improved from one week to the next. This process informs students of the potential need for change. Similar questions asked of the students are also asked of the standardized patients and faculty. The questions pertain to whether the students displayed signs of empathy, recognized that the patient was

Figure 24-1. Frontal view of standardized patient.

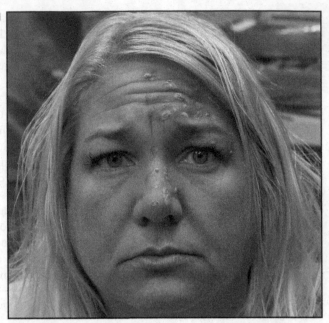

Figure 24-2. Side view of standardized patient.

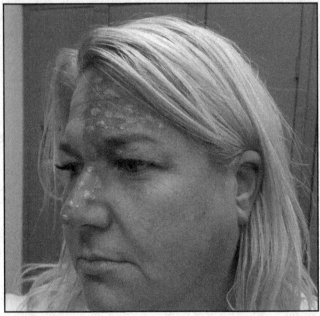

homeless, asked if the patient had health insurance, determined if the patient had access to transportation, and appropriately addressed the patient's financial concerns. In addition, the students are asked to rank their level of comfort in providing empathy to the patient and navigating resources for a patient who is homeless and uninsured. As course coordinators, we report back to the class during a formalized debrief session. During this session, we communicate how students responded to the self-reflections and how their perceptions aligned with the views of the standardized patients and observations made by the faculty.

Debrief

Debriefing, a specific form of feedback, is well referenced in the literature as one of the most important aspects of simulation (Gardner, 2013; Motola et al., 2013). Because debriefing and feedback are critical in ensuring effective learning in simulation, feedback is provided to our students from several sources. First, students receive immediate feedback from a faculty member who observed the event live, along with written feedback from the standardized patients, followed by a formal debrief session. Having dedicated time for feedback immediately following the event allows faculty the opportunity to explore actions observed during the encounter, provide direct feedback to the pair of students, and ensure learning objectives are met. In the formal debrief session, there is guided discussion as a class in a nonthreatening manner where course coordinators solicit students' reactions, analyze the case, highlight what went well, and identify areas for improvement. Additionally, we ask the students to share what could be done differently next time. Debriefing affords students the opportunity to enhance their ability to reflect, self-correct, and apply acquired knowledge and skills to future practice.

APPLICATION TO CROSS-DISCIPLINARY CONTEXTS

Simulation in health care education provides students with the means to experience meaningful and relevant clinical experiences, participate in self-reflection, and apply knowledge gained to future practice (Gardner, 2013). Using evidence-based practices in simulation can be applied to other clinically based disciplines and can be tailored to the needs of the program. Current literature supports the use of simulation in several health professions, such as medicine, nursing, pharmacy, physical therapy, speech-language pathology, dental, etc. (Coerver et al., 2017; Multak et al., 2015).

Simulation-based clinical scenarios lend themselves nicely in an IPE activity focused on promoting effective interprofessional collaboration in the areas of role identification, teamwork, and communication. The clinical scenario discussed would work well with students from medicine, including physician assistants and nurse practitioners, ophthalmology/optometry, social work, and pharmacy. For instance, a physician assistant student could complete the history and physical, consult with the ophthalmology/optometry student about their concerns regarding the patients' sight-threatening condition, together verify proper medication management with the pharmacy student, and as a team, discuss the lack of health insurance/payment for prescriptions, with the student from social work. Another example would be to design a simulated clinical scenario around a standardized patient who plays the role of a patient who had a stroke for a team consisting of physical therapy, occupational therapy, and speech-language pathology students. Additional elements, such as the need for wound care, nursing, nutritional support, and mental/behavioral health, could be added to include students from medicine, nursing, dietetics, psychiatry, and social work.

While this case would serve well as an IPE event, we see that this simulated clinical event would apply to any discipline interested in assessing their students' empathetic communication. Given the importance of empathy in health care, education aimed at developing empathetic skills is indeed beneficial for all health care students. Demonstrating empathy is an ability that many students overestimate (Floyd et al., 2015). As future health care professionals interacting with patients, this may be a favorable pedagogical approach for other programs to evaluate their students' empathetic abilities, not only from faculty observation, but from a standardized patient's perspective as well.

The focus of our course places a greater emphasis on the noncognitive attributes, such as empathy, than the cognitive factors often assessed in simulation-based education. Starting with a medical diagnosis and adding complex layers to the case creates opportunities to assess students not only on empathy, but also on oral communication, teamwork, critical thinking, and cultural competence. Some examples include a clinical scenario with a patient who lives in a rural setting with limited access to care and resources, an angry patient due to a medical error, a patient with special needs, or

Table 24-2

Plus/Delta Debriefing Model Example

+	Δ

a patient who lives alone and is blind secondary to uncontrolled diabetes requiring insulin. These clinical scenarios are designed to push students outside of their comfort zones and create simulated clinical encounters that reflect what students will encounter in clinical practice.

Much of this discussion has centered around simulation-based education during the didactic phase of training. Future considerations for simulation-based education include augmenting traditional clinical education with simulation-based clinical experiences. The use of simulation is applicable to all health care professions and can improve patient care through deliberate practice (Gaba, 2004; Guinane & Molloy, 2013). Studies have found simulation-based education with deliberate practice superior in achievement of goals and clinical skills acquisition compared to traditional clinical education (Guinane & Molloy, 2013; McGaghie et al., 2011). Simulation is designed to integrate, not replace, the need for actual patient care experience into the existing curriculum to enhance and supplement traditional clinical education to achieve learning outcomes. Simulation complements clinical education as it offers students the opportunity not only to master skills, but also to experience uncommon or rare presentations that may otherwise not be encountered through traditional clinical education. Given the benefits of simulation in health care education, this approach might be especially helpful for disciplines facing a shortage of clinical rotation sites to ensure students receive high quality education and programs have the means to assess competency.

ADDITIONAL RESOURCES

The resources provided may offer programs the tools to enhance simulation in existing curriculum.

- Plus/Delta Debriefing Model (Table 24-2): The plus (+) column represents what went well and the delta (Δ) column indicates areas for improvement or things that could be done differently (Garder, 2013; Motola et al., 2013). The plus/delta model can be completed by students and/or the faculty. This method allows the facilitator to identify key points to discuss during the debrief. Table 24-2 was adapted based on this model and is used in the Clinical Simulation course.

- Institute for Healthcare Improvement: Institute for Healthcare Improvement Open School offers online courses that can be incorporated into the existing curriculum with topics that focus on quality improvement, patient safety, person-centered care, leadership, and the triple aim. These online courses are an excellent way to supplement a course with material that introduces or reinforces concepts aligned with the objectives and goals of the simulated events:
  - http://www.ihi.org/education/IHIOpenSchool/Courses/Pages/default.aspx

- Moulage: Moulage for either standardized patients or high-fidelity mannequins:
  - www.moulage.net
- Supplemental Articles:
  - Fox, L., Onders, R., Hermansen-Kobulnicky, C. J., Nguyen, T. N., Myran, L., Linn, B., & Hornecker, J. (2018). Teaching interprofessional teamwork skills to health professional students: A scoping review. *Journal of Interprofessional Care, 32*(2), 127-135.
  - Mandel, E. D., & Schweinle, W. E. (2012). A study of empathy decline in physician assistant students at completion of the first didactic year. *Journal of Physician Assistant Education, 23*(4), 16-24.
  - McTighe, A. J., DiTomasso, R. A., Felgoise, S., & Hojat, M. (2016). Correlation between standardize patients' perceptions of osteopathic medical students and students' self-rated empathy. *The Journal of the American Osteopathic Association, 116*(10), 640-646.
  - Teng, V. C., Nguyen, C., Hall, K. T., Rydel, T., Sattler, A., Schillinger, E., Weinlander, E., & Lin, S. (2017). Rethinking empathy decline: Results from an OSCE. *The Clinical Teacher, 14*(6), 441-445.
  - Ruiz-Moral, R., Pérula de Torres, L., Monge, D., García Leonardo, C., & Caballero, F. (2017). Teaching medical students to express empathy by exploring patient emotions and experiences in standardized medical encounters. *Patient Education and Counseling, 100*(9), 1694-1700.
  - Schweller, M., Costa, F. O., Antônio, M. Â., Amaral, E. M., & de Carvalho-Filho, M. A. (2014). The impact of simulated medical consultations on the empathy levels of students at one medical school. *Academic Medicine, 89*(4), 632-637.

REFERENCES

Cleland, J. A., Abe, K., & Rethans, J. J. (2009). The use of simulated patients in medical education: AMEE Guide No 42. *Medical Teacher, 31*(6), 477-486.

Coerver, D., Multak, N., Marquardt, A., & Larson, E. H. (2017). The use of simulation in physician assistant programs: A national survey. *The Journal of Physician Assistant Education, 28*(4), 175-181.

Fanning, R. M., & Gaba, D. M. (2007). The role of debriefing in simulation-based learning. *Simulation in Healthcare, 2*(2), 115-125.

Floyd, K., Generous, M. A., Clark, L., Simon, A., & Mcleod, I. (2015). Empathy between physician assistant students and standardized patients: Evidence of an inflation bias. *The Journal of Physician Assistant Education, 26*(2), 93-98.

Gaba, D. M. (2004). The future vision of simulation in health care. *Quality and Safety in Health Care, 13*(Suppl. 1), i2-i10. http://dx.doi.org/10.1136/qshc.2004.009878

Gardner, R. (2013). Introduction to debriefing. *Seminars in Perinatology, 37*(3), 166-174.

Gormley, G., Sterling, M., Menary, A., & McKeown, G. (2012). Keeping it real! Enhancing realism in standardised patient OSCE stations. *The Clinical Teacher, 9*(6), 382-386.

Guinane, S., & Molloy, L. (2013). Training on demand: A solution to clinical education through simulation. *The Journal of Physician Assistant Education, 24*(4), 32-36.

Huang, G. C., Sacks, H., Devita, M., Reynolds, R., Gammon, W., Saleh, M., Gliva-McConvey, G., Owens, T., Anderson, J., Stillsmoking, K., Cantrell, M., & Passiment, M. (2012). Characteristics of simulation at North American medical schools and teaching hospitals: An AAMC-SSH-ASPE-AACN collaboration. *Simulation in Healthcare, 7*(6), 329-333.

Issenberg, S. B., McGaghie, W. C., Petrusa, E. R., Lee Gordon, D., & Scalese, R. J. (2005). Features and uses of high-fidelity medical simulations that lead to effective learning: A BEME systematic review. *Medical Teacher, 27*(1), 10-28.

Kneebone, R., Nestel, D., & Bello, F. (2017). Learning in a simulated environment. In J. A. Dent, R. M. Harden, & D. Hunt (Eds.), *A practical guide for medical teachers* (5th ed., pp. 92-100). Elsevier.

Kolb, D. A. (1984). *Experiential learning: Experience as the source of learning and development.* Prentice-Hall.

McGaghie, W., Issenberg, S. B., Cohen, E. R., Barsuk, J. H., & Wayne, D. B. (2011). Does simulation-based medical education with deliberate practice yield better results than traditional clinical education? A meta-analytic comparative review of the evidence. *Academic Medicine, 86*(6), 706-711. https://doi.org/10.1097/ACM.0b013e318217e119

McGaghie, W. C., Issenberg, S. B., Petrusa, E. R., & Scalese, R. J. (2010). A critical review of simulation-based medical education research: 2003-2009. *Medical Education, 44*(1), 50-63. https://doi.org/10.1111/j.1365-2923.2009.03547.x

Motola, I., Devine, L. A., Chung, H. S., Sullivan, J. E., & Issenberg, S. B. (2013). Simulation in healthcare education: A best evidence practical guide. AMEE Guide No. 82. *Medical Teacher, 35*(10), 1511-1530.

Multak, N., Newell, K., Spear, S., Scalese, R., & Issenberg, B. (2015). A multi-institutional study using simulation to teach cardiopulmonary physical examination and diagnosis skills to physician assistant students. *The Journal of Physician Assistant Education, 26*(2), 70-76.

Paterson, C., & Chapman, J. (2013). Enhancing skills of critical reflection to evidence learning in professional practice. *Physical Therapy in Sport, 14*(3), 133-138.

Rudolph, J. W., Simon, R., Raemer, D. B., & Eppich, W. J. (2008). Debriefing as formative assessment: closing performance gaps in medical education. *Academic Emergency Medicine, 15*(11), 1010-1016. https://doi.org/10.1111/j.1553-2712.2008.00248.x

Stephenson, E., & Poore, J. (2016). Tips for conducting the pre-brief for a simulation. *Journal of Continuing Education in Nursing, 47*(8), 353-355.

Spies, C., Seale, I., & Botma, Y. (2015). Adult learning: What nurse educators need to know about mature students. *Curationis, 38*(2), 1494.

Stokes-Parish, J. B., Duvivier, R., & Jolly, B. (2017). Does appearance matter? Current issues and formulation of research agenda for moulage in simulation. *Simulation in Healthcare, 12*(1), 47-50.

Vandyk, A. D., Lalonde, M., Merali, S., Wright, E., Bajnok, I., & Bavies, B. (2018). The use of psychiatry-focused simulation in undergraduate nursing education: A systematic search and review. *International Journal of Mental Health Nursing, 27*(2), 514-535. https://doi.org/10.1111/inm.12419

Zorn, J., Snyder, J., & Guthrie, J. (2018). Use of moulage to evaluate student assessment of skin in an objective structured clinical examination. *The Journal of Physician Assistant Education, 29*(2), 99-103.

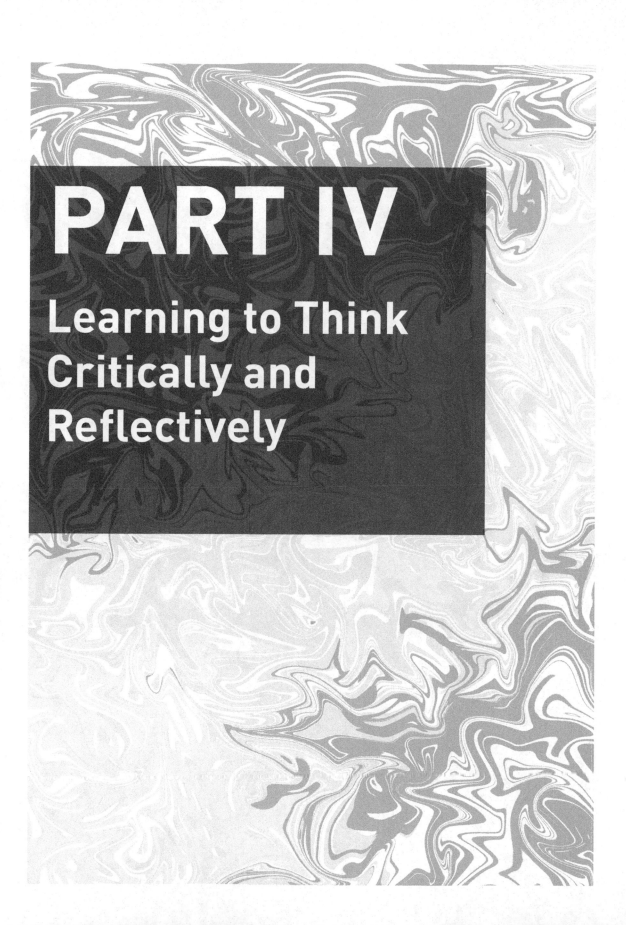

PART IV
Learning to Think Critically and Reflectively

25

Preparing Communication Sciences and Disorders Students for the Graduate Application Process

Ann R. Beck, PhD; Heidi Verticchio, MS;
and Scott Seeman, PhD

Description of Teaching/Learning Context

In Fall 2018, we offered an independent study on the graduate admission process to senior-level undergraduate students majoring in Communication Sciences and Disorders (CSD). The purpose of this independent study was to facilitate students' ability to begin and complete their applications for graduate school in speech-language pathology and audiology with as little stress as possible. The independent study met for 50 minutes a week during the Fall 2018 semester. In class we provided an overview of the general components of the graduate applications; taught students how to navigate and use the CSD Centralized Application System; helped students determine which graduate programs to consider; covered program statistics of graduate schools to which our students frequently applied; and discussed how to request letters of recommendation, compile portfolios of experiences/achievements, and compose resumes, personal statements, and essays. To cover these topics, we demonstrated how to navigate the system in class, required students to complete components of the CSD Centralized Application System by specified dates, lectured and held whole-class and small-group discussions about specific components of the process, assigned groups of students to study and present information to the class about various speech-language pathology and audiology graduate programs, and used peer review of resumes and portfolios.

In addition to the above topics, we aimed to reduce students' levels of stress and negative aspects of perfectionism and to increase their self-compassion. We did this primarily by engaging students in a mindfulness practice. In the remainder of this chapter, we discuss stress, perfectionism, self-compassion, and mindfulness. We review evidence about the positive effects of a mindfulness

Friberg, J. C., Visconti, C. F., & Ginsberg, S. M. (Eds.). *Evidence–Based Education in the Classroom: Examples From Clinical Disciplines* (pp. 223-231).

practice for CSD students and describe how we used a mindfulness practice in class and the outcomes of the practice. Finally, we discuss the importance of application of the mindfulness practice used in this independent study to coursework in other clinically related programs.

REVIEW OF LITERATURE

Everyday life contains many stressors. Some level of manageable stress is positive and helps people grow and learn. Stress that becomes overwhelming and chronic, however, can have detrimental effects on individuals' mental and physical well-being (McCall, 2007). College students are often presented with significant stressors (e.g., increased academic demands, new social and physical environments, financial concerns). If they are not able to manage their stress well, not only can their mental and physical well-being be decreased, but their ability to focus and learn in the educational setting can be negatively affected (Lieberman et al., 2018; Ross, 2011).

A trait that is associated with stress is perfectionism. Perfectionism is a multidimensional disposition that is composed of both healthy and unhealthy aspects (Hill & Curran, 2016; Suh et al., 2017). Individuals with healthy, or adaptive, perfectionism tend to have lower levels of stress, whereas those with unhealthy, or maladaptive, perfectionism have higher levels of stress (Ashby & Gnilka, 2017). Furthermore, students with healthy perfectionism tend to be satisfied with their lives and have positive self-esteem and self-efficacy (Noble et al., 2014). These students set high standards for themselves and are realistic about them. If they do not meet the standards set, they are not overly distressed and can view this as a learning opportunity (Christman, 2012). These students also tend not to procrastinate and to use active, task-oriented coping strategies (Noble et al., 2014).

Conversely, students who demonstrate unhealthy perfectionism tend toward depression and anxiety (Christman, 2012). Being perfectionists, they too set high standards for themselves, yet often perceive themselves as not being able to meet their goals, which causes them distress (Noble et al., 2014). They might also engage in behaviors that could hinder their academic success such as procrastinating, overcommitting, and being disagreeable and aggressive (Christman, 2012).

Brown (2012) believes that all individuals fall somewhere on a continuum of perfectionism. She stated that no matter where we are on the continuum, to ensure perfectionism does not have a negative effect, "we have to make the long journey from 'What will people think?' to 'I am enough'" (p. 131). One of the paths that can start people on that journey is the development of self-compassion. Individuals who have high levels of self-compassion tend to engage in self-care behaviors (e.g., eating well, exercising appropriately; Neff & Faso, 2015) and face difficult situations in a calm manner (Yang et al., 2016).

One component of self-compassion is mindfulness (Neff, 2011). Mindfulness, the ability to pay attention purposefully and nonjudgmentally in the present moment (Kabat-Zinn, 1994, p. 4), has been documented to increase mindfulness practitioners' compassion, empathy, and kindness and to produce positive changes in the areas of their brains responsible for how they view their worlds (Kingsland, 2016). Additionally, Kingsland (2016) reported that the practice of mindfulness has been documented to be highly effective in treating anxiety disorders, substance abuse, and chronic pain.

Communication Sciences and Disorders Students and Mindfulness

The evidence on the positive effects of mindfulness led Beck and her colleagues to study mindfulness and CSD students. A consistent finding in their early studies (Beck et al., 2015; Beck & Verticchio, 2014) was that CSD students demonstrated elevated levels of stress. Results of a recent study (Beck et al., 2020) also documented that not only were stress levels of CSD students elevated, but a majority of the students were perfectionistic and many of them were categorized as maladaptive perfectionists.

To help students learn to manage stress, increase self-compassion, and decrease negative aspects of perfectionism, Beck and colleagues (2017) engaged one group of CSD students in a short meditative mindfulness practice once a week for a semester. Another group of CSD students served as a control group and did not participate in the practice. The practice began with a short series of yoga-based stretches followed by 5 minutes of focused breathwork and 2 minutes of journaling about anything that might have arisen for the student during the practice. This practice aimed to develop awareness of the body and of the calming effects of the breath, both of which targeted reduction in physical and mental stress. Journaling is also a contemplative practice (Germer, 2009) that can increase students' psychological well-being (Khramtsova & Glasscock, 2010). Self-reported measures of perceived stress, perfectionism, and self-compassion, as well as biological measures of stress indicated that, as compared to the control group, the students who practiced mindfulness had statistically significant decreases in perceived and biological levels of stress and in negative aspects of perfectionism. Their self-compassion also increased significantly.

Application of Mindfulness to the Graduate Application Process

While anecdotal evidence led us to believe that the graduate admission process was stressful for students, Beck and colleagues (2020) documented that it is one of the primary stressors for CSD undergraduate students, especially seniors. Based on the evidence cited earlier, we also recognized that participating in a mindfulness practice was one way of helping CSD students manage stress and negative aspects of perfectionism and increase their self-compassion. Because one of the primary goals of our independent study was to help students manage the stress of the graduate application process as effectively as possible, we incorporated a mindfulness practice into the independent study.

ORIGINAL DATA

Our participants were the 33 senior-level CSD students who voluntarily registered for the independent study. After obtaining approval from the institutional review board, we took pretest and posttest measures to determine the effects of participating in the independent study and the mindfulness practice. The pretest measures we conducted documented students' beginning levels of stress, self-compassion, and perfectionism. On the first day of class, we asked students to complete the Self-Compassion Scale (SCS; Neff, 2003; Neff 2019) and the Almost Perfect Scale–Revised (APS-R; Slaney, 2015; Slaney et al., 2001). The SCS is a frequently used measure of self-compassion (Germer, 2009) and the APS-R was designed specifically to measure the perfectionism of college students (Slaney et al., 2001). Both the SCS and the APS-R have been found to be psychometrically sound tests (Beck et al., 2020). The SCS has six subscales that yield a total SCS score. For this independent study, we analyzed the total SCS score. The APS-R has three subscales: Standards, Discrepancy, and Order. The Standards subscale measures expectations regarding performance, the Discrepancy subscale measures the difference between performance expectations and evaluations of performance, and the Order subscale measures the importance of neatness and structure. The Order subscale does not add information about type of perfectionism, so we did not analyze responses to it for this independent study.

We also asked students to complete a questionnaire we created to measure how confident they were about completing various aspects of the graduate application, how stressful they believed the process to be, what aspects of the process they perceived to be the most stressful, if they engaged in stress management, and, if so, what their stress management practice was. Additionally, we asked students to indicate how self-compassionate they believed themselves to be and to define mindfulness.

During the first week of the semester, we asked students to sign up for measures of heart rate variability (HRV), a biological measure of stress levels. During periods of rest, heart rate varies relatively quickly in synchrony with the breathing cycle. During periods of stress, heart rate tends to be higher and less variable. Therefore, HRV is higher during periods of rest and lower during periods of stress. We took three measures of HRV: normalized high frequency power, standard deviation for normalized R-to-R, and normalized low frequency power. We conducted HRV measurements in a research laboratory in the building in which the independent study was held. The sessions took approximately 15 minutes. First, baseline HRV measures were taken. Then, HRV measures were taken during stress-inducing n-back and Stroop tasks (i.e., recalling previously shown stimuli and naming colors printed in either the color of the printed word or a color different from the printed word, respectively).

On the last day of class, students again completed the SCS, APS-R, and author-created questionnaire. They were also asked to sign up for measures of HRV during the last week of the semester. The same procedures used in the pretest sessions were used in the posttest sessions.

APPLICATION OF LITERATURE/DATA

On the first day of the independent study, students were given the assignments of reading part one of Rogers' (2016) book, *The Mindful Twenty-Something: Life Skills to Handle Stress…and Everything Else*, and completing a self-care plan (ReachOut.com, 2019). Both these assignments were due the next class period. Students were also to keep a reflective journal, which was to be a record of their thoughts, experiences, and impressions of the topics and activities covered in class. Students were to write in their journal two to five times a week throughout the semester. The journal was due on the last day of class.

We began the second day of class with a 12- to 15-minute mindfulness practice based on that used by Beck and colleagues (2017). The remainder of the class was devoted to a discussion of mindfulness and self-care. We also engaged in the 12- to 15-minute mindfulness practice at the beginning of the sixth, 10th, and 16th class periods. Before each of these classes, students read sections two, three, and four of Rogers' book, respectively, and came to class ready to discuss one main thought from each of the chapters contained in the assigned sections. Thus, four of the class sessions, one per month, were dedicated to engaging in and discussing mindfulness and stress management. All other classes began with 5 minutes of breath work and 2 minutes of journaling following the prompt to write about whatever came up for the student during the breathwork.

Outcomes

Stress Measures

Due to scheduling conflicts, only 17 of the 33 students (51%) completed both pretest and posttest HRV measures. The result of their measurements indicated that two (standard deviation for normalized R-to-R and normalized low frequency power) of the three biological measures of stress were significantly improved in the posttest session as compared to the pretest session. The other measure, normalized high frequency power, did not change. Given that posttest measures were taken at the end of a semester, when the students were taking finals, finishing final class projects, and finalizing their graduate applications, we consider this remarkable. Additionally, students' responses to the questionnaire item regarding how stressful they believed the graduate application process to be decreased significantly from pretest to posttest; at the beginning of the semester, students rated the process as highly stressful, but by the end of the semester, their perceptions of the overall stressful nature of the process decreased to a more moderate level.

We were also interested in the aspects of the process students found most stressful. At the beginning of the semester, the most frequent item students indicated as stressful was "all aspects of the process." They believed that the process was overwhelming, and the amount of organization required to get it all done added to their sense of stress. Many students also indicated that completing personal statements/essays and feeling inadequate when comparing themselves to others were stressors caused by the process. At the end of the semester, the aspect of the process most frequently cited as most stressful was the personal statements/essays. This was due primarily to the large number of different statements and essays students had to write. The majority of students applied to multiple schools and each school typically had a unique topic to which they required students to respond. The number of students who listed the nature of the process overall and the personal concern of not feeling adequate as stressful decreased.

We also asked students to rate their confidence in completing various aspects of the application. We found students' confidence in their ability to complete all aspects of the graduate application process increased significantly from the beginning to the end of the semester. This outcome, combined with the outcome regarding aspects of the process students considered stressful, suggests that the independent study was successful in helping students increase their confidence about being able to complete the graduate application while decreasing the stress they associated with most of the components in the application process.

An interesting finding was that the number of students who reported engaging in stress management practices increased from 18 in the beginning of the semester to 28 by the end of the semester. Furthermore, the number of different practices cited by students increased. The most frequently cited practices at the beginning of the semester were time management, exercise, and prayer. At the end of the semester, the top-listed stress management practice was mindfulness/meditation/breathwork, followed by exercise, active leisure time activities (e.g., singing, reading, listening to music, painting), yoga, prayer, and time for self.

These outcomes suggest that the creation of a self-care plan and participation in and discussion of mindfulness practices increased students' self-initiated engagement in activities aimed at managing their stress and caring for themselves. The increase in students who engaged in mindfulness/meditation/breathwork and yoga indicates that the practices done in class were not only accepted by the students but also adopted by them for personal use outside of class.

Self-Compassion and Mindfulness Measures

Analysis of pretest and posttest measures of SCS scores and of students' responses to the questionnaire item asking them to rate their level of self-compassion both indicated statistically significant increases in students' self-compassion. Students perceived themselves to be more self-compassionate at the end of the semester as compared to the beginning of the semester.

A comparison of students' definitions of mindfulness from the beginning of the semester to the end of the semester indicated an increase in awareness and acceptance of self and in the importance of being nonjudgmental. At the beginning of the semester, 39% of the students defined mindfulness as being aware of the mind (i.e., control/adjust mind, emotions, thoughts, desires). The next most frequently given definition was being aware of things around you. This definition was followed closely by the definitions of being aware of/responsive to responsibilities (i.e., manage/adjust schedule or be aware of actions and consequence), being aware of self (allowing time for self, care for self, accept self), and relaxing/managing stress. No student defined mindfulness as being nonjudgmental. At the end of the semester, 39% of the students continued to define mindfulness as being aware of the mind. This definition was closely followed by being aware of self and being nonjudgmental. Definitions of being aware of things around you, being aware of/responsive to responsibilities, and relaxing/managing stress were given by only two to four students, a decrease from pretest to posttest.

Perfectionism

A person can be categorized as an adaptive perfectionist, a maladaptive perfectionist, or a nonperfectionist by comparing their score on the APS-R Standards subscale to their score on the APS-R Discrepancy subscale (Rice & Ashby, 2007). We classified students using the guidelines given by Rice and Ashby (2007) and found a similar number of the students were classified as adaptive perfectionists at the beginning (48%) and the end of the semester (52%). Fewer students, however, were classified as maladaptive perfectionists at the end of the semester (32%) than they were at the beginning of the semester (48%).

Analysis of the pretest and posttest APS-R Standards and of the pretest and posttest APS-R Discrepancy scores indicated no significant difference occurred in either set of scores across the semester. The means for the pretest and posttest Standards scores were both higher than the cut-off score set by Rice and Ashby (2007) for perfectionism. Participation in our independent study did not affect the high standards students set for their performance. We considered this to be a positive finding because higher Standards scores have been associated with positive psychological outcomes (Rice et al., 2006). While not significant, the mean for the posttest Discrepancy score was lower than that found for the pretest Discrepancy score. A lower Discrepancy score indicates greater congruence between a person's expectation of their performance and the person's evaluation of their performance. The change in Discrepancy scores was in the desired direction.

Relationship Between Self-Compassion and Perfectionism

One aspect of self-compassion is understanding our common humanity (Neff, 2011). Neff (2011) indicated that this is what allows people to understand that, as humans, we are all imperfect and "our humanity can never be taken away from us, no matter how far we fall" (p. 69). Another component of self-compassion is being kind to oneself rather than judging one's self harshly. Developing this aspect should also help students accept times when they fail to meet goals and to view these instances as learning opportunities rather than failures. Thus, we hypothesized that students who had higher levels of self-compassion would also have lower levels of concern about not meeting the goals they set for themselves (i.e., APS-R Discrepancy scores), and that students with lower levels of self-compassion would have higher Discrepancy scores.

To determine if such a relationship existed, we calculated a Pearson correlation coefficient between SCS scores and APS-R Discrepancy scores. Statistically significant negative correlations were found between the pretest SCS and Discrepancy scores and between posttest SCS and Discrepancy scores; students who had lower levels of self-compassion tended to judge their ability to meet the standards they set for themselves more critically. Students with higher Discrepancy scores also were students who were classified as maladaptive perfectionists (Rice & Ashby, 2007). Ashby and Gnilka (2017) found maladaptive perfectionists tended to have significantly higher levels of perceived stress than adaptive perfectionists. Additionally, students who demonstrate maladaptive perfectionism are more likely to behave in ways that interfere with their academic success (Christman, 2012) and to use more avoidant coping strategies than other students (Noble et al., 2014). Conversely, the significant negative correlations we found between SCS and Discrepancy scores of the students in our independent study also indicate that students who had higher measures of self-compassion tended to have less of a gap between their expectations for their performance and their evaluation of their performance. This suggests that the more we can help students develop self-compassion, the more accepting they might become of their attempts to meet the high standards they set for themselves, even if they are not entirely successful in doing so. Higher levels of self-compassion might then help diminish the presence of maladaptive perfectionistic traits in students and ameliorate the negative effects of not meeting set goals.

Conclusion

The outcomes of this independent study indicate that providing students with appropriate scaffolding around the graduate application process and engaging them in a mindfulness practice and discussions of the importance of mindfulness and self-care were effective ways of decreasing the stress associated with completing graduate applications and increasing students' confidence in their ability to complete all aspects of the application appropriately. We also documented improvements in biological markers of stress and increases in self-compassion and participation in a variety of stress management practices. While APS-R scores did not change significantly across the semester, there was a downward trend in mean Discrepancy scores and a decrease in number of students classified as maladaptive perfectionists. The mindfulness practice used in this independent study was also well accepted by the students who voluntarily enrolled in the class. In evaluations of the independent study, only one student indicated that perhaps less time could be spent on the mindfulness and stress management aspects of the course. Interestingly, we offered the independent study again in Fall 2019, and 35 of our 70 CSD seniors enrolled.

APPLICATION TO CROSS-DISCIPLINARY CONTEXTS

Helping students develop mindfulness to manage stress and increase self-compassion are important goals for clinical programs other than CSD. Not only can these traits help students in clinically oriented programs maintain their overall mental and physical well-being, but they can also serve them well in their professional lives. If health care practitioners are not able to manage stress appropriately, negative outcomes in terms of both client care and attrition from the profession can result (deVibe et al., 2013).

Additionally, health care practitioners often work with individuals who are experiencing difficult life events. To provide high-quality care to an individual who is suffering, the practitioner must be able to take that person's perspective and show the person empathy, without becoming overwhelmed by the person's suffering. A practitioner who is mindful and self-compassionate is more likely to be able to do this than someone with a lesser degree of self-compassion (Neff, 2011). Furthermore, as Duarte and colleagues (2016) indicated, without self-compassion, empathy can be a "double-edged sword" (p. 2) because it can result in practitioner compassion fatigue (i.e., exhaustion and professional burnout with the possibility of symptoms similar to posttraumatic stress disorders; Neff, 2011).

After reviewing mindfulness training offered to dental and medical students and residents in 14 different medical schools, Dobkin and Hutchinson (2013) concluded that this type of training is "beneficial in terms of reducing negative emotions and stress, as well as enhancing mindfulness, empathy, and self-compassion" (p. 769). Our findings support this conclusion, and we believe the addition of mindfulness training to any clinical curriculum would be beneficial to students during their training and into their professional lives.

ADDITIONAL RESOURCES

- A description of stress and perfectionism levels of CSD students:
  - Beck, A., Verticchio, H., & Miller, A. (2020). Levels of stress and characteristics of perfectionism in CSD students. *Teaching and Learning in Communication Sciences and Disorders, 4*(1), Article 3.
- A description of a mindfulness practice that was effective for helping CSD students manage stress and negative aspects of perfectionism and for increasing their self-compassion:
  - Beck, A., Verticchio, H., Seeman, S., Milliken, E., & Schaab, H. (2017). A mindfulness practice for communication sciences and disorders undergraduate and speech-language pathology graduate students: Effects on stress, self-compassion and perfectionism. *American Journal Speech-Language Pathology, 26,* 893-907. https://doi.org/10.1044/2017_AJSLP-16-0172
- A description of the importance of recognizing characteristics of perfectionism and how instructors can help students decrease negative perfectionism:
  - Christman, E. (2012). Understanding maladaptive perfectionism in college students. *Nurse Educator, 37*(5), 202-205.
- A book that describes self-compassion and many ways of developing it:
  - Germer, C. K. (2009). *The mindful path to self-compassion: Freeing yourself from destructive thoughts and emotions.* The Guilford Press.

- A book that describes the mindfulness-based stress reduction program:
  - Kabat-Zinn, J. (2013). *Full catastrophe living: Using the wisdom of your body and mind to face stress, pain, and illness.* Bantam Books Trade Paperback.
- A website with many resources on self-compassion, including an online version of the SCS:
  - Neff, K. (2019). *Self-compassion.* https://self-compassion.org/
- A book describing the importance of self-compassion and many techniques for developing it:
  - Neff, K. (2011). *Self-compassion: Stop beating yourself up and leave insecurity behind.* HarperCollins.
- A book on mindfulness for college students:
  - Rogers, H. B. (2016). *The mindful twenty-something: Life skills to handle stress... and everything else.* New Harbinger Publications.

REFERENCES

Ashby, J. S., & Gnilka, P. B. (2017). Multidimensional perfectionism and perceived stress: Group differences and test of a coping mediation model. *Personality and Individual Differences, 119,* 106-111. https://doi.org/10.1016/j.paid.2017.07.012

Beck, A., Seeman, S., Verticchio, H., & Rice, J. (2015). Yoga as a technique to reduce stress experienced by CSD graduate students. *Contemporary Issues in Communication Sciences and Disorders, 42,* 1-15.

Beck, A., & Verticchio, H. (2014). Facilitating speech-language pathology graduate students' ability to manage stress: A pilot study. *Contemporary Issues in Communication Sciences and Disorders, 41,* 24-38.

Beck, A., Verticchio, H., & Miller, A. (2020). Levels of stress and characteristics of perfectionism in CSD students. *Teaching and Learning in Communication Sciences and Disorders, 4(1),* Article 3.

Beck, A., Verticchio, H., Seeman, S., Milliken, E., & Schaab, H. (2017). A mindfulness practice for CSD undergraduate and SLP graduate students: Effects on stress, self-compassion and perfectionism. *American Journal Speech-Language Pathology, 26,* 893-907. https://doi.org/10.1044/2017_AJSLP-16-0172

Brown, B. (2012). *Daring greatly: How the courage to be vulnerable transforms the way we live, love, parent, and lead.* Gotham Books.

Christman, E. (2012). Understanding maladaptive perfectionism in college students. *Nurse Educator, 37(5),* 202-205.

deVibe, M., Solhaug, I., Tyssen, R., Friborg, O., Rosenvinge, J. H., Sorlie, T., & Bjorndal, A. (2013). Mindfulness training for stress management: A randomized controlled study of medical and psychology students. *Medical Education, 13,* Article 107. https://doi.org/10.1186/1472-6920-13-107

Dobkin, P. L., & Hutchinson, T. A. (2013). Teaching mindfulness in medical school: Where are we now and where are we going? *Medical Education, 47,* 768-779. https://doi.org/10.1111/medu.12200

Duarte, J., Pinto-Gouveia, J., & Cruz, B. (2016). Relationships between nurses' empathy, self-compassion and dimensions of professional quality of life: A cross-sectional study. *International Journal of Nursing Studies, 60,* 1-11. http://dx.doi.org/10.1016/j.ijnurstu.2016.02.015

Germer, C. K. (2009). *The mindful path to self-compassion: Freeing yourself from destructive thoughts and emotions.* The Guilford Press.

Hill, A. P., & Curran, T. (2016). Multidimensional perfectionism and burnout: A meta-analysis. *Personality and Social Psychology Review, 20,* 269-288. https://doi.org/10.1177/1088868315596286

Kabat-Zinn, J. (1994). *Wherever you go there you are.* Hyperion.

Khramtsova, I., & Glasscock, P. (2010). Outcomes of an integrated journaling and mindfulness program on a US university campus. *Revista de psihologie, 56(3-4),* 208-217.

Kingsland, J. (2016). *Siddhartha's brain: Unlocking the ancient science of enlightenment.* HarperCollins.

Lieberman, R., Raisor-Becker, L., Sotto, C., & Reddle, E. (2018). Investigation of graduate student stress in speech language pathology. *Teaching and Learning in Communication Sciences and Disorders, 2(2),* Article 6.

McCall, T. (2007). *Yoga as medicine: The yogic prescription for health and healing.* Bantam.

Neff, K. (2003). The development and validation of a scale of measure self-compassion. *Self and Identity, 2,* 223-250. https://doi.org/10.1080/15298860309027

Neff, K. (2011). *Self-compassion: Stop beating yourself up and leave insecurity behind.* HarperCollins.

Neff, K. (2019). Self-compassion. https://self-compassion.org/

Neff, K. D., & Faso, D. J. (2015). Self-compassion and well-being in parents of children with autism. *Mindfulness, 6(4),* 938-947.

Noble, C. L., Ashby, J. S., & Gnilka, P. B. (2014). Multidimensional perfectionism, coping, and depression: Differential prediction of depression symptoms by perfectionism type. *Journal of College Counseling, 17,* 80-94. https://doi.org/10.1002/j.2161-1882.2014.00049.x

ReachOut.com. (2019). Developing a self-care plan. https://schools.au.reachout.com/articles/developing-a-self-care-plan

Rice, K. G., & Ashby, J. S. (2007). An efficient method for classifying perfectionists. *Journal of Counseling Psychology, 54,* 72-85. https://doi.org/10.1037/0022-0167.54.1.72

Rice, K. G., Leever, B. A., Christopher, J., & Porter, J. D. (2006). Perfectionism, stress, and social (dis)connection: A short-term study of hopelessness, depression, and academic adjustment among honors students. *Journal of Counseling Psychology, 53,* 524-534. https://doi.org/10.1037/0022-0167.53.4.524

Rogers, H. B. (2016). *The mindful twenty-something: Life skills to handle stress...and everything else.* New Harbinger Publications.

Ross, E. (2011). Burnout and self-care in the practice of speech pathology and audiology: An ecological perspective. In R. J. Fourie (Ed.), *Therapeutic processes for communication disorders* (pp. 213-228). Psychology Press.

Slaney, R. B. (2015). *Almost Perfect Scale–Revised.* http://kennethwang.com/apsr/scales/APS-R_96.pdf

Slaney, R. B., Rice, K. G., Mobley, M., Trippi, J., & Ashby, J. S. (2001). The revised almost perfect scale. *Measurement and Evaluation in Counseling and Development, 34,* 130-145.

Suh, H., Gnilka, P. B., & Rice, K. G. (2017). Perfectionism and well-being: A positive psychology framework. *Personality and Individual Differences, 111,* 25-30. http://dx.doi.org/10.1016/j.paid.2017.01.041

Yang, Y., Zhang, M., & Kou, Y. (2016). Self-compassion and life satisfaction: The mediating role of hope. *Personality and Individual Differences, 98,* 91-95. https://dx.doi.org/10.1016/j.paid.2016.03.086

26

A FRAMEWORK FOR ENHANCING CRITICAL THINKING WITHIN HEALTH SCIENCE COURSES

Tim Brackenbury, PhD, CCC-SLP
and Mary-Jon Ludy, PhD, RDN, FAND

DESCRIPTION OF TEACHING/LEARNING CONTEXT

Critical thinking is a cognitive act that applies analysis and reasoning to answer complex questions and guide decision making (Dwyer et al., 2014). It is an important skill to address in the classroom, but instructors can find themselves at a loss for best practices (Folkins, 2016; Halx & Reybold, 2005; Nicholas & Raider-Roth, 2011, 2016). This chapter provides an evidence-based framework for enhancing college students' critical thinking skills across health disciplines.

Critical thinking is an essential component of clinical practice in the health professions (Huang et al., 2014; Sharples et al., 2017). Providers must draw upon the body of evidence-based literature to guide patients and the interdisciplinary medical team to make informed health decisions. Critical thinking skills can reduce the frequency of diagnostic and management errors that occur in patient care (Harasym et al., 2008). Among students in health disciplines, critical thinking skills are positively associated with academic success (Ross et al., 2013).

The course, FN 4400: Research Methods in Nutrition, Foods, and Dietetics, at Bowling Green State University (Bowling Green, Ohio) was recently redesigned to improve students' critical thinking skills and address their common concerns about research (see Earley, 2014). To do so, we developed an evidence-based framework for teaching critical thinking and incorporated it into the FN 4400 course. The framework consists of the following four themes:

Friberg, J. C., Visconti, C. F., & Ginsberg, S. M. (Eds.). *Evidence-Based Education in the Classroom: Examples From Clinical Disciplines* (pp. 233-240).
© 2021 Taylor & Francis Group.

1. Design and integration: Critical thinking needs to be addressed in the design of courses and integrated throughout course activities and assignments.

2. Routine application: Careful consideration and routine application are required for introducing students to critical thinking and motivating them to use it.

3. Modeling the process: Instructors need to model the process of critical thinking, with an emphasis on how different conclusions can be reached and justified.

4. Risk taking and creativity: Assignments and assessments of students' critical thinking should allow space for risk taking and creativity.

REVIEW OF LITERATURE

There is considerable literature on teaching critical thinking within disciplinary courses. The research consists primarily of experimental and quasi-experimental studies that examine changes in students' critical thinking skills before and after teaching experiences, typically in comparison to those of a control group. Outcome measures include standardized tests of critical thinking and tasks developed by educators and researchers. Health care professions, especially nursing, play a prominent role in this literature.

Meta-analyses and systematic reviews have shown reliable positive effects of teaching critical thinking within college courses (Abrami et al., 2015; Tiruneh et al., 2014). For example, Harris and Welch Bacon's (2019) review of 154 studies in health care professions identified improvements in critical thinking, problem solving, and/or decision making in 84% of investigations that used active learning methods. The results from studies examining specific teaching methods, however, have varied. Two approaches that have shown particular promise and are highly relevant to critical thinking within health professions are problem-based learning (PBL) and evidence-based teaching (EBT).

PBL is a learner-centered approach that promotes student inquiry through efforts that address complex, real-world issues (Savery, 2006). As the first step in PBL, students are presented with multifaceted problems to motivate understanding and application of the course objectives and content (Hung, 2009). The problems can include case studies, ethical dilemmas, simulations, and role-playing (Abrami et al., 2015). Instructors in PBL serve as facilitators and tutors, guiding students through stimulating questions, providing "just-in-time" feedback, and delivering encouragement. Developed from medical science education, PBL addresses critical thinking skills through student collaborations that analyze problems and their origins, evaluate potential solutions, and create defensible plans of action. Most of the studies identified across systematic reviews and meta-analyses reveal significant improvements in critical thinking skills following PBL (Carvalho et al., 2017; Harris & Welch Bacon, 2019; Kowalczyk, 2011; Tiruneh et al., 2014).

EBT is an educational offshoot of evidence-based medicine/practice. It focuses on the knowledge and skills for incorporating research literature, clinician expertise, and client values to address educational and professional issues. EBT incorporates PBL by presenting students with perplexing clinical cases that are not easily solvable, such as determining the optimal course of treatment for an atypical patient or addressing a controversy within the field. EBT connects with critical thinking through activities such as finding and evaluating evidence, examining one's own experiences and biases, and collecting and incorporating clients' opinions (Petty, 2009; Schwartz & Gurung, 2012). Cui and colleagues (2018) reviewed nine studies that examined evidence-based nursing, a form of EBT. Significant improvements in overall critical thinking and its subdomains (e.g., inferences, interpretations, truth-seeking) were reported among students who received training in evidence-based nursing compared to those who did not.

Along with individual approaches like PBL and EBT, there is evidence that combining approaches facilitates critical thinking development. For example, Abrami and colleagues (2015) found that "authentic instruction" (i.e., PBL) and classroom dialogue, but not direct mentorship, uniquely contributed to critical thinking development. Significantly higher effect sizes, however, were observed when authentic instruction was combined with dialogue, and when all three factors were intermixed. There are additional positive effects on students' critical thinking when teaching models address multiple components of thought and practice (Anderson & Reed, 2013; Ralston & Bays, 2015).

General strategies for teaching critical thinking have also been examined. These include whether critical thinking skills should be taught explicitly or implicitly, and if they should be addressed within the course content or as a separate unit. Abrami and colleagues' (2015) analysis of effect sizes from 684 experimental studies on teaching critical thinking found significant individual positive effects for (1) explicit instruction within the content, (2) explicit instruction outside of the content, (3) implicit critical thinking experiences within the content, and (4) explicit separate instruction followed by implicit experiences (see also Ennis, 1989). No significant differences were observed between strategies, suggesting that instructors can use the strategy that best fits their experiences and circumstances.

APPLICATION OF LITERATURE/DATA

As a whole, the literature demonstrates that critical thinking can be effectively taught within disciplinary courses in the health professions. Using an evidence-based approach, we applied the research literature, our own teaching experiences and those of our colleagues, and students' input to develop our critical thinking framework. This section provides details on the framework's four interactive components, as well as examples of how they were incorporated into the course.

Design and Integration

Component Overview

Critical thinking needs to be considered and incorporated throughout the design of the course. It should be an essential element of the experience, infused within the daily sessions, assignments, and assessments. This can be achieved by designing the class around a critical thinking–based theme that complements the topic of the course and aligns with students' interests in a manner that is clearly relevant to their future professional practice. Similarly, including critical thinking in the course goals clearly demonstrates its importance. The problem-solving nature of critical thinking, for example, can be incorporated into goals for improving students' understanding of foundational knowledge by applying important terms in meaningful contexts, analyzing and evaluating different forms of evidence, and developing clinical reasoning and decision-making skills.

FN 4400 Application

To motivate an early interest in the course and stimulate critical thinking about the importance of course content in the professional setting, an engaging syllabus is used (Ludy, Brackenbury, et al., 2016; the course syllabus may be viewed at https://tinyurl.com/FN4400Syllabus). This is distributed to students electronically prior to the first class. It includes pictures of students and faculty from the program who are engaged in research activities (e.g., conference presentation, laboratory-based data collection). To demonstrate relevance, learning objectives are explicitly linked to programmatic accreditation standards (Accreditation Council for Education in Nutrition and Dietetics, 2017) and many required readings are from disciplinary journals (see Byerley et al., 2017). In recent years, readings from popular press books were incorporated (e.g., Hanna-Attisha, 2018; Skloot, 2010).

Throughout the course, junior- and senior-level research methods students conduct health assessments on first-year college students as part of an ongoing research study that is linked with a learning community. Assessment variables include common health markers that are evaluated in clinical nutrition practice (e.g., blood pressure, body composition, cholesterol, fitness). Prior to conducting assessments on first-year students, research methods students receive training from and demonstrate proficiency to graduate students and faculty in nutrition and exercise science (Ludy, Tucker, et al., 2016). Assessments are conducted twice during the semester. In addition to collecting the data, research methods students are involved in preliminary data analysis and communicating the results back to the first-year students in the learning community. The research methods students have responded favorably to this model of incorporating critical thinking into the course, as demonstrated by the following comment from a recent course evaluation:

> The hands-on approach within FN 4400 should stay the same. It was very beneficial to have that experience with the health study, and I personally learned a lot from it. Having this experience helped me understand how to work with human subjects and learn from trial and error.

Routine Application

Component Overview

Students should be provided with repeated small and large activities that invite critical thinking as a routine part of the course experience. Our preference is to identify and define critical thinking (i.e., applying analysis and reasoning to answer complex questions and guide decision making) at the very start of the course and refer to it throughout the semester. This includes introducing and applying key terms and skills associated with critical thinking, such as assumptions, confirmation bias, value preferences, evidence, and self-reflection.

FN 4400 Application

The culminating assignment in the research methods course is preparation and review of a federal-style grant proposal. Instead of a single high-point value assignment, the grant proposal process is divided into multiple low-stakes assignments with regular feedback and numerous opportunities for revision. Students have seven low-stakes assignments related to grant writing, including developing research questions, identifying key references, summarizing the background literature, planning the methods, and justifying a budget. Each low-stakes submission includes revisions based on feedback from previous submissions. Likewise, after receiving feedback from the instructor and graduate assistants, students engage in a low-stakes peer critique prior to participating in a full federal-style grant panel review. One student's comment that relates to routine application was, "I loved how the grant proposal was broken up into sections each week. It made it simple and I was not overwhelmed. We had the right amount of time to work on each section."

Modeling the Process

Component Overview

Instructors are good at describing complex professional situations and the choices they would make. However, they do not always include the "behind-the-scenes" details about how the conclusion was determined, such as the other possibilities considered, why certain possibilities were eliminated, additional information needed and how it was acquired, conclusions that other professionals might choose, and deciding what to do when more than one conclusion appears to be appropriate.

FN 4400 Application

To reduce anxiety and nervousness about the process of receiving and responding to critical feedback, the instructor shares reviewer feedback from previous grant and manuscript submissions that demonstrate both imperfections and differing viewpoints. Additionally, past students in this course voluntarily return to present their undergraduate research projects and share rough drafts of manuscripts that they plan to submit to peer-reviewed professional journals. Current FN

4400 students provide critical feedback to past students using guided prompts (e.g., concerning the scientific merit, clarity of goals and writing, discussion of findings in the context of previous literature, greatest strength, single improvement that would have the greatest impact). This serves as a mutually beneficial process. Current students have the opportunity to learn peer review skills and build confidence in the process, subsequently using the same guided prompts to provide low-stakes reviews to their classmates. Past students model the process of accepting and integrating feedback prior to manuscript submission, ultimately being successful at having their manuscripts accepted for publication in professional journals (Lechner et al., 2019; Mansperger et al., 2020; Traxler et al., 2020). Collectively, these activities provide students with a model for critically evaluating and discussing the work of their peers. A student commented that, "It was super beneficial how we had so much feedback from each other, the professor, and older dietetics students."

Risk Taking and Creativity

Component Overview

Critical thinking in the classroom is a risky endeavor for many students. Not fully understanding the problem, misapplying information, making false assumptions, and giving a wrong answer can all be frustrating and embarrassing. Creating a classroom environment that allows for risk taking and creativity addresses these issues while demonstrating the process and power of critical thinking. Throughout this process, the instructor reinforces all of the ideas shared, accurate or inaccurate, as valuable steps in critical thinking. To maximize risk taking and creativity, few points or other negative consequences are associated with these activities.

FN 4400 Application

To encourage risk taking and creativity throughout the grant proposal process, students are assigned to small groups based on similar research interests and varied skillsets. Prior to group assignments, students complete a survey. They rank their research interests from a number of faculty areas of expertise (e.g., food insecurity, sports nutrition), so that if they decide to pursue undergraduate research opportunities, they can find mentorship. They rank self-perceived skills, including creativity, math, and writing. They also rank preferred group roles, including people manager, project manager, and recorder. Each group has a common research interest and students were assigned primary responsibilities based on their self-perceived skills and preferred group roles. For example, one three-member group had a shared interest in diabetes with assigned roles as math/recorder, creativity/people manager, and writing/project manager. The rationale is that students will be more likely to take risks because they know that group members have all the skills necessary to succeed, combined with multiple opportunities for revision (as described in the Routine Application section earlier). A student appreciated "the process put in place to form our groups for the Grant Proposal project. I feel that that worked well in forming groups of people with different strengths but similar interests." Another student liked "the way the groups are assigned. I would have not picked the members that were in my group originally—but I would not change who I ended up with since we all worked evenly and well together." Two of the eight groups from the most recent course have gone on to pursue undergraduate research funding based on the grant topics they explored in FN 4400.

APPLICATION TO CROSS-DISCIPLINARY CONTEXTS

We have successfully applied this teaching critical thinking framework to a number of courses outside of FN 4400 (e.g., https://tinyurl.com/3110Syllabus), and believe that it can be used in classes across health disciplines. This section contains general ideas for applying these in a cross-disciplinary context.

Design and Integration

Critical thinking and its related skills can be designed as themes that complement the course topic. Examples of such themes include facing challenges, learning from others, appreciating differences, and professional thinking. Once a theme is identified, it should be integrated into the course goals, teaching and learning activities, and feedback and assessment. For example, a course designed around appreciating differences can include goals such as:

- You (the student) will identify and consider the points of view of different professions toward clinical assessment and intervention.
- You will incorporate clients' personal and cultural views in your intervention planning.
- You will identify your own preconceptions and how they can negatively influence your professional decisions.

Classroom activities focused on appreciating differences should emphasize the multiple ideas that relate to the problem and how they each contribute to a comprehensive understanding of the issue. Likewise, evaluations and feedback should focus on the process of identifying and considering different ideas in decision making.

Routine Application

A simple way to build routine application into a course is to follow a similar structure for each unit. In some of our classes, for example, we follow the principles of PBL by starting new units with a clinically relevant problem that is strongly connected to the topic and is approximately 80% solvable with the students' current knowledge and skills. After considering the issue, they identify what they know, what they would like to know, and multiple potential solutions. They turn to the course readings to address all three of these topics and submit reading worksheets describing the relevant information, the confusing information, and how both might help address the issue. The instructor leads small and large group classroom discussions that address these issues and introduce other relevant information. Assignments provide similar cases to be analyzed, to promote comparisons and generalization. Final conclusions to the original problem are developed, as well as compared and contrasted with each other and the initial solutions.

Modeling the Process

Storytelling of past clinical decision making is a common method for modeling critical thinking. This is useful but may not be as influential as directly demonstrating critical thinking in real-time along with the students. Engaging in critical thinking activities such as those described earlier changes the instructor's role from the course's source of knowledge to a fellow problem-solver. It is especially helpful if the instructor can step back from their preconceived solution and take on the mindset of a less experienced professional. As an active participant, the instructor shares their initial questions, collects and incorporates information from other sources, considers and learns from the students' ideas, and reaches reasonable conclusions. Doing so models the critical thinking process, demystifies clinical decision making, debunks the notion of a "one-true correct response," and provides meaningful opportunities for EBT.

Risk Taking and Creativity

Working in small, in-class groups provides students with an intimate setting to brainstorm and work through their initial ideas. These can be shared in a nonthreatening way by having each group write their initial conclusions, solutions, and rejected ideas on the board. The instructor leads a whole class discussion comparing and contrasting the groups' ideas. Strong ideas are recognized, and weak ideas are acknowledged for their contribution to better understanding. Near the end of the conversation, each student walks around the room and places a checkmark by the three ideas that they like the best overall. This facilitates a final discussion to plan the next steps. The advantage of a structure like this is that students get to share their ideas and be creative without fear of personal embarrassment or penalty for being incorrect.

ADDITIONAL RESOURCES

- Additional helpful resources for enhancing students' critical thinking skills include:
  - A repository of books, research, and professional development opportunities:
    - https://www.criticalthinking.org/
  - A process for designing a critical thinking–based course:
    - https://www.thecriticalthinkinginitiative.org/
- An overview of teaching critical thinking within health disciplines:
  - Finn, P., Brundage, S. B., & DiLollo, A. (2016). Preparing our future helping professionals to become critical thinkers: A tutorial. *Perspectives of the ASHA Special Interest Groups, 1*(SIG 10), 43-68.
- An integrated approach to designing college courses:
  - Fink, L. D. (2013). *Creating significant learning experiences: An integrated approach to designing college courses* (2nd ed.). Jossey-Bass Inc.
- Examples of how components of this framework connect with motivation and engagement principles from video game design:
  - Folkins, J. W., Brackenbury, T., Kraus, M., & Haviland, A. (2016). Enhancing the therapy experience using principles of video game design. *American Journal of Speech-Language Pathology, 25,* 111-121.
- A discussion of how critical thinking fits within disciplinary teaching:
  - Brackenbury, T., Folkins, J. W., & Ginsberg, S. M. (2014). Examining educational challenges in communication sciences and disorders from the perspectives of signature pedagogy and reflective practice. *Contemporary Issues in Communication Sciences and Disorders, 41*(1), 70-82.

REFERENCES

Abrami, P. C., Bernard, R. M., Borokhovski, E., Waddington, D. I., Wade, C. A., & Persson, T. (2015). Strategies for teaching students to think critically: A meta-analysis. *Review of Educational Research, 85*(2), 275-314. http://doi.org/10.3102/0034654314551063

Accreditation Council for Education in Nutrition and Dietetics. (2017). Accreditation Standards for Nutrition and Dietetics Didactic Programs (DPD). *Academy of Nutrition and Dietetics.* https://www.eatrightpro.org/acend/accreditation-standards-fees-and-policies/2017-standards

Anderson, P. R., & Reed, J. R. (2013). The effect of critical thinking instruction on graduates of a college of business administration. *Journal of Higher Education Theory and Practice, 13*(3/4), 149-167. http://na-businesspress.homestead.com/JHETP/ReidJR_Web13_3__4_.pdf

Byerley, L., Lane, H., Ludy, M. J., Vitolins, M. Z., Anderson, E., Niedert, K., Pennington, K., Yang, J., & Abram, J. K. (2017). Ethical considerations for successfully navigating the research process. *Journal of the Academy of Nutrition and Dietetics, 117*(8), 1302-1307. http://doi.org/10.1016/j.jand.2017.02.011

Carvalho, D. P., Azevedoa, I. C., Cruza, G. K., Mafra, G. A., Rego A. L., Vitor, A. F., Santos, V. E. P., Cogo, A. L. P., & Ferreira Júnior, M. A. (2017). Strategies used for the promotion of critical thinking in nursing undergraduate education: A systematic review. *Nurse Education Today, 57,* 103-107. https://doi.org/10.1016/j.nedt.2017.07.010

Cui, C., Li, Y., Geng, D., Zhang, H., & Jin, C. (2018). The effectiveness of evidence-based nursing on development of nursing students' critical thinking: A meta-analysis. *Nurse Education Today, 65,* 46-53. https://doi.org/10.1016/j.nedt.2018.02.036

Dwyer, C. P., Hogan, M. J., & Stewart, I. (2014). An integrated critical thinking framework for the 21st century. *Thinking Skills and Creativity, 12,* 43-52. http://doi.org/10.1016/j.tsc.2013.12.004

Earley, M. A. (2014). A synthesis of the literature on research methods education. *Teaching in Higher Education, 19*(3), 242-253. http://doi.org/10.1080/13562517.2013.860105

Ennis, R. A. (1989). Critical thinking and subject specificity: Clarification and needed research. *Educational Researcher, 18*(3), 4-10. http://doi.org/10.3102/0013189X018003004

Folkins, J. W. (2016) Are we asking the right questions about pedagogy in communication sciences and disorders? *Contemporary Issues in Communication Sciences and Disorders, 43,* 77-86. https://pubs.asha.org/doi/pdf/10.1044/cicsd_43_S_77

Halx, M. D., & Reybold, L. E. (2005). A pedagogy of force: Faculty perspectives of critical thinking capacity in undergraduate students. *The Journal of General Education, 54*(4), 293-315. https://www.jstor.org/stable/27798029

Hanna-Attisha, M. (2018). *What the eyes don't see: A story of crisis, resistance, and hope in an American city.* Random House.

Harasym, P. H., Tsai, T. C., & Hemmati, P. (2008). Current trends in developing medical students' critical thinking abilities. *The Kaohsiung Journal of Medical Sciences, 24*(7), 341-355. http://doi.org/10.1016/S1607-551X(08)70131-1

Harris, N., & Welch Bacon, C. E. (2019). Developing cognitive skills through active learning: A systematic review of health care professions. *Athletic Training Education Journal, 14*(2), 135-148. http://doi.org/10.4085/1402135

Huang, G. C., Newman, L. R., & Schwartzstein, R. M. (2014). Critical thinking in health professions education: Summary and consensus statements of the Millennium Conference 2011. *Teaching and Learning in Medicine, 26*(1), 95-102. http://doi.org/10.1080/10401334.2013.857335

Hung, W. (2009). The 9-step problem design process for problem-based learning: Application of the 3C3R model. *Educational Research Review, 4*(2), 118-141. https://doi.org/10.1016/j.edurev.2008.12.001

Kowalczyk, N. (2011). Review of teaching methods and critical thinking skills. *Radiology Technology, 83*(2), 120-132. http://www.radiologictechnology.org/content/83/2.toc

Lechner, T. E., Gill, E. M., Drees, M. J., Hamady, C. M., & Ludy, M. J. (2019). Prevalence of disordered eating and muscle dysmorphia in college students by predominant exercise type. *International Journal of Exercise Science, 12*(4), 989-1000. https://digitalcommons.wku.edu/ijes/vol12/iss4/

Ludy, M., Brackenbury, T., Folkins, J. W., Peet, S. H., Langendorfer, S. J., & Beining, K. (2016). Student impressions of syllabus design: Engaging versus contractual syllabus. *International Journal for the Scholarship of Teaching and Learning, 10*(2), Article 6. https://digitalcommons.georgiasouthern.edu/ij-sotl/vol10/iss2/6/

Ludy, M., Tucker, R. M., Crum, A., & Young, C. (2016). Engaging undergraduate nutrition students in research: A graduate student mentorship approach. *Journal of the Academy of Nutrition and Dietetics, 116*(9), A64. https://doi.org/10.1016/j.jand.2016.06.227

Mansperger, J. A., Morgan, A. L., Kiss, J. E., & Ludy, M. J. (2020). The story of Josie: From involvement to influence. *Learning Communities Research and Practice, 8*(2), 1-12. https://washingtoncenter.evergreen.edu/lcrpjournal/vol8/iss2/2/

Nicholas, M. N., & Raider-Roth, M. (2011). *Approaches used by faculty to assess critical thinking—Implications for general education.* Paper presented at the ASHE Annual Conference, Seattle, WA. https://files.eric.ed.gov/fulltext/ED536592.pdf

Nicholas, M. N., & Raider-Roth, M. (2016). A hopeful pedagogy to critical thinking. *International Journal for the Scholarship of Teaching and Learning, 10*(2), 1-10. https://eric.ed.gov/?id=EJ1134753

Petty, G. (2009). *Evidence-based teaching: A practical approach* (2nd ed.). Nelson Thornes Ltd.

Ralston, P. A., & Bays, C. L. (2015). Critical thinking development in undergraduate engineering students from freshman through senior year: A 3-cohort longitudinal study. *American Journal of Engineering Education, 6*(2), 85-98. https://eric.ed.gov/?id=EJ1083228

Ross, D., Loeffler, K., Schipper, S., Vandermeer, B., & Allan, G. M. (2013). Do scores on three commonly used measures of critical thinking correlate with academic success of health professions trainees? A systematic review and meta-analysis. *Academic Medicine, 88*(5), 724-734. http://doi.org/10.1097/ACM.0b013e31828b0823

Savery, J. R. (2006). Overview of problem-based learning: Definitions and distinctions. *Interdisciplinary Journal of Problem-Based Learning, 1*(1), 9-20. http://doi.org/10.7771/1541-5015.1002

Schwartz, B. M., & Gurung, R. A. (2012). *Evidence-based teaching for higher education.* American Psychological Association.

Sharples, J. M., Oxman, A. D., Mahtani, K. R., Chalmers, I., Oliver, S., Collins, K., Austvoll-Dahlgren, A., & Hoffmann, T. (2017). Critical thinking in healthcare and education. *BMJ, 357,* j2234. https://doi.org/10.1136/bmj.j2234

Skloot, R. L. (2010). *The immortal life of Henrietta Lacks.* Crown Publishing.

Tiruneh, D. T., Verbugh, A., & Elen, J. (2014). Effectiveness of critical thinking instruction in higher education: A systematic review of intervention studies. *Higher Education Studies, 4*(1), 1-17. http://doi.org/10.5539/hes.v4n1p1

Traxler, E. A., Morgan, A. L., Kiss, J. E., & Ludy, M. J. (2020). Animated case study videos: A creative approach for exploring health in the high school to college transition. *Health Promotion Practice, 21*(1), 16-19. https://doi.org/10.1177/1524839919874053

27

Linking Art and Visual Thinking Strategies to Teach Clinical Observation Skills

Jennifer C. Friberg, EdD, CCC-SLP, F-ASHA

Description of Teaching/Learning Context

Recently, I was assigned to teach a course focused on assessment practices for speech-language pathology graduate students. The first semester I taught this course started out reasonably well, with students demonstrating increasing competency (and confidence) as emerging diagnosticians. However, as the semester progressed, it became evident that my students' clinical observation skills were actually quite weak, which was a huge surprise to me. Through a variety of large and small group activities, I noted that my students engaged in clinical observations of patients quite shallowly, identifying symptoms and behaviors, rather than looking deeply and systematically at the entire communication context to understand patients' strengths and needs. I reflected on why this might be, then asked the class how they learned to observe patients within various communication contexts. Most students could not recall being explicitly taught such skills. They reported that they had no systematic method for conducting clinical observations. Rather, they endeavored to simply record what seemed notable to them regarding a patient's communication skills.

While I feel as though there are times as a course instructor that it is acceptable to identify changes/additions to content to address in future iterations of a course, this was not one of those times. I felt compelled to find a way to integrate the teaching of clinical observation skills and strategies to my students before the semester ended, rather than waiting to integrate such content into the course in future academic terms. Thus, I undertook a literature review to identify evidence-informed approaches to teaching comprehensive clinical observation skills. Finding few resources in my discipline of speech-language pathology, I focused my search on other health care fields, as observing patients is a (relatively) ubiquitous skill in medicine, nursing, dietetics, counseling, etc.

Friberg, J. C., Visconti, C. F., & Ginsberg, S. M. (Eds.). *Evidence-Based Education in the Classroom: Examples From Clinical Disciplines* (pp. 241-248).

This chapter describes outcomes from my literature search, outlines how I applied outcomes from research to address a problem in my assessment course, and presents results from original data collected to determine whether the application of this evidence-informed approach to teaching actually helped to improve students' competency in clinical observation.

REVIEW OF LITERATURE

Visual thinking strategies (VTS) were developed as a standardized method to encourage discussion and engagement with art in meaningful ways across a variety of perspectives (Housen & Yenawine, 2001; Visual Thinking Strategies, n.d.). It is quite common for museum guides, for instance, to use VTS to facilitate discussion about art with patrons, many of whom have little experience with talking about works of art. Most people who use VTS are seeking to deepen visual literacy, generally described as the ability to interpret and process things seen with other sensory inputs (Hailey et al., 2015). Hailey and colleagues (2015) posit that these skills may need to be explicitly taught, as "the culture at large seems to assume that somehow, perhaps because of our constant bombardment with images, visual literacy will simply happen without specific instruction" (p. 50).

VTS relies on the application of a predictable structure using the following three questions, asked in the same sequence in the same manner for each new observational situation, to jumpstart thinking and/or discussions from an observer's own unique perspective (Visual Thinking Strategies, n.d.):

1. What is going on in this picture?
2. What makes you say that?
3. What else can we find?

Because VTS allows for a systematic investigation of visual phenomena, this technique has been successfully utilized in numerous health-related disciplines to teach observation skills to students (Beck et al., 2017; Boudreau et al., 2008; Poirier et al., 2019; Wellbery & McAteer, 2015). While art and patient assessment could seem an incongruous pairing, VTS is a method of improving visual literacy to promote critical thinking, something necessary for effective assessment of patients (Reilly et al., 2005). By adopting VTS questions for use in clinical contexts, students can learn to think systematically and critically about the diagnostic process (Moorman & Hensel, 2016).

Moorman and colleagues (2017) described a process of using VTS as students observe works of art with a trained museum guide as a way of learning a systematic approach to clinical observation, with the hope of transitioning these skills to clinical contexts. Study of student learning as a result of this intervention indicated that students perceived gains in observational, cognitive, interpersonal, and intrapersonal skills. Other similar studies have had positive outcomes as well, with students perceiving growth as diagnosticians as a result of VTS-based learning experiences (Beck et al., 2017; Boudreau et al., 2008; Poirier et al., 2019; Wellbery & McAteer, 2015).

APPLICATION OF LITERATURE/DATA

Using a framework suggested by Moorman and Hensel (2016) for inspiration, I designed a purposeful intervention for using VTS questions to teach students to conduct high-quality clinical observations. The purpose for this intervention was twofold: to facilitate students' transfer of VTS questions from art-based contexts to clinically based contexts and to encourage the development of comprehensive clinical observation skills for students seemingly lacking competency in this area.

Introduction of Visual Thinking Strategies Intervention

A trained guide from a regional museum offered to assist in the implementation of this VTS intervention. This guide was able to work with his museum to secure large-scale gallery-style copies of three works of art and smaller, printed copies of another four paintings. Copies of the large-scale artworks were brought to campus and hung in the classroom just prior to a 2-hour long class meeting. Desks and tables were pushed to the side of the room to create a gallery-type feel for the classroom. When students arrived, they were told that class would begin with a discussion related to specific works of art led by a museum guide. The guide led students from one picture to the next in a single large group, asking students to respond to the art using the VTS questions he commonly used during tours at his own museum:

- What is going on in this picture?
- What do you see that makes you say that?
- What else do you see when you look at the picture?

Because he found it to be a useful addition to expand on established VTS questions, the guide added a fourth question to his interactions with students: What other questions do you have about this picture?

Students responded to these questions during the walking tour of the three large artworks, then (after helping to rearrange the classroom) worked in smaller groups of three to four students, looking critically at the smaller copies of four additional works of art. The guide directed each group to apply VTS questions to make observations of the pictures they were given within their small groups for discussion, then facilitated a large group discussion for students to share their impressions of the art in question. This part of the VTS intervention lasted approximately 75 minutes.

Transition of Visual Thinking Strategies Intervention Questions From Art to Clinic

The next step in the VTS intervention was to encourage my students, now experienced in applying VTS questions to the observation of art, to consider how VTS questions might be transitioned to apply to clinical context. It is important to note that at no time during the work students did with the museum guide did I mention that the aim of this intervention was to improve competency with clinical observation skills. I could have revealed that VTS questions could transfer directly to clinical observations, but I wanted my students to make that cognitive leap themselves, as research on teaching and learning has been quite clear that when students have to engage metacognitive skills to make such connections, learning is deeper (Bransford et al., 2000).

I began a whole class discussion asking students how VTS questions might apply to the practice of speech-language pathology, asking students where they might be applied to assessment in particular. It was not long into the discussion that students identified clinical observations as being particularly well-suited to the use of VTS questions, though students acknowledged that the VTS questions would need to be adapted for such use. At that point, I tasked students with adapting VTS questions for use in clinical contexts. The class negotiated one final set of VTS questions that we adopted for clinical observations (Table 27-1). This portion of the VTS intervention lasted approximately 5 to 10 minutes.

Following the drafting of VTS questions for clinical contexts, students were given the opportunity to practice the use of their questions to complete an observation of a 5-minute video of a pediatric patient engaged in diagnostic therapy. Students were asked to make note of all they felt was important to know about the client and the communication context. Students uniformly indicated that they felt the VTS intervention was interesting and valuable; however, because I felt it was important to understand students' learning as a result of this process, I collected data before, during, and after the implementation of the VTS intervention. The structure for and outcomes of this study are described in the following section.

TABLE 27-1

Transfer of Visual Thinking Strategies Question to the Clinical Context

VISUAL THINKING STRATEGIES QUESTION FOR ARTS-BASED CONTEXT	VISUAL THINKING STRATEGIES QUESTION FOR CLINICAL CONTEXT
What is going on in this picture?	What is going on with and around this client?
What do you see that makes you say that?	What do you see that makes you say that?
What else do you see?	Take a closer look. What more can you see?
What questions do you still have?	Now that you have observed the client, what other questions do you have?

ORIGINAL DATA

Predominantly, research on the use of VTS to aid in teaching clinical observation skills has utilized indirect data sources (e.g., student perceptions), which can lack objectivity in measuring learning as they speak to student preference rather than actual student learning (Vanderbilt University Center for Teaching, 2013). Thus, I designed a study to determine if the VTS intervention led to immediate and/or sustained changes in students' clinical observation skills. This work was approved by my institution's human subjects review board. Each of my 30 students provided consent for participation in this study.

The study was undertaken in four distinct phases: pre-VTS intervention, VTS intervention, post-VTS intervention 1, and post-VTS intervention 2. Each of these phases are described in Table 27-2.

Learning Outcomes

Student learning as a result of this VTS experience was measured in two ways: direct measures of complexity of clinical observations and student reflection on the VTS experience.

Complexity of Clinical Observations

Because my initial motivation to engage in the development and implementation of this intervention emerged from my anecdotal observation that students' clinical observations were relatively shallow, I wanted to measure the impact of the VTS intervention on the complexity of students' clinical observations. To accomplish this, students' clinical observations from pre-VTS intervention, post-VTS intervention 1, and post-VTS intervention 2 phases were analyzed. Each observation was broken down into individual statements that were assigned to one of four categories: description of client's communication, description of other behaviors, description of communication context, or evidence (this was any sort of documentation or quantification of a behavior). Analyses were completed to determine whether student observations included an increase in the number of categories selected by the student after the VTS intervention. Data indicate that students made and maintained gains as a result of the VTS intervention (Table 27-3).

TABLE 27-2

Measuring the Impact of the Visual Thinking Strategies Intervention

STUDY PHASE	DESCRIPTION OF PHASE	DURATION OF PHASE
Pre-VTS intervention	In the class meeting, immediately prior to the implementation of the VTS intervention, students were asked to perform a clinical observation of a pediatric client engaged in a diagnostic language therapy session. Students were asked to watch a 5-minute video clip of the session and note anything they felt was important to know about the client or the communication context. These observations were archived for later comparison.	5 to 10 minutes
VTS intervention	The VTS intervention was implemented as described previously in this chapter. This phase included the whole class gallery experience and small group VTS practice with large group sharing.	75 minutes
Post-VTS intervention 1	Students watched a 5-minute video clip of a diagnostic language therapy session (featuring a different context but the same client as was part of the observation in pre-VTS intervention phase) and noted anything they felt was important to know about the client or the communication context. These observations were archived for later comparison. Students answered three open-ended reflection questions (in writing) to discuss their learning as part of the VTS intervention.	5 to 10 minutes
Post-VTS intervention 2	Students watched a 5-minute video clip of a diagnostic language therapy session (featuring a different context but the same client as was part of the observation in pre-VTS intervention and post-VTS intervention 1 phases) and noted anything they felt was important to know about the client or the communication context. These observations were archived for later comparison.	5 to 10 minutes

TABLE 27-3

Mean Scores for Complexity of Clinical Observations

PHASE	MEAN CATEGORIES (STANDARD DEVIATION) REPRESENTED IN CLINICAL OBSERVATIONS
Pre-VTS intervention	1.4 (0.45)
Post-VTS intervention 1	3.1 (0.47)
Post-VTS intervention 2	3.0 (0.58)

Student Reflection of the Visual Thinking Strategies Intervention

During the post-VTS intervention 1 phase of the study, students were asked to describe what they learned as part of their VTS intervention experiences by writing responses to three reflection questions. Content analysis of these responses yielded five themes that were noted consistently in student reflections, each of which is described in Table 27-4. Satisfied that this intervention was successful, I plan to utilize it again in the future to teach clinical observation skills to my students.

APPLICATION TO CROSS-DISCIPLINARY CONTEXTS

This particular approach to clinical observation can be readily applied to other clinical fields, as the learning experience of observing art while practicing the use of standard VTS questions, has no direct disciplinary content. Rather, it is the process of using VTS questions that would need to be customized to fit unique needs of separate clinical fields' content. Based on my experience using this pedagogy, I learned that it is important to make the process of adapting VTS questions to fit clinical contexts explicit to students. Quite honestly, the use of VTS to teach clinical observation could skip the arts-based experience completely. It would be possible to systematically teach VTS questions specific to clinical contexts only (e.g., provide a list of clinically based VTS questions for students to learn and use). That said, the experience of applying VTS questions to something unexpected (art) and transferring the process of using VTS questions to clinical contexts may very well be what engaged my students and helped them take ownership of their learning processes.

With the advent of various technologies and the move toward interprofessional educational models in clinically based disciplines, the potential uses and applications for a VTS framework for teaching clinical observation are numerous. VTS could be used to prepare students for clinical observations that occur via live, video, or simulated experiences. Students representing different disciplines could use VTS to compare and contrast what they find notable through their own professional lenses during clinical observations. Essentially, VTS could be applied to any situation where students need to process—and practice the process of—collecting information visually and systematically.

ADDITIONAL RESOURCES

Related Websites

- VTS homepage (created by the founders of VTS):
  - https://vtshome.org
- *What are Visual Thinking Strategies:*
  - https://voicethread.com/blog/what-are-visual-thinking-strategies/

Suggested Readings

- Blanding, M. (2019). Museum studies: Art unleashes emotions and discussion among new doctors. *Harvard Medicine.* https://hms.harvard.edu/magazine/art-medicine/museum-studies
- Jasani, S. K., & Saks, N. S. (2013). Utilizing visual art to enhance the clinical observation skills of medical students. *Medical Teacher, 35*(7), 1327-1331.
- Naghshineh, S., Hafler, J. P., Miller, A. R., Blanco, M. A., Lipsitz, S. R., Dubroff, R. P., Khoshbin, S., & Katz, J. T. (2008). Formal art observation training improves medical students' visual diagnostic skills. *Journal of General Internal Medicine, 23*(7), 991-997. https://doi.org/10.1007/s11606-008-0667-0

TABLE 27-4

Outcomes From Qualitative Analysis of Post-Intervention Student Reflections

THEME	DESCRIPTION OF THEME	QUOTES FROM STUDENT REFLECTIONS
The "big picture" phenomenon	An understanding that the client is more than a collection of symptoms	"My 'aha' moment was physically looking closer to the pictures to see the details then stepping back to see how those little elements interacted with each other. This directly correlated with observing clients where we need to consider the little things we see and then see how those things interact to make the individual client." "Clinical observation isn't just looking once and knowing it all, just like was the case with the paintings."
Investing time in the client	A realization that high-quality observations require time and thought	"This made me feel okay about not knowing the 'right' answer immediately and showed me the importance of taking my time with observation and diagnosis." "I think I will look at my patients now with more depth across more factors and considerations."
Understanding processes	Use and practice with a systematic process for observation was helpful to clarify how to observe comprehensively	"VTS helped me feel more guided in my observations and feel like I know what to look at, as well as what to consider regarding what I see." "Part of clinical observation is thinking about all the things that impact a client, even those things that don't bring attention to themselves."
Understanding context	Observation of more than just the client is important to understand the client's strengths and needs	"I really liked the 'What else do you see?' question, as it pushed me to look at a client from different perspectives." "I realized how much the context surrounding an observation can change the information I gather from it."
Seeking additional evidence	Evidence is necessary to contextualize observations	"The question 'What makes you say that?' allows for deeper connections and meanings to emerge and makes us think about what we are using to back up our observations." "VTS made me think that it would be really important to do more than one observation to understand my patient's needs."

REFERENCES

Beck, C., Gaunt, H., & Chiavaroli, N. (2017). Improving visual observation skills through the arts to aid radiographic interpretation in veterinary practice: A pilot study. *Veterinary Radiology Ultrasound, 58*(5), 495-502.

Boudreau, J. D., Cassell, E. J., & Fuks, A. (2008). Preparing medical students to become skilled at clinical observation. *Medical Teacher, 30,* 857-862.

Bransford, J. D., Brown, A. L., & Cocking, R. R. (2000). *How people learn: Brain, mind, experience, and school.* National Academy Press.

Hailey, D., Miller, A., & Yenawine, P. (2015). Understanding visual literacy: The visual thinking strategies approach. In D. M. Baylen & A. D'Alba (Eds.)., *Essentials of teaching and integrating visual and media literacy: Visualizing learning.* Springer.

Housen, A., & Yenawine, P. (2001). *VTS curriculum.* Visual Understanding in Education.

Moorman, M., & Hensel, D. (2016). Using visual thinking strategies in nursing education. *Nurse Educator, 41*(1), 5-6.

Moorman, M., Hensel, D., Decker, K. A., & Busby, K. (2017). Learning outcomes with visual thinking strategies in nursing education. *Nursing Education Today, 51,* 127-129.

Poirier, T. I., Newman, K., & Ronald, K. (2019). An exploratory study using visual thinking strategies (VTS) to improve observational skills. *American Journal of Pharmaceutical Education, 84*(4), 7600. https://dx.doi.org/10.5688%2Fajpe7600

Reilly, M., Ring, J., & Duke, L. (2005). Visual thinking strategies: A new role for art in medical education. *Family Medicine, 37*(4), 250-252.

Vanderbilt University Center for Teaching. (2013). *Gathering evidence: Making student learning visible.* https://my.vanderbilt.edu/sotl/files/2013/09/4SoTLEvidence.pdf

Visual Thinking Strategies. (n.d.). Visual thinking strategies. www.vtshome.org

Wellbery, C., & McAteer, R. A. (2015). The art of observation: A pedagogical framework. *Academic Medicine, 90*(12), 1625-1630.

28

EFFECTIVE AND EFFICIENT ASSESSMENT OF REFLECTIVE JOURNALS

April Garrity, PhD, CCC-SLP; Casey Keck, PhD, CCC-SLP; and Keiko Ishikawa, PhD, CCC-SLP

DESCRIPTION OF TEACHING/LEARNING CONTEXT

Service-learning experiences are regarded as an instructional paradigm that facilitates engagement, deep learning, and critical thinking skills. Service learning includes a significant reflective component, which is believed to be critical to the transformative nature of these learning experiences. Many theories have hypothesized the nature of the relationship between reflection and learning, whereas other theories propose different types of reflection. Although we acknowledge the importance of reflection in learning, assessing students' reflections is often a complicated and time-consuming task.

Communication Help for Adults After Stroke (CHATS) is a service-learning experience that was established in 2009 with an existing community-based stroke survivors' group. Graduate speech-language pathology students participating in CHATS develop and facilitate fun, interactive weekly modules, typically focused on functional communication for activities of daily living, with the members of the group. Activities emphasize the use of any available functional communicative modality—including speaking, writing, drawing, and gesturing—in conversation. Students submit weekly reflective journals based on their CHATS experiences. The purpose of the journals is to facilitate deeper engagement with the experience, hence, transformative learning.

Friberg, J. C., Visconti, C. F., & Ginsberg, S. M. (Eds.). *Evidence-Based Education in the Classroom: Examples From Clinical Disciplines* (pp. 249-259). © 2021 Taylor & Francis Group.

REVIEW OF LITERATURE

As educators in clinical professions, we are responsible for teaching our students discipline-specific content, while simultaneously assisting them in developing the strong critical thinking skills that are necessary for successful clinical practice. Over the past century, scholars have offered theoretical frameworks to explain the nature of critical thinking, as well as guidance for teaching and assessing this collection of skills (Bloom & Krathwohl, 1956; Dewey, 1916, 1938; Kolb, 1984; Schön, 1983, 1987). While these frameworks are different in some ways, all of them include the concept of reflection as an underlying component of the development of critical thinking.

Service Learning and Reflection

One method educators may use to foster higher-order thinking in their students is service learning, a pedagogical approach in which didactic learning objectives are integrated with real-world experience through hands-on service provision. A goal of service learning is to provide bidirectional advantages, such that students are learning and applying knowledge in a highly engaged manner and that those who are being served benefit from this application of knowledge and skill. Service-learning experiences provide students with opportunities to engage in community service within an instructional framework of discipline-specific learning objectives. The service-learning context is structured to help students develop critical thinking skills, as well as a sense of both personal and civic responsibility. Specifically, students involved in service learning are expected to use a number of critical thinking skills relative to their experiences, including planning for effective service provision, evaluating the effects of services, solving problems that arise in real time, and reflecting on the experience as a whole. Ideally, the reflection component encourages students to draw on their prior content knowledge, as well as their values and beliefs, to synthesize and assimilate new knowledge and skills gained from the service-learning experience. In other words, reflective practice is a critical component of service learning because it gives meaning to these experiences, fostering transformative learning, and cultivating proficiency in content knowledge and clinical application (Kerka, 2002; Schön, 1983, 1987).

Although acknowledged as a valuable learning activity, the use of reflective practice in a written or journal-style format may be difficult for busy college instructors to incorporate into their courses, owing primarily to the difficulties related to the assessment of such assignments. As with any written assignment, assessment of reflective journals requires a significant time commitment on the part of the instructor. Another dilemma, the somewhat subjective nature of these journals (Bourner, 2003), calls for a systematic assessment process based on a reliable assessment tool (Boud, 2001; Woodward, 1998).

Theoretical Frameworks of Reflection Processes

The pursuit of an efficient and reliable assessment tool begins with an understanding of the seminal theoretical frameworks of three scholars. Boud and colleagues (1985) and Mezirow (1990) proposed assessment frameworks based on the degree to which an individual reflects, whereas Schön's (1987) three-level framework is based on when the reflection takes place.

Boud and colleagues' (1985) theoretical framework includes the descriptors returns to experience, attends to feelings, and re-evaluates the experience. Returning to the experience is considered the lowest level of reflection and represents an objective retelling of the events of the experience. Attending to feelings is characterized by the individual's awareness of emotions evoked by and associated with the events of the experience. An integration of the objective and subjective components, such as an interpretation of why one had certain emotions or beliefs regarding the events of the experience, particularly in light of prior or newly gained knowledge, would be described as a re-evaluation of the experience.

Mezirow (1990) proposed a reflection framework with the holistic categories of nonreflection and reflection. Reflection must include, at a minimum, the content (what happened) and/or process (why/how it happened) of the experience. A third holistic category, critical reflection, then, occurs when one recognizes how prior knowledge or beliefs are changed in light of the experience. Critical reflection, conceptualized as the level of reflection at which the most transformative learning occurs, encompasses an examination of premise (presuppositions).

Schön (1987) also delineated three types of reflection. However, rather than degree of reflection, this framework relies on chronology, which is theoretically analogous to the quality or depth of reflection as described in the other two frameworks discussed here. Schön's (1987) descriptors are reflection *in* action, reflection *on* action, and reflection *for* action. Reflection in action is characterized by observations of what is happening during the experience at an objective level. Reflection on action represents contemplation of an experience after it has occurred. Reflection on action includes the consideration of recently learned concepts within the context of the experience. Reflection for action requires the individual to integrate values and beliefs, along with knowledge and experience, to plan for and predict aspects of future experiences.

APPLICATION OF LITERATURE

A great deal of the research into assessment of students' written reflections has focused on evaluating whether the students demonstrate, through their writing, that they have met the didactic learning outcomes of a given course. However, given that theories of reflection generally assert that the most meaningful and transformative learning occurs when students engage in deep, integrative reflection, educators also need to be able to determine whether this type of profound learning is occurring among their students.

Methods of reflective journal assessment have been examined in a variety of student populations, including those in the clinical health professions. These studies have focused on various frameworks, including the seminal frameworks described here, as well as other frameworks, some with relatively few types of ratings and others with multiple rating levels. At least two studies have found that combining the Boud and colleagues (1985) and Mezirow (1990) frameworks have yielded moderate to high levels of interrater agreement and/or interrater reliability (Williams et al., 2000; Wong et al., 1995). In these studies, reflective journals were rated on no more than a 6-point scale. Other studies, however, have employed more comprehensive frameworks with additional rating levels.

Plack and colleagues (2005) developed a framework with two dimensions (one discrete and one holistic) and examined its reliability when used to evaluate the reflection journals of physical therapy students. The discrete dimension integrated all three of the seminal frameworks described here in their evaluation of the reflective journals' text (words, sentences, and paragraphs) for themes related to time, content, and stage of reflection. Schön's (1987) descriptors (reflection in action, reflection on action, and reflection for action) were used to assess the time aspect of the framework. The content ratings were based on Mezirow's (1990) framework and included content reflection, process reflection, and premise reflection. Finally, reflective journals were assessed for stage, based on the work of Boud and colleagues (1985), to indicate the degree of a student's engagement with the experience and the extent to which they integrated concepts and constructed meaning. These ratings were returns to experience, attends to feelings, and re-evaluates the experience. The holistic dimension, also based on Mezirow (1990), assessed each reflective journal for the depth of reflection, and included the descriptors nonreflection, reflection, and critical reflection. Thus, each reflective journal was given four different ratings (one each for time, content, and stage of reflection, and one holistic rating related to the depth of reflection).

Hill and colleagues (2012) also used Plack and colleagues' (2005) comprehensive framework to assess reflective journals of speech-language pathology students. Both studies yielded moderate to high levels of interrater agreement. On the other hand, studies that used a framework with fewer rating levels (Williams et al., 2000; Wong et al., 1995) rather than a comprehensive, integrated one, also achieved moderate to high levels of agreement. The similarity in their findings seems to suggest that the more comprehensive framework does not necessarily yield significantly greater agreement or reliability.

As busy faculty members at a teaching-intensive institution, our goal is to use a reliable rubric that requires a reasonable time commitment. Although the authors of most of these studies do not report the time commitment associated with assessing the reflective journals with the various frameworks, it would stand to reason that a framework with fewer rating levels should be less time consuming. Therefore, informed by previous work on the topic, we set out to determine whether we could develop a reliable and efficient assessment rating framework for reflective journals.

ORIGINAL DATA

To evaluate usability, as measured by interrater agreement, the reflection rubric was piloted in two phases. Phase 1 consisted of two raters, Rater A and Rater B, using the rubric to independently rate a subset of student journals. Interrater agreement for the rubric ratings were low and variable (mean = 43%; range = 19% to 50%). These poor results were unexpected and prompted a revision of the rubric that included clarifying the nonreflection, reflection, and critical reflection rating criteria and adding passage examples from the subset of journals that exemplified each rating. Phase 2 of piloting included a third rater, Rater C, using the revised rubric from Phase 1 to rate a portion of student journals (Garrity et al., 2019).

To evaluate the objectivity and reliability of the revised rubric (used in Phase 2 of piloting), a preliminary study was conducted. Raters A, B, and C used the revised rubric to analyze the remaining student journals (students $n = 33$, journals $n = 198$). Prior to rating the remaining journals, the raters participated in a brief training to familiarize themselves with the revised rubric criteria and representative examples of each criterion (Garrity et al., 2019). The training consisted of the three raters' completing relevant readings, jointly and independently rating student journals, and discussing the ratings. The training was abbreviated because the raters were already familiar with the rating framework, having used it previously during the piloting phases.

After training, raters used the revised rubric to independently rate the remaining journals as nonreflection, reflection, and critical reflection. Raters were required to extract passages from the students' journals that supported ratings of reflection or critical reflection. Ratings of nonreflection did not require the extraction of supportive passages because these journals did not contain evidence of reflection.

The raters' ratings were evaluated for agreement and reliability. Agreement was measured through manual calculations of percent agreement, and reliability was calculated using a statistical test of interrater agreement. Results suggested poor interrater agreement among the three raters. Reliability was statistically tested between rater pairs (i.e., A and B, A and C, and B and C) and among the three raters. Results indicated poor interrater reliability between rater pairs and among all three raters (Garrity et al., 2019).

A secondary agreement analysis was conducted to identify which reflection ratings were applied inconsistently by the raters. This secondary analysis focused on "disagreement journals," in which two raters had the same ratings, but a third rater had a different rating. Three agreement comparisons were conducted: reflection versus nonreflection, critical reflection versus nonreflection, and critical reflection versus reflection. The journals in which all three raters had different ratings (i.e., one rater rated the journal as nonreflection, another rated it as reflection, and the other rated it as critical reflection) were included as part of the critical reflection versus reflection comparison. Agreement results suggested that raters were least consistent at distinguishing between ratings of critical reflection and reflection, with interrater agreement among all three raters near chance (52%; Garrity et al., 2019).

The raters' disagreement journals were evaluated to determine potential reasons for the inconsistent agreement results. To complete this subsequent analysis, the three raters independently reviewed and rated again the disagreement journals based solely on the extracted passages. The raters then discussed the ratings and passages until consensus was reached by at least two raters. Through analysis of the extracted passages and consensus discussions, it became apparent that a major shortcoming of the rubric was that it did not operationally define or provide clear examples of the reflection and critical reflection ratings, which led to difficulty distinguishing these ratings from one another (Garrity et al., 2019).

APPLICATION OF DATA

Based on the results of the preliminary study, the reflection rubric was revised to further clarify how ratings of reflection and critical reflection are distinct from one another. This revision consisted of developing additional reflection and critical reflection criteria. These criteria emerged from qualitative observations of typical differences between journal passages rated as critical reflection and those rated as reflection in the previous study. The distinction between reflection and critical reflection seemed to be related to the concept of general experience or general knowledge as opposed to specific experience or specific knowledge. In other words, journals rated as critical reflection considered the CHATS experience based on discipline-specific knowledge related to the service-learning situation. Those journals rated as reflection considered the CHATS experience based on a general understanding of the service-learning situation, one that typically functioning adults would notice, regardless of their educational or occupational background. The rubric is provided in Table 28-1.

To evaluate objectivity and reliability of the revised rubric, the first two authors of this chapter used the revised rubric to independently rate another 30 students' journals. This phase included three rating events. Each rating event consisted of the raters rating students' journals that had not previously been rated. During the first rating event, 20 students' journals were rated. During the second and third events, five students' journals ($n = 10$) were rated. Following each rating event, the raters discussed the disagreement journals until consensus was reached on the ratings, and then the accepted ratings were confirmed by the extracted passages.

Additionally, 15 of the 30 students' journals were randomly selected and evaluated for intrarater reliability. Intrarater ratings were completed during each of the three rating events described earlier. Each intrarater event consisted of five students' journals being randomly selected and rated again by each rater. Completing this additional reliability measure was important given the teaching/learning context in which the rubric is meant to be used (i.e., by an instructor individually evaluating students' reflective journals).

The raters' independent ratings of the 30 students' journals were evaluated for interrater agreement. Of the 30 students' journals that were rated, 23 students' journals (journal $n = 137$) were included in the interrater agreement evaluations. Seven students' journals were excluded from the analysis because of concerns that some of their journals were self-plagiarized as well as because of missing data. Interrater reliability was measured statistically through Cohen's kappa and percent agreement. Cohen's kappa results indicated interrater reliability for all ratings was weak ($k = 0.44$, 95% CI [.29 to .60], $p < .05$), whereas the percent agreement between raters was moderate (75.2%; McHugh, 2012).

TABLE 28-1

Revised Reflection Rubric

RATING	DEFINITIONS/CRITERIA
Nonreflection	No evidence of reflection is present within the journal. May see description of experiences with no evidence of evaluation/questioning of the experience.[a]
Reflection	Evidence of reflection is present in the journal. Writer reflects to better understand the situation, decides how best to perform, or writes beyond describing/reporting experiences.[a] Writer provides a label and description for emotions evoked by the experience, and/or writer draws conclusions based on general experience or knowledge (not discipline-specific and/or related to the individuals who were involved in CHATS).[b]
Critical reflection	Evidence of critical reflection is present within the journal. The writer explores the existence of the problem, where the problem stems from, or the assumptions underlying the problem; or the writer will critique their experiences/assumptions and may begin to show evidence of modifying their own biases or assumptions.[a] The writer provides specific details and/or examples of how/what will be modified, and/or writer draws conclusions based on discipline-specific experience or knowledge of communication/cognitive/swallowing disorders that they have learned through the CHATS experience or outside of it (e.g., classroom discussion). The writer may give examples and/or highlight what they have learned.[b]

[a]Definitions adapted from Plack, M. M., Driscoll, M., Blissett, S., McKenna, R., & Plack, T. P. (2005). A method for assessing reflective journal writing. *Journal of Allied Health, 34*(4), 199-208.
[b]Definitions developed by the authors for previous analyses (Garrity & Bradshaw, 2016) and the current analyses.

The rater's intrarater ratings of the randomly selected 15 students' journals were evaluated for agreement and reliability. Intrarater agreement was measured manually through calculations of percent agreement. Intrarater reliability was measured statistically through intraclass correlation coefficient (ICC). The results indicated strong intrarater agreement (85.6%) and 87.7% agreement (McHugh, 2012). ICC results indicated moderate intrarater reliability (ICC = .59, 95% CI [.44 to .71], F [89, 90] = 3.91, p < .005; ICC = .69, 95% CI [.5 to .78], F [89, 90] = 5.37, p < .005; McHugh, 2012).

Figures 28-1 and 28-2 illustrate interrater and intrarater agreement across all iterations of the rubric. The interrater and intrarater analyses suggest that our assessment rubric is improving, but it has not yet reached a sufficient level of interrater reliability. On the other hand, the intrarater reliability analyses revealed moderate reliability and strong percent agreement. We interpret this as a success and are encouraged that this rubric will serve as at least a starting point for other educators attempting to independently and objectively assess their students' written reflections. Those who use it might find that additional refinements are required for it to be as effective as possible for other applications. For instance, our initial reliability analyses (Garrity et al., 2019) led us to define reflection levels on our rubric with specific reference to the service-learning context in which they were being written. This refinement ultimately led to improved interrater agreement. In addition, the intrarater agreement, which is arguably more important for instructors' classroom use, was strong when we applied the revised, more context-bound rubric. This suggests that the most effective reflection assessment frameworks might be those that are specifically tailored in some way to the experience, the discipline, or some combination thereof.

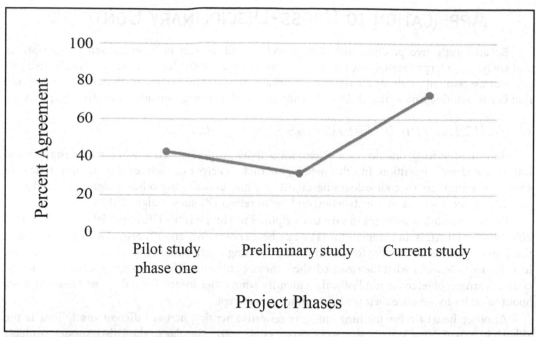

Figure 28-1. Interrater agreement across rubrics.

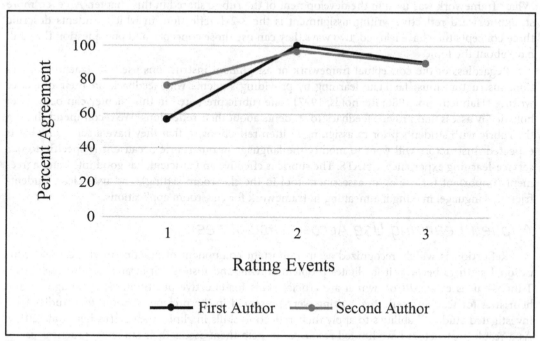

Figure 28-2. Intrarater agreement across rubrics.

APPLICATION TO CROSS-DISCIPLINARY CONTEXTS

Because reflective practice, including reflective writing, can facilitate students' descriptions and analytical interpretations of learning experiences (Boud, 2001; Jarvis, 1992, 2001), effective and efficient assessment methods for reflective journals are applicable to many disciplines for use in a number of activities, including didactic learning, applied learning, and administrative purposes.

Didactic Learning Use Across Disciplines

Reflective writing practice as a classroom activity is most effective when it is designed and implemented with intention. In other words, instructors across disciplines should align reflective writing assignments to course learning objectives, just as with any other assignment, and they should provide students with instruction on how to reflect (Ziomek-Daigle, 2017).

One framework instructors in various disciplines might use is the DEAL model (Ash & Clayton, 2004, 2009). DEAL is an acronym for (1) describe, (2) examine, and (3) articulate learning. These three steps provide a structure for students when writing a reflection. First, students describe their learning experience or what they learned; then, they examine how this learning experience relates to course learning objectives; and lastly, they identify what other information they may need to learn about in order to advance their understanding of a concept.

Another heuristic for teaching students reflective writing across different disciplines is the What? So What? Now What? framework (Rolfe et al., 2001). Similar to the DEAL model, students describe what happened during the learning experience; then, they discuss why the experience was meaningful; and lastly, how they will advance and/or apply their learning. The What? So What? Now What? framework was used in the development of the rubric shared in this chapter. An even more straightforward reflective writing assignment is the 3-2-1 reflection, in which students describe three concepts they have learned, two ways they can use those concepts, and one question they still have about the topic.

Regardless of the conceptual framework or assignment instructions used for teaching reflection, instructors must facilitate learning by providing students with feedback on their reflective writing (Hahnemann, 1986; Reynolds, 1997). The rubric presented in this chapter can be used to holistically assess and provide feedback to students about their reflections. We recommend sharing the rubric with students prior to assigning written reflections so that they have a sense of what is expected. Instructors will want to modify the language of our rubric because it is specific to our service-learning experience, CHATS. The rubric is effective and efficient, has good intrarater agreement (important for use as an assessment tool in the classroom setting), and uses clear, student-friendly language, making it a meaningful framework for classroom applications.

Applied Learning Use Across Disciplines

Reflection is widely recognized as an important component of practice in clinical and educational settings because it facilitates problem solving and fosters self-awareness (Benade, 2015; Tsingos-Lucas et al., 2016), which are crucial skills for effective practitioners. Although several heuristics for teaching reflective writing were presented in the previous section, few studies have investigated students' abilities to apply their reflection skills in clinic practice (Fisher et al., 2015). As a result, instructors have limited resources to help them assess their students' practical use of reflection. The rubric we developed and tested here was created specifically for use in clinical practice within a service-learning experience, so it is particularly well-suited to assessing and providing feedback to students about reflective writing in an applied learning context, regardless of discipline.

Instructors will likely need to revise the rubric's criteria slightly to fit the discipline and applied learning situation. Although the language in the rubric criteria is general enough to be utilized across disciplines, instructors may need to modify the context and skills targeted in the rubric. For example, instead of communication and cognition for speech-language pathology students and the CHATS experience, instructors will need to substitute the specific practicum skills required for a given context (e.g., community clinic, Head Start classroom, nonprofit hospital pharmacy, inpatient rehabilitation hospital).

Administrative Use Across Disciplines

Another possible application of this type of rubric, and one that we are beginning to investigate ourselves, is the assessment of materials and/or media other than written reflections. Specifically, in our case, we are interested in determining if assessment of reflection levels might differentiate between prospective speech-language pathology graduate students who are more likely to be successful in a rigorous clinical graduate program and those who are less likely to be successful in the program. In other words, are there measurable relationships between evidence of reflection on specifically designed qualitative application materials (e.g., personal essays, interviews) and levels of academic and clinical success in graduate school?

Considering the significant theoretical relationship among reflection, cognitive ability, and learning, we predict that applicants with stronger reflective skills would be stronger graduate students. Current literature suggests that the typical quantitative admissions measures, such as GPA and GRE scores, are related to participants' subsequent cognitive and noncognitive/behavioral performance in graduate programs (Fonteyne et al., 2017; Halberstam & Redstone, 2005). Identifying and characterizing the nature of these relationships might be particularly important for competitive programs, including many health professions disciplines, because it could guide admissions decisions toward applicants who are more likely to be successful in these programs.

ADDITIONAL RESOURCES

A number of excellent resources related to reflection, rubrics, and service learning are available online. In addition to those listed in the References, a selection of such resources is available in the following sections.

Reflection

- The Service Learning Reflection Toolkit includes a summary of research on reflection and learning as well as numerous ideas and activities for incorporating reflection activities into the classroom. This is an excellent, practical resource for instructors looking to start using reflections:
  - Gateway Technical College. (2013). *Service-learning reflection toolkit.* https://www.gtc.edu/sites/default/files/files/documents/Service_Learning_Reflection_Toolkit.pdf
- A resource developed by instructional designers, this resource outlines the benefits of reflective journaling, describes several different types of reflections, and provides a visual representation of the reflection cycle. It also includes some additional useful resources:
  - Northern Illinois University Center for Innovative Teaching and Learning. (2012). Reflective journals and learning logs. https://www.niu.edu/citl/resources/guides/instructional-guide/reflective-journals-and-learning-logs.shtml

- The author of this post on McGill University's Teaching and Learning Services' blog studies reflective journaling in postsecondary classrooms. She cites a number of benefits of reflective journal writing and cites research findings that support these benefits:
  - Van Wallraven, C. (2017, April 8). The benefits of reflective journal writing. *Teaching and Learning @ McGill University*. https://teachingblog.mcgill.ca/2017/04/11/the-benefits-of-reflective-journal-writing/

Rubrics

- Assessment of Learning in Undergraduate Education (VALUE) rubrics have been developed to capture meaningful learning across disciplines. This resource includes links to 16 different VALUE rubrics that cover the categories of intellectual and practical skills (e.g., critical thinking, oral communication), personal and social responsibility (e.g., civic engagement, ethical reasoning), and integrative and applied learning:
  - Association of American Colleges & Universities. (2018). VALUE rubrics. https://www.aacu.org/value-rubrics

Service-Learning

- This seminal article introduces the Comprehensive Action Plan for Service-Learning, a framework for the development and implementation of service learning:
  - Bringle, R., & Hatcher, J. (1996). Implementing service-learning in higher education. *Journal of Higher Education, 67*(2), 221-239.
- This website offers numerous resources for those involved in community-based teaching and learning, including Knowledge Hubs for learning more about service learning and syllabi that have been curated from service-learning courses around the country:
  - Campus Compact: https://compact.org
- Required reading for those involved in service learning. This book is a comprehensive manual on service learning and all of its components. The chapters cover topics such as critical reflection, developing and sustaining partnerships for service learning, designing and assessing service-learning experiences, and administrative issues:
  - Jacoby, B. (2015). *Service-learning essentials: Questions, answers and lessons learned.* Jossey-Bass Inc.

REFERENCES

Ash, S., & Clayton, P. (2004). The articulated learning: An approach to guided reflection and assessment. *Innovative Higher Education, 29,* 137-154. https://doi.org/10.1023/B:IHIE.0000048795.84634.4a

Ash, S., & Clayton, P. (2009). Generating, deepening, and documenting learning: The power of critical reflection in applied learning. *Journal of Applied Learning in Higher Education, 1,* 25-48.

Benade, L. (2015). Teachers' critical reflective practice in the context of twenty-first century learning. *Open Review of Educational Research, 2,* 42-54. https://doi.org/10.1080/23265507.2014.998159

Bloom, B., & Krathwohl, D. (1956). *Taxonomy of educational objectives: The classification of educational goals, by a committee of college and university examiners. Handbook I: Cognitive Domain.* Longmans, Green.

Boud, D. (2001). Using journal writing to enhance reflective practice. *New Directions Adult Continuing Education, 90,* 9-18.

Boud, D., Keogh, R., & Walker, D. (1985). Promoting reflection in learning. In D. Boud, R. Keogh, & D. Walker (Eds.), *Reflection: Turning experience into learning* (pp. 18-40). Koran Page.

Bourner, T. (2003). Assessing reflective learning. *Education Training, 45,* 267-272.

Dewey, J. (1916). *Democracy and education: An introduction to the philosophy of education.* Macmillan.

Dewey, J. (1938). *Experience and education.* Macmillan.

Fisher, P., Chew, K., & Leow, Y. (2015). Clinical psychologists' use of reflection and reflective practice within clinical work. *Reflective Practice, 6,* 731-743. https://doi.org/10.1080/14623943.2015.1095724

Fonteyne, L., Duyck, W., & De Fruyt, F. (2017). Program-specific prediction of academic achievement on the basis of cognitive and non-cognitive factors. *Learning and Individual Differences, 56,* 34-48.

Garrity, A., Keck, C., Bradshaw, J. L., & Ishikawa, K. (2019). Toward the development of a quick, reliable assessment tool for reflective journals. *Teaching and Learning in Communication Sciences and Disorders, 3*(2), 1-19.

Hahnemann, B. (1986). Journal writing: A key to promoting critical thinking in nursing students. *Journal of Nursing Education, 25,* 213-215.

Halberstam, B., & Redstone, F. (2005). The predictive value of admissions materials on objective and subjective measures of graduate school performance in speech-language pathology. *Journal of Higher Education Policy and Management, 27,* 261-272.

Hill, A., Davidson, B., & Theodoros, D. (2012). Reflections on clinical learning in novice speech-language therapy students. *International Journal of Language and Communication Disorders, 47,* 413-426.

Jarvis, P. (1992). Reflective practice and nursing. *Nurse Education Today, 12,* 174-181.

Jarvis, P. (2001). Journal writing in higher education. *New Directions for Adult and Continuing Education, 90,* 79-86.

Kerka, S. (2002). Journal writing as an adult learning tool. Practice application brief No. 22. *ERIC Clearinghouse on Adult, Career, and Vocational Education. Office of Educational Research and Improvement.* ERIC Number ED470782.

Kolb, D. (1984). *Experiential learning: Experience as the source of learning and development.* Prentice Hall.

McHugh, M. L. (2012). Interrater reliability: The kappa statistic. *Biochemia Medica, 22*(3), 276-282.

Mezirow, J. (1990). *Fostering critical reflection in adulthood: A guide to transformative and emancipatory learning.* Jossey-Bass Inc.

Plack, M., Driscoll, M., Blisset, S., Mckenna, R., & Plack, T. P. (2005). A method for assessing reflective journal writing. *Journal of Allied Health, 34*(4), 199-208.

Reynolds, S. (1997). Journal writing in nursing. In G. Poirrier (Ed.), *Writing-to-learn: Curriculum strategies for nursing and other disciplines.* National League for Nursing Press.

Rolfe, G., Freshwater, D., & Jasper, M. (2001) *Critical reflection in nursing and the helping professions: A user's guide.* Palgrave Macmillan.

Schön, D. (1983). *The reflective practitioner: How professionals think in action.* Basic Books.

Schön, D. (1987). *Educating the reflective practitioner: Toward a new design for learning in the professions.* Jossey-Bass Inc.

Tsingos-Lucas, C., Bosnic-Anticevich, S., Schneider, C., & Smith, L. (2016). The effect of reflective activities on reflective thinking ability in an undergraduate pharmacy curriculum. *American Journal of Pharmaceutical Education, 80,* Article 65. https://doi.org/10.5688/ajpe80465

Williams, R., Sundelin, G., Foster-Seargeant, E., & Norman, G. (2000). Assessing the reliability of grading reflective journal writing. *Journal of Physical Therapy Education, 14,* 23-26.

Wong, F., Kember, D., Chung, L., & Yan, L. (1995). Assessing the level of student reflection from reflective journals. *Journal of Advanced Nursing, 22,* 48-57.

Woodward, H. (1998). Reflective journals and portfolios: Learning through assessment. *Assessment and Evaluation in Higher Education, 23,* 415-423.

Ziomek-Daigle, J. (2017). Using reflective writing practices to articulate student learning. *Journal of Creativity in Mental Health, 2,* 262-270. https://doi.org/10.1080/15401383.2016.1187581

29

ENHANCING SELF-DIRECTED LEARNING AND METACOGNITION WITH GUIDED REFLECTION

Leslie A. Hoffman, PhD
and Audra F. Schaefer, PhD

DESCRIPTION OF TEACHING/LEARNING CONTEXT

The beginning of medical school can be a challenging time for medical students. As expected, most medical students are bright individuals, which means that many did not have to study very hard to perform well in their undergraduate courses. As a result, some medical students arrive in medical school without well-established study strategies and habits, leaving them overwhelmed as they adjust to the pace and rigor of medical school coursework. Even more concerning is that many medical students lack metacognitive awareness, meaning they do not realize that they do not know how to study or that their study strategies are ineffective until after they have performed poorly on an examination.

In 2016, Indiana University School of Medicine (Indianapolis, Indiana) introduced a guided reflection exercise for our first-year medical students in the Human Structure course, which is taught during the first semester of medical school. Human Structure is a semester-long course that integrates gross anatomy, histology, embryology, and radiological imaging. The purpose of the guided reflection was to introduce students to the process of self-directed learning (SDL) by asking them to think about their study strategies in preparation for the first Human Structure examination, and how they determined whether those strategies were effective.

This chapter discusses the effectiveness of the reflective exercise on enhancing medical students' metacognitive awareness of their study strategies and SDL skills. We will present a qualitative analysis of students' reflection responses as it relates to their examination performance, as well as a quantitative analysis of students' SDL skills, as measured by a validated survey instrument.

Friberg, J. C., Visconti, C. F., & Ginsberg, S. M. (Eds.). *Evidence-Based Education in the Classroom: Examples From Clinical Disciplines* (pp. 261-267).
© 2021 Taylor & Francis Group.

REVIEW OF LITERATURE

Medical education places a heavy emphasis on preparing students to become not only competent practitioners but also lifelong learners who are able to continue to learn effectively throughout their practice. In order to engage in lifelong learning, students must become self-directed in their learning. The Liaison Committee on Medical Education (LCME), which is the accrediting body for allopathic medical schools in the United States, requires that medical schools provide students with opportunities to engage in SDL in the medical curriculum. The LCME defines SDL as any activity that requires students to (1) assess their learning needs; (2) identify, analyze, and synthesize relevant information; and (3) appraise the credibility of their information sources (Association of American Medical Colleges & the American Medical Association, 2020).

SDL is more broadly defined as "a process in which individuals take the initiative, with or without the help of others, in diagnosing their learning needs, formulating learning goals, identifying human and material resources for learning, choosing and implementing appropriate learning strategies, and evaluating learning outcomes" (Knowles, 1975, p. 18). The concept of SDL arose from adult learning theory, which states that adults are motivated to learn when it addresses a specific need or can be applied to real-world situations and that adults prefer a self-directed approach that affords them some level of control over their own learning (Knowles et al., 2005).

While Knowles' definition focuses on the external processes of SDL, such as setting learning goals, selecting resources, and implementing learning strategies, there is an equally critical cognitive component of SDL that involves the following: (1) self-monitoring to ensure that the chosen approach effectively addresses the learning need; (2) self-evaluation to determine whether the learning goals have been met; and (3) self-reflection, which is a metacognitive awareness of the learning process that includes not only how much learning has occurred but also how and why the learning strategies utilized were effective or not effective. Indeed, Brookfield argued that SDL is only fully realized when external activities and internal reflective dimensions are fused (Brookfield, 1985, 1986).

While not always explicitly discussed in designing SDL activities, the aspects of SDL that involve introspection from the learner are highly important. As clarified by Husmann and colleagues (2018), self-regulated learning is a subcomponent of SDL in which learners utilize skills necessary to achieve specific, smaller learning goals. Achieving these goals relies on students' awareness of learning strategies that work best for them in a given situation, as well as their abilities to plan their time and resource use and assess the effectiveness of strategies along the way. This awareness and skillset of planning and assessing progress are collectively referred to as *metacognition*. Metacognition has been studied across multiple disciplines, and its importance is clear. Many students enter college, and even graduate or professional school, with poorly developed metacognitive skills, but students who are successful learners, regardless of subject, are able to effectively integrate metacognition in their learning process (Kaplan et al., 2013). Fortunately, research has also shown that, as instructors, we can shape our teaching practices, course goals, and assessment methods to help facilitate the development of our students' metacognitive skills, therefore, promoting learning (Ross et al., 2006; Tanner, 2012).

An example of an activity instructors can implement to improve metacognition and SDL skills is an examination wrapper, which is a structured reflective activity that prompts students to practice key metacognitive skills after they get back their graded examinations (Lovett, 2013). The reflective exercise implemented in the Human Structure course is a modified examination wrapper. Examination wrappers typically ask students three types of questions: (1) how they prepared for the exam, (2) what kinds of errors they made on the exam, and (3) what they might do differently to prepare for the next exam (Lovett, 2013). The main goal of an examination wrapper is to encourage student reflection on the learning process and self-monitoring to foster metacognitive development.

APPLICATION OF LITERATURE/DATA

During the Human Structure course, students were required to complete a two-part reflective assignment in conjunction with the first examination of the course. While a typical examination wrapper asks students to reflect on their examination preparation after receiving their graded examination, we chose to divide the reflective activity into a pre-examination and post-examination reflection so we could ask students to reflect on their examination preparation and level of confidence before the examination without the bias of knowing how they performed. We felt that this modification would provide us with better insight into students' metacognitive awareness of their examination preparedness.

The reflection prompts for each part of the assignment are included in Appendix. Part 1, the pre-examination reflection, was submitted prior to the first Human Structure examination. The pre-examination reflection prompted students to identify their strengths and weaknesses regarding the content, and to describe how they identified their learning needs, how they addressed those learning needs, and which resources they found to be most and least helpful in preparing them for the upcoming examination. They were also asked to provide an assessment of their level of confidence going into the examination, and what grade they were aiming to achieve. About 1 week after receiving their examination grades, students submitted a post-examination reflection, which asked them to reflect on their examination performance and how they planned to modify their study strategies in preparation for the next examination. Students were again asked which resources they intended to use in the remainder of the course.

The intention of the examination wrapper was to guide students through the process of SDL, as it is defined by the LCME, and to promote students' metacognitive awareness of their study strategies and how they know whether they are studying effectively or not. Additionally, asking students to explicitly reflect at multiple points along the way can help to model the idea that they should regularly evaluate their learning and use what they learn to shape future learning goals and plans to achieve those goals.

ORIGINAL DATA

We then conducted a qualitative analysis of the students' pre- and post-examination reflections to examine how students prepared for the examination, whether their perception of their preparedness was consistent with their actual examination performance, and what adjustments, if any, they planned to make to their study strategies based on their examination performance. The qualitative analysis found that students who performed poorly on the first Human Structure examination tended to overestimate their preparedness for the examination and predicted that they would perform much better than they actually did. In short, the students thought they knew the content, but when tested, realized that they did not. This overconfidence among students who are "unskilled and unaware of it" has been termed the Dunning-Kruger effect (Kruger & Dunning, 1999).

The Dunning-Kruger effect illustrates a deficiency in students' metacognitive awareness, which can lead to overconfidence in one's knowledge or abilities and an inability to identify areas of weakness. In medicine, metacognitive skills are critical for practicing physicians to monitor their own performance and identify areas of weakness or incompetence, which can lead to medical errors that may cause harm to patients. Unfortunately, studies have found that many physicians seem to have limited capacity for assessing their own performance (Davis et al., 2006). This lack of metacognitive awareness among physicians highlights the need for medical schools to teach and assess metacognitive skills so that medical students learn how to monitor and assess their own performance.

By examining the study strategies employed by both low- and high-performing students, we were able to identify the most effective study strategies, as well as common pitfalls, that we could then use to advise struggling students to help them improve their performance on future exams. We found that low-performing students tended to use more passive study methods, such as rewatching lecture recordings, rereading notes, or reviewing flashcards. These methods often give students a false sense of preparedness because they are able to recognize terms and concepts when they see or hear them, as discussed by one low-performing student who wrote, "I took the easy way out when learning the muscles, thinking I could just read over the charts in textbooks and I'd remember them fine." But these methods do not incorporate the metacognitive processes that allow students to monitor and assess their progress. One low-performing student realized this error too late: "I thought that I had been studying before by simply reviewing the slides, but when I started quizzing myself, I quickly realized that what I had been doing was grossly insufficient. I knew that I was in deep trouble and that this exam was not going to go as well as I wanted." Low-performing students also tended to become overwhelmed with learning small details and missed important concepts (i.e., "I was too focused on trying to learn everything and failed to pick up on a few main points").

In contrast, high-performing students tended to use more active learning strategies such as writing or drawing out the content from memory, creating tables or charts, talking through the content (either alone or with another student), and quizzing themselves. These activities required the students to actively retrieve information from memory rather than simply recognize it. This process of retrieval is a means of self-assessment that enables students to actively monitor their progress to determine whether they actually know the content. These methods also provide students with feedback regarding the effectiveness of their study strategies and allow them to adjust as needed. High-performing students also focused more on big-picture concepts, functions, and clinically important relationships: "I focused on the larger picture and seeing the connections between overall ideas and concepts. This helped to place everything into perspective, especially for the clinical-type questions. Focusing less on memorizing small details and understanding the reasons behind why things occur was very helpful."

When asked to discuss changes that students intended to make to their study strategies in response to their first examination score, the high-performing students often discussed making minor changes in terms of their content focus or time allotment (i.e., "put a lot more effort into studying histology"; "I will spend more time studying on the cadavers"), but their overall strategies tended to remain the same. Low-performing students, on the other hand, often discussed making drastic changes to their study strategies, as illustrated by the following quotes: "I really think I need to overhaul my method of studying"; "I will completely change my studying approach." Some students even realized that they did not know how to study or did not have a clear approach to studying: "I didn't have much of an approach to the first exam"; "I had no idea how to properly study in medical school."

In addition to the qualitative analysis, we also wanted to understand how students' SDL skills develop throughout medical school. We assessed medical students' development of SDL skills using the Self-Directed Learning Instrument (SDLI; Cheng et al., 2010). The SDLI measures four domains of SDL: (1) learning motivation, (2) planning and implementing, (3) self-monitoring, and (4) interpersonal communication. Students completed the SDLI at the beginning of the semester and again at the end.

We found that students' SDLI scores increased significantly during the first semester of medical school, and that the increase was largely driven by improvements in the planning and implementing domain. This domain includes activities such as setting learning goals, using learning strategies, and selecting appropriate resources. This suggests that students' study habits change and evolve as they adjust to the pace and rigor of medical school coursework. Students become more deliberate and focused regarding the content they are studying, which enables them to study more efficiently and effectively, and they are better able to discern which resources are most beneficial to their learning.

Although some low-performing students expressed great uncertainty about their study skills at the beginning of the Human Structure course, most showed improvement in their examination scores throughout the remainder of the semester, which demonstrates that these students were able to improve their study strategies over time. This is consistent with the improvements we observed in the planning and implementing domain of the SDLI.

The qualitative analysis of the pre- and post-examination reflections suggests that examination wrappers are an effective method for promoting metacognition among medical students. Improvements in metacognitive skills may be particularly beneficial to lower performing students, as it will enable them to better recognize areas of weakness so they can adjust their study strategies to improve their learning and performance. These metacognitive processes are a key component that will enable students to become self-directed learners.

APPLICATION TO CROSS-DISCIPLINARY CONTEXTS

SDL is an important competency in many health care professions. In addition to the LCME, the accrediting bodies of many other health professions require educational programs to prepare students for self-directed, lifelong learning, including dental education, physical therapy, and occupational therapy, to name a few. Examination wrappers are among many activities that can be implemented and have been successfully used in many higher education contexts to promote metacognitive skills (Pate et al., 2019; Soicher & Gurung, 2017). The pre- and post-examination reflection described here can be applied to any education program to encourage SDL and metacognition, and such reflections can be modified by instructors to promote reflection of specific aspects of the SDL process. Tanner's article (2012) is a useful resource for instructors, giving a variety of suggestions for questions that instructors can ask students to prompt reflection in different stages of learning. The reflective activity described in this chapter could also be adapted for use in a clinical setting to promote reflection on clinical skills and patient encounters. In fact, applying diagnostic reflection activities, in which medical residents reflect on the diagnosis of recent cases, has been shown to improve diagnostic accuracy in first and second-year residents (Mamede et al., 2010). It stands to reason that such an activity would be beneficial for clinicians of any variety. The findings of our qualitative analysis can be used by educators in any discipline to proactively provide students with advice regarding effective study strategies and to encourage them to monitor their progress through self-assessment and self-reflection.

ADDITIONAL RESOURCES

- The *Improve With Metacognition* blog discusses the processes of teaching and learning, with an emphasis on metacognition. Posts discuss these processes in all stages of formal education, as well as outside of the traditional academic environment:
  - https://www.improvewithmetacognition.com/category/blog/
- How do students become self-directed learners? This chapter presents research that supports the use of SDL to promote metacognition and offers practical advice for designing learning activities to guide students through the SDL process:
  - Ambrose, S. A., Bridges, M. W., DiPietro, M., Lovett, M. C., & Norman, M. K. (2010). *How learning works: Seven research-based principles for smart teaching* (1st ed.). Jossey-Bass Inc.

REFERENCES

Association of American Medical Colleges, & American Medical Association. (2020). LCME functions and structure of a medical school: Standards for accreditation of medical education programs leading to the MD degree. *Liaison Committee on Medical Education*. http://lcme.org/publications/

Brookfield, S. (1985). Analyzing a critical paradigm of self-directed learning: A response. *Adult Education Quarterly, 36*, 60-64.

Brookfield, S. D. (1986). *Understanding and facilitating adult learning*. Jossey-Bass Inc.

Cheng, S. F., Kuo, C. L., & Lee-Hsieh, J. (2010). Development and preliminary testing of a self-rating instrument to measure self-directed learning ability of nursing students. *International Journal of Nursing Studies, 47*, 1152-1158.

Davis, D. A., Mazmanian, P. E., Fordis, M., Harrison, R., Thorpe, K. E., & Perrier, L. (2006). Accuracy of physician self-assessment compared with observed measures of competence: A systematic review. *JAMA, 296*, 1094-1102.

Husmann, P. R., Hoffman, L. A., & Schaefer, A. F. (2018). Unique terms or are we splitting hairs? Clarification of self-directed versus self-regulated learning and related terms. *Medical Science Educator, 28*(4), 777-783. https://doi.org/10.1007/s40670-018-0626-2

Kaplan, M., Silver, N., Lavaque-Manty, D., & Meizlish, D. (2013). *Using reflection and metacognition to improve student learning: Across the disciplines, across the academy*. Stylus.

Knowles, M. S. (1975). *Self-directed learning: A guide for learners and teachers*. Cambridge.

Knowles, M. S., Swanson, R. A., & Holton, E. F. (2005). *The adult learner: The definitive classic in adult education and human resource development* (6th ed.). Routledge.

Kruger, J., & Dunning, D. (1999). Unskilled and unaware of it: How difficulties in recognizing one's own incompetence lead to inflated self-assessments. *Journal of Personality and Social Psychology, 77*(6), 1121-1134.

Lovett, M. C. (2013). Make exams worth more than the grade: Using exam wrappers to promote metacognition. In M. Kaplan, N. Silver, D. LaVague-Manty, & D. Meizlish (Eds.), *Using reflection and metacognition to improve student learning: Across the disciplines, across the academy* (pp. 18-52). Stylus.

Mamede, S., van Gog, T., & van den Berge, K. (2010). Effect of availability bias and reflective reasoning on diagnostic accuracy among internal medicine residents. *JAMA, 304*(11), 1198-1203.

Pate, A., Lafitte, E. M., Ramachandran, S., & Caldwell, D. J. (2019). The use of exam wrappers to promote metacognition. *Currents in Pharmacy Teaching and Learning, 11*, 492-498.

Ross, M. E., Green, S. B., Salisbury-Glennon, J. D., & Tollefson, N. (2006). College students' study strategies as a function of testing: An investigation into metacognitive self-regulation. *Innovative Higher Education, 30*(5), 361-375.

Soicher, R. N., & Gurung, R. A. R. (2017). Do exam wrappers increase metacognition and performance? A single course intervention. *Psychology Learning & Teaching, 16*(1), 64-73.

Tanner, K. D. (2012). Promoting student metacognition. *CBE-Life Sciences Education, 11*, 113-120.

APPENDIX: PRE- AND POST-EXAMINATION REFLECTION PROMPTS

Part 1: Pre-Examination Reflection

Part 1 of this reflective exercise guides you to engage in the process of SDL by prompting you to reflect on your strengths and potential limitations, to use this information to close gaps in your understanding, and to consider and weigh the quality or usefulness of learning resources. As you continue in your preparation for the first examination, you have the opportunity to assess your level of confidence and predict how you expect to perform on the upcoming examination.

1. With respect to the upcoming examination, identify the two areas/topics in which you feel *best* prepared.
2. With respect to the upcoming examination, identify the two areas/topics in which you feel *least* prepared.
3. How did you determine what you needed to learn for this examination? How did you go about addressing your learning needs?
4. Which resources have you found to be most helpful for addressing your learning needs? Which have been least helpful?
5. How confident do you feel about performing well on the first exam? (Select one)
   [Not confident at all   Low confidence   Moderate confidence   High confidence]
6. What percentage score are you aiming to achieve on the upcoming examination? (Select one)
   [92% to 100%   85% to 91%   70% to 84%   < 70%]

Part 2: Post-Examination Reflection

Part 2 of this reflective exercise asks you to confirm whether your confidence going into the first examination was accurate and realistic, and whether your performance met your expectations. This information will be helpful to both you and faculty instructors in considering any revisions that may need to be made in study strategies in advance of the second examination. Continued practice and implementation of these skills will increase your confidence as an autonomous learner. These are foundational elements in your development as a lifelong learner.

1. Were you satisfied with your performance on the first examination? Why or why not?
2. Reflecting on your approach to learning the material for the first examination and your score, what approaches will you preserve in your approach to the second examination and what approaches will you modify or eliminate?
3. Going forward, how will you decide what resources to rely on to most effectively learn the content of the Human Structure course?

30

HELPING STUDENTS HELP THEMSELVES
Fostering Undergraduate Metacognition

Polly R. Husmann, PhD
and Audra F. Schaefer, PhD

DESCRIPTION OF TEACHING/LEARNING CONTEXT

Basic Human Anatomy is a large undergraduate anatomy course that is taught every fall, spring, and summer at Indiana University in Bloomington, Indiana. This systems-based course has both lecture and laboratory components. The lecture is set up as a single large lecture that meets for 50 minutes, three times each week, in a traditional lecture hall with auditorium-style immovable seats. Lecture exams are given during a separate time block so that all students may take the exam simultaneously in various rooms to allow for spacing between students. The exam itself includes 45 to 50 multiple-choice questions. The laboratory component is set up as 12 separate sections that meet for 105 minutes twice a week. During the laboratory time, students are instructed by two graduate student associate instructors and one undergraduate teaching assistant using physical models of the anatomy, a virtual microscope for histology, and two cadavers that have been purposely dissected so that students may see demonstrations of most body systems. Students sit facing two large projection screens and chalkboards in three rows of long tables with one desktop computer available for each pair of students. At the beginning of each laboratory session, one of the graduate students will give a brief (15- to 20-minute) overview of the day's materials and point out relevant models or bones around the room. Following this introduction, students are instructed to read through their laboratory guide for the Basic Human Anatomy course (a text created in-house with all the necessary terms listed in bold font and discussions of which models adequately demonstrate the structures). Students are encouraged to work with a partner or two at a self-directed pace throughout the session and may leave the classroom whenever they feel that they have mastered the material. At some point during the session, the two graduate student associate instructors invite the students to come in

Friberg, J. C., Visconti, C. F., & Ginsberg, S. M. (Eds.). *Evidence-Based Education in the Classroom: Examples From Clinical Disciplines* (pp. 269-278).

small groups (8 to 12) to view a demonstration of the relevant structures on the cadavers. Laboratory exams are given during regular class times, though each section will be split into two groups for the exam to allow for adequate spacing between students. The laboratory exams are purely identification of structures with students rotating through the room to answer questions at each of the 20 stations. Each station is set up with two questions and the student has 1 minute to answer both questions before a timer beeps to indicate that it is time to move to the next station. Students may not return to any previous stations and approximately half the questions are changed between each section so that students cannot reliably reveal to students in later sections what was on the exam.

The student population of the Basic Human Anatomy course is comprised predominantly of students planning to enter health care–related fields, such as medicine, nursing, optometry, occupational therapy, physical therapy, physician assistant, or other programs. The largest of these populations is the pre-nursing cohort. Many of our pre-nursing students take this course the first year of their undergraduate education as a prerequisite to get into nursing school. Pre-nursing students are expected to do very well in this course to have a good chance of obtaining admission into a very competitive nursing program. This pressure adds to the stress of an already-challenging course. As first-year students, they are also often still adjusting to life outside of their parents' house. As a whole, the difficulty of this course has led to a withdrawal rate that ranges from 8% to 13% depending on the semester (O'Loughlin, 2002), with many of these students retaking the course a second time to achieve a sufficient course grade to remain enrolled in their program of study or to apply for professional school. Perhaps not surprisingly, nursing students make up the largest proportion of students who end up repeating the course, as they need to achieve a high course grade to be a competitive applicant into nursing school (Schutte, 2016).

In an effort to improve student learning, the Basic Human Anatomy course had previously been revamped in the fall of 2000 to incorporate more interactive learning exercises into what had been a very traditional large lecture (O'Loughlin, 2002). The incorporation of these activities correlated with the exam scores that were significantly higher than previous years on three of the four exams. The transition also correlated with increased students demonstrating mastery of the material (i.e., achieving As in the course) and passing the course (i.e., receiving As, Bs, or Cs), as well as more positive instructor evaluations (O'Loughlin, 2002). Based on these results, the learning activities have continued to be a prominent component of the course since that time. In more recent years, additional activities have also been added to further improve student engagement, metacognition, and active study strategies.

REVIEW OF LITERATURE

In 2016, Gooding and colleagues published 12 tips for applying the scholarship of teaching and learning to education, particularly in the health sciences. Two of their recommendations were (1) to provide opportunities for retrieval practice and (2) to promote metacognition as a means to improve student outcomes. These two guidelines directly relate to how we have continued to improve our Basic Human Anatomy course.

Metacognition

Metacognition is part of a larger phenomenon known as *self-regulated learning*. However, metacognition itself may also be broken down into subcomponents, including knowledge of cognition and regulation of cognition (see the following for more detail on these constructs: Husmann et al., 2018; Livingston, 2003; Schraw et al., 2006; Terrell, 2006). Knowledge of cognition essentially describes the different types of information students hold (or know) about how they learn, various learning strategies, how to use those strategies, and when it is appropriate to use those strategies. Regulation of cognition involves the planning for learning, implementing strategies, and then determining whether the methods in use are effectively helping the student work toward their learning goals through regular monitoring and self-assessment. This ability to self-assess has consistently been shown to correlate with improved performance (de Bruin et al., 2017; Garrett et al., 2007; Hall et al., 2016; Handel & Dresel, 2018; Nietfeld et al., 2006; Ohtani & Hisasaka, 2018; Sawdon & Finn, 2014).

Yet, previous research has shown that students from multiple student populations struggle with producing an accurate appraisal of what they know (Burman et al., 2014; Costabile et al., 2013; de Bruin et al., 2017; Garrett et al., 2007; Hall et al., 2016; Kruger & Dunning, 1999; Lundeberg & Mohan, 2009; Naug et al., 2011; Ross et al., 2006). As one might expect, this difficulty in monitoring their own learning has then been found to negatively affect academic success (Burman et al., 2014; Costabile et al., 2013; Ross et al., 2006; Tobias & Everson, 2009). Nonetheless, most researchers agree that these self-assessment skills can be improved with instruction (Callender et al., 2016; de Bruin et al., 2017; Fernandez & Jamet, 2017; Hall et al., 2016; Kruger & Dunning, 1999; Manlove et al., 2007; Miller & Geraci, 2011; Nietfeld et al., 2006; Schraw, 2007).

Retrieval Practice

In addition to promoting metacognition, Gooding and colleagues (2016) also recommend providing students with opportunities for retrieval practice. Retrieval practice refers to the act of forcefully recalling the information rather than simply recognizing the information upon review of a text or notes. This practice has been found to produce substantial benefits in information retention in the medical sciences, including anatomy (Dobson & Linderholm, 2015; Dobson et al., 2017), and in other fields (Karpicke & Bauernschmidt, 2011; Karpicke & Blunt, 2011; Roediger & Karpicke, 2006). These studies have shown that students who study via retrieval practice consistently perform significantly higher than their peers who repeatedly review the information for the same amount of time. These trends remain present even though the students who are using retrieval practice often predict that they will perform worse on assessment than their peers who repeatedly review the information. Furthermore, additional studies have also found evidence that the benefits of repeated retrieval on outcomes may actually be mediated by self-regulation processes (Fernandez & Jamet, 2017). Thus, we aimed to encourage the use of both self-regulation and retrieval practice among our students in the hopes that it might benefit their metacognitive skills for all classes and, specifically, their outcomes in the Basic Human Anatomy course.

Supplemental Instruction

One of the ways that colleges and universities have attempted to help students gain mastery of their metacognition and to learn study skills, particularly in the context of course content, has been through supplemental instruction. Supplemental instruction was originally designed at the University of Missouri–Kansas City (Blanc & Martin, 1994). In its original format, supplemental instruction sessions are held outside of regular class time and led by students who previously took the course and performed well. Often these student leaders work with course directors to prepare supplemental instruction sessions that follow along closely with content progression in the main course. Over the past 25 years, supplemental instruction has been implemented in numerous institutions to aid students in traditionally difficult courses (30% failure rate or greater), as it is proactive, assisting students from the beginning of a course instead of a response to poor performance on the first examination, and student participation is voluntary, allowing students to attend as many supplemental instruction sessions as they choose. It has been shown that students who participate in supplemental instruction tend to earn higher average course grades and experience lower failure and withdrawal rates than students who do not attend supplemental instruction (Etter et al., 2001; Rye et al., 1993), as well as decreased levels of anxiety and increased feelings of support (Bronstein, 2008). Some institutions have designed courses that closely mimic the original supplemental instruction format in an effort to support students in science courses and found students who completed such courses also tended to successfully complete the corresponding science course with higher grades and retention rates (Belzer et al., 2003; Hopper, 2011). The structure of supplemental instruction and these formal courses became models for the development of a supplemental learning skills course aimed at promoting student success in the Basic Human Anatomy course.

ORIGINAL DATA

Improving Learning Skills in Anatomy Course

The regularity with which students in the Basic Human Anatomy course were repeating the class was noted by graduate student associate instructors teaching the lab sessions. Students also frequently commented that although they thought they studied enough, their exam grade did not reflect the time and effort they put into preparing. With the intent of helping to reduce the frequency of students repeating this course and helping those who were repeating, two graduate students codeveloped a new 1-credit hour undergraduate supplemental instruction course that would teach students study skills in the context of what they were concurrently learning in the Basic Human Anatomy course. The course, Improving Learning Skills in Anatomy, would be geared toward both repeating students and students in their first Basic Human Anatomy course enrollment who self-identified as needing assistance with how best to study anatomy. One of the major course goals that was established for the Improving Learning Skills in Anatomy course was improving student metacognition. Specifically, students would recognize different ways they learn effectively and introduce these approaches into their studies. Although the intent of the Improving Learning Skills in Anatomy course was not to become a weekly review session for the other courses' content, another goal for the Improving Learning Skills in Anatomy course was for students to explain and differentiate major body systems. Being able to understand and explain anatomy content in an accurate manner would serve as a means for students to determine if their current study methods were effective. In-class activities would revolve heavily around giving students experience implementing study methods in the context of the material currently being taught in the Basic Human Anatomy course.

The first time the supplemental course was offered was the summer session of 2010. With each semester after this, the course continued to be offered concurrently with the Basic Human Anatomy course, with enrollment increasing to around 40 students per semester. In the following semesters, the course activities evolved based on student feedback, logistical factors (including increasing student enrollment in the course and changes to the Basic Human Anatomy class assignments), and lessons learned by instructors. Two course activities became the primary approaches for achieving the goal of improving student metacognition: weekly journal entries/blog posts and study logs. Through the blog function in the online course management system, instructors were able to provide weekly prompts that students were required to respond to before the next class session. Prompts typically involved some aspect of self-assessment of study strategies, planning and time management, and reflection on Basic Human Anatomy course exams. Study logs were assigned 3 days prior to Basic Human Anatomy lecture exams, and 1 log was completed each of these 3 days. Students recorded where and when they studied, as well as how productive they were for each 30-minute increment on a scale of 1 to 4 (1 = nonproductive, 4 = high productivity; study logs adapted from Angelo & Cross, 1993). Most semesters, students followed up study logs by writing a brief reflection on why they were or were not productive and what they learned about their study habits from completing the logs.

As instructors gained experience with providing reflective writing prompts for the blog posts, it was noted that students' responses became increasingly insightful regarding their learning. Additionally, thematic analysis of students' posts was conducted to identify patterns in students' responses to the prompts from three semesters' worth of blog posts. This analysis revealed trends in which early in the semester, students would spend more time discussing specific learning methods they were trying but little about whether those methods were effective for their learning. Additionally, it was common to find discussion that suggested deficient metacognitive skill as students felt confident in their preparation for an exam, but their exam grade was lower than expected/desired. In other words, students were uncertain about what was necessary for them to be successful or lacked awareness of when their study methods were not helpful. Both blogs and study logs revealed difficulties surrounding time management, in that students either recognized that they were not using their time well or discussed how they struggled to stick to effective time management strategies. As a result of time management being a major theme in student discussions in the blogs and study logs, a new activity was introduced: study plans. Instructors noticed that when students were asked directly to outline a study plan, including how they would manage distractions, students gave more details about how they intended to use their time than they previously discussed in their posts. Students also were asked to follow up on how well they stuck to their plans and why they were more or less successful. As the semester progressed, it was observed that students shifted their focus to discussing how well various study methods worked for them, as well as increasing confidence in their preparedness and ability to do well on exams. While it is difficult to attribute all of this improved awareness and confidence to the activities of the Improving Learning Skills in Anatomy course, it is a positive trend to see in students, as high levels of confidence in their ability to do well and effective monitoring of learning processes are consistently linked to academic success (Garrett et al., 2007; Zimmerman & Martinez-Pons, 1990). The Improving Learning Skills in Anatomy course has continued to be offered each semester, and as of the 2019 fall semester, enrollment has reached 60 students because students increasingly realize the benefits of this course.

LearnSmarts

Unfortunately, less than 15% of the students enrolled in the Basic Human Anatomy course are able to benefit from the activities of the Improving Learning Skills in Anatomy course, and often (or so it has been hypothesized) the students who most need the activities in the supplemental course are unlikely to enroll. Thus, in the fall of 2011, the Basic Human Anatomy course also began using online LearnSmart modules through the McGraw-Hill Connect website associated with our textbook (McKinley et al., 2017). It was hoped that these modules would help the students to practice retrieval of the material throughout the course instead of attempting to passively review or "cram" the material just before the exam. Each LearnSmart module is designed to focus on one chapter or part of a chapter of the text. For each module, students are given practice questions in any of the following formats: multiple choice, fill in the blank, matching, rank order, and/or multiple answer. For each question, students must answer the question and also indicate how confident they are in that answer using the following options: I Know It, Think So, Unsure, or No Idea. After the student has completed the questions, the program was then set to automatically provide feedback because online platforms that provide immediate feedback to students have been associated with improved abilities to self-assess (de Bruin et al., 2017; El Saadawi et al., 2010; Manlove et al., 2007; Schraw, 2007; Schraw et al., 2006; Winne & Nesbit, 2009). However, no analysis of the effects of these modules was completed until Fall 2017.

During the Fall 2017 semester, four to nine LearnSmart modules were given to students to complete in each block of the course. These numbers varied based on the number of chapters from the text included in that block. Each module usually had around 40 questions, though one was as short as nine questions and one as large as 77 questions. These modules were available beginning at the start of the block, but they must be turned in within approximately 1 week from the day the content was covered in lecture. After the examination for the block was completed, the instructors would then choose two of the available LearnSmart modules to count for extra credit. Up to two points of extra credit were awarded for completion of the module. Thus, a total of 16 extra credit points were available (4 blocks x 2 Learnsmarts per block x 2 points per LearnSmart) out of 800 points available in the course.

On the back end of the software, instructors were able to view the number of students who had not started each module and the number of students that had completed each module. If a student began a module, the program was set to automatically submit any completed questions once the deadline for the module was reached, so that students could receive partial credit even if they ran out of time to complete the entire module. The program also provided running percentages for each student on the number of questions that fell into the four following metacognitive categories: correct and aware, correct and unaware, incorrect and aware, or incorrect and unaware. These were based on the students' responses to their confidence in their answer. In addition to the completion and metacognitive percentages, the platform also provided basic statistics of each module for all students, the basic statistics of each student for all modules, and basic item statistics for each question.

We began the analysis by looking at how many LearnSmart practice questions our students were completing. On average, students were completing over 800 practice questions on the LearnSmart platform throughout the semester (student $n = 377$), suggesting that students were utilizing this resource quite regularly. Students' metacognitive awareness scores (% correct and aware + % incorrect and aware) on these questions generally ranged from the high 40s to the mid-90s with higher scores indicating better metacognitive skills for each block and overall for the course. Pearson correlations were run comparing the number of questions completed and the metacognitive awareness scores on those questions with the final point totals in the class. Both correlations were found to be statistically significant with $r = .523$, $p < .0001$ and $r = .200$, $p < .001$, respectively. However, the relationship between the number of questions completed and the metacognitive awareness scores was not found to be statistically significant ($r = -.074$, $p = .157$). Thus, indicating that, while both completing the questions and being metacognitively aware were associated with the final point totals in the class, the act of completing the questions did not significantly change students' metacognitive awareness.

APPLICATION OF LITERATURE/DATA

Our goal for this research was to improve study strategies and metacognitive skills in students in our Basic Human Anatomy course. This goal was based on the demonstrated importance of metacognition for academic success as seen in previous literature (Burman et al., 2014; Costabile et al., 2013; de Bruin et al., 2017; Ohtani & Hisaska, 2018; Ross et al., 2006; Schraw, 2007). In particular, we aimed to apply the science of learning, as presented by Gooding and colleagues (2016), to our classroom via activities involving self-regulation and retrieval practice. Implementation of an optional study skills course (Improving Learning Skills in Anatomy) revealed a positive effect on students. The class activities provided instructors with insight into the metacognitive skills of students, and therefore, provided opportunities to address gaps in these skills. Assessment of LearnSmart modules revealed that the number of practice questions a student completed and the percentage of those questions on which the student was aware are both correlated with their outcome in the course. Unfortunately, the number of practice questions completed did not correlate with any improvement in the percentage of questions on which the student was metacognitively aware.

These results were consistent with O'Loughlin's (2002) previous work in the Basic Human Anatomy course, showing the positive effects of active learning processes and engaging with the course material outside of the classroom. However, previous literature had also shown that feedback provided through electronic assessments correlated with increases in metacognition (de Bruin et al., 2017; Schraw, 2007; Schraw et al., 2006) and that repeated recall may even mediate self-regulation processes (Fernandez & Jamet, 2017). Yet these conclusions are not consistent with our results. One possible explanation for this discrepancy may include differences in the granularity of the measurements that are being used. Rovers and colleagues (2019) recently described the importance of types and levels of measurements when discussing self-regulated learning. Looking at Fernandez and Jamet (2017), they used a summative self-assessment, instead of individual question-level assessments, and a think-aloud protocol, instead of a single Likert scale question. Thus, these different levels of measurement may relate to the discrepancies that we are seeing here.

Nonetheless, there is some previous research that aligns well with these outcomes. El Saadawi and colleagues (2010) used a computer-based program to provide students with immediate feedback on content learning and "feeling of knowing" accuracy. Their study found that some students became reliant on this feedback instead of developing metacognitive skills of their own.

APPLICATION TO CROSS-DISCIPLINARY CONTEXTS

While these activities were implemented specifically in a large undergraduate anatomy course, their applicability to other fields is untold. Although the Improving Learning Skills in Anatomy course was taught through the lens of anatomy, such an approach could be implemented in numerous courses and learning settings. Courses similar to the Improving Learning Skill in Anatomy have been developed at other institutions (Belzer et al., 2003; Hopper, 2011), and although there are benefits to having a separate course, this is not always feasible. Instructors can certainly still incorporate activities into their teaching of regular course content to also help improve student metacognition and study skills. Something as simple as demonstrating a study approach, such as creating a flow chart, into our teaching of the material may help students to understand content and gain practice with an approach they may not have tried on their own. Student awareness of their own deficits in study strategies is clearly an issue that is not limited to anatomy students. Reflection has consistently been shown to be a powerful tool for improving metacognition, and instructors can incorporate reflective activities into their regular courses to help raise students' awareness of their learning processes (Fonteyn & Cahill, 1998; Schraw, 1998). For resources that describe activities that instructors could implement into their courses to promote reflection and metacognition, see the Additional Resources section.

The use of LearnSmart modules in other large, introductory sciences courses, such as biology (James, 2012) and chemistry (Thadani & Bouvier-Brown, 2016), has also been evaluated. In an introductory biology class, James (2012) found that LearnSmart completion rates were correlated with exam scores in the course. However, she did not find the metacognitive data within the program to significantly correlate with outcomes in the course, yet, she still recommends using this data for student self-reflection or during individual student consultations with instructors. In general chemistry, Thadani and Bouvier-Brown (2016) did not find any learning benefits to the use of LearnSmart modules. However, when they provided metacognitive scaffolding questions for students to better understand the metacognitive data from the LearnSmart platform, significant learning gains were found. These results are fairly similar to ours in that there may be some overall correlations with outcomes, but metacognitive skills did not demonstrate improvement with the LearnSmart modules alone.

Outside of large, introductory science, technology, engineering, and math courses, LearnSmart modules are also available for some business, humanities, social science, and language courses (https://www.edsurge.com/product-reviews/mcgraw-hill-learnsmart/compare/aleks-highered). Unfortunately, data from these courses do not seem to be as well reported as those in science, technology, engineering, and math fields. One report that was found evaluated the use of LearnSmart modules in a course on interpersonal communication (Gearhart, 2016). Gearhart reports that students who used the LearnSmart modules performed slightly better than students who did not use the LearnSmart modules, but not enough to be statistically significant. However, the metacognitive data was not reported. All these studies, taken in concert with our own assessments, suggest that LearnSmart modules (or other similar programs) may provide students with opportunities for spaced retrieval practice and practice self-monitoring their learning, both of which have been shown to correlate with better course outcomes (de Bruin et al., 2017; Garrett et al., 2007; Hall et al., 2016; Handel & Dresel, 2018; Nietfeld et al., 2006; Ohtani & Hisasaka, 2018; Sawdon & Finn, 2014) and material retention (Dobson & Linderholm, 2015; Dobson et al., 2017; Karpicke & Bauernschmidt, 2011; Karpicke & Blunt, 2011; Roediger & Karpicke, 2006). However, the metacognitive data provided by these programs requires further development. While not as much research has been published on this aspect of the LearnSmart program, those data which have been shown here, as well as by James (2012) and Thadani and Bouvier-Brown (2016), suggest that, if these data are to prove useful, additional resources are required. Thus, for the Basic Human Anatomy course, we will continue looking for other ways that we might improve our students' metacognitive skills and effective study strategies, such as the resources listed in the following section.

ADDITIONAL RESOURCES

- Angelo and Cross describe a variety of activities that instructors could implement in regular courses to promote reflection, such as a muddiest point exercises in which students write down the topic that is most confusing from that class session for future investigation or instructor feedback:
  - Angelo, T. A., & Cross, K. P. (1993). *Classroom assessment techniques: A handbook for college teachers* (2nd ed.). Jossey-Bass Inc.
- Tanner also provides excellent examples of reflective questions that instructors can ask students to prompt reflection along the various stages of cognitive regulation:
  - Tanner, K. D. (2012). Promoting student metacognition. *CBE-Life Sciences Education, 11,* 113-120.
- Nilson provides a variety of activities to help students monitor their learning, such as exam review assessments that may help students to determine what types of mistakes they commonly make or which content they tend to struggle with on exams:
  - Nilson, L. B. (2013). *Creating self-regulated learners: Strategies to strengthen students' self-awareness and learning skills.* Stylus.

ACKNOWLEDGMENT

Polly R. Husmann would like to acknowledge Theodore Smith for his help in collecting some of these data.

REFERENCES

Angelo, T. A., & Cross, K. P. (1993). *Classroom assessment techniques: A handbook for college teachers* (2nd ed.). Jossey-Bass Inc.

Belzer, S., Miller, M., & Shoemaker, S. (2003). A supplemental study skills course designed to improve introductory students' skills for learning biology. *The American Biology Teacher, 65*(1), 30-40. https://doi.org/10.2307/4451430

Blanc, R., & Martin, D. C. (1994). Supplemental instruction: Increasing student performance and persistence in difficult academic courses. *Academic Medicine, 69*(6), 452-454. http://dx.doi.org/10.1097/00001888-199406000-00004

Bronstein, S. B. (2008). Supplemental instruction: Supporting persistence in barrier courses. *Learning Assistance Review, 13*(1), 31-45. https://files.eric.ed.gov/fulltext/EJ818225.pdf

Burman, N. J., Boscardin, C. K., & Van Schaik, S. (2014). Career-long learning: Relationship between cognitive and metacognitive skills. *Medical Teacher, 36*(8), 715-723. https://doi.org/10.3109/0142159X.2014.909010

Callender, A. A., Franco-Watkins, A. M., & Roberts, A. S. (2016). Improving metacognition in the classroom through instruction, training, and feedback. *Metacognition & Learning, 11*, 215-235. https://doi.org/10.1007/s11409-015-9142-6

Costabile, A., Cornoldi, C., De Beni, R., Manfredi, P., & Figliuzzi, S. (2013). Metacognitive components of student's difficulties in the first year of university. *International Journal of Higher Education, 2*(4), 165-171. https://doi.org/10.5430/ijhe.v2n4p165

de Bruin, A. B. H., Kok, E. M., Lobbestael, J., & de Grip, A. (2017). The impact of an online tool for monitoring and regulating learning at university: Overconfidence, learning strategy, and personality. *Metacognition & Learning, 12*, 21-43. https://doi.org/10.1007/s11409-016-9159-5

Dobson, J. L., & Linderholm, T. (2015). Self-testing promotes superior retention of anatomy and physiology information. *Advances in Health Sciences Education, 20*, 149-161.

Dobson, J. L., Perez, J., & Linderholm, T. (2017). Distributed retrieval practice promotes superior recall of anatomy information. *Anatomical Sciences Education, 10*, 339-347. https://doi.org/10.1002/ase.1668

El Saadawi, G. M., Azevedo, R., Castine, M., Payne, V., Medvedeva, O., Tseytlin, E., Legowski, E., Jukic, D., & Crowley, R. S. (2010). Factors affecting feeling-of-knowing in a medical intelligent tutoring system: The role of immediate feedback as a metacognitive scaffold. *Advances in Health Science Education, 15*, 9-30. https://doi.org/10.1007/s10459-009-9162-6

Etter, E. R., Burmeister, S. L., & Elder, R. J. (2001). Improving student performance and retention viz supplemental instruction. *Journal of Accounting Education, 18*(4), 355-368. https://doi.org/10.1016/S0748-5751(01)00006-9

Fernandez, J., & Jamet, E. (2017). Extending the testing effect to self-regulated learning. *Metacognition & Learning, 12*, 131-156. https://doi.org/10.1007/s11409-016-9163-9

Fonteyn, M. E., & Cahill, M. (1998). The use of clinical logs to improve nursing students' metacognition: A pilot study. *Journal of Advanced Nursing, 28*(1), 149-154. https://doi.org/10.1046/j.1365-2648.1998.00777.x

Garrett, J., Alman, M., Gardner, S., & Born, C. (2007). Assessing students' metacognitive skills. *American Journal of Pharmaceutical Education, 71*(1), 1-14.

Gearhart, C. (2016). Does LearnSmart connect students to textbook content in an Interpersonal Communication course? Assessing the effectiveness of and satisfaction with LearnSmart. *International Journal of Teaching and Learning in Higher Education, 28*(1), 9-17. https://files.eric.ed.gov/fulltext/EJ1106331.pdf

Gooding, H. C., Mann, K., & Armstrong, E. (2016). Twelve tips for applying the science of learning to health professions education. *Medical Teacher, 39*(1), 26-31. https://doi.org/10.1080/0142159X.2016.1231913

Hall, S. R., Stephens, J. R., Seaby, E. G., Andrade, M. G., Lowry, A. F., Parton, W. J. C., Smith, C. F., & Border, S. (2016). Can medical students accurately predict their learning? A study comparing perceived and actual performance in neuroanatomy. *Anatomical Sciences Education, 9*(5), 488-495. https://doi.org/10.1002/ase.1601

Handel, M., & Dresel, M. (2018). Confidence in performance judgment accuracy: The unskilled and unaware effect revisited. *Metacognition & Learning, 13*, 265-285. https://doi.org/10.1007/s11409-018-9185-6

Hopper, M. (2011). Student enrollment in a supplement course for anatomy and physiology results in improved retention and success. *Journal of College Science Teaching, 40*(3), 70-79. https://eric.ed.gov/?id=EJ921524

Husmann, P. R., Hoffman, L. A., & Schaefer, A. F. (2018). Unique terms or are we splitting hairs? Clarification of self-directed versus self-regulated learning and related terms. *Medical Science Educator, 28*(4), 777-783. https://doi.org/10.1007/s40670-018-0626-2

James, L. A. (2012). Evaluation of an adaptive learning technology as a predictor of student performance in undergraduate biology [Master's thesis, Appalachian State University]. NC Docks. https://libres.uncg.edu/ir/asu/f/James,%20Lauren_2012_Thesis.pdf

Karpicke, J. D., & Bauernschmidt, A. (2011). Spaced retrieval: Absolute spacing enhances learning regardless of relative spacing. *Journal of Experimental Psychology: Learning, Memory, and Cognition, 37*, 1250-1257. https://doi.org/10.1037/a0023436

Karpicke, J. D., & Blunt, J. R. (2011). Retrieval practice produces more learning than elaborative studying with concept mapping. *Science, 331*, 772-775. https://doi.org/10.1126/science.1199327

Kruger, J., & Dunning, D. (1999). Unskilled and unaware of it: How difficulties in recognizing one's own incompetence lead to inflated self-assessments. *Journal of Personality and Social Psychology, 77*(6), 1121-1134.

Livingston, J. A. (2003). *Metacognition: An overview.* https://files.eric.ed.gov/fulltext/ED474273.pdf

Lundeberg, M., & Mohan, L. (2009). Context matters: Gender and cross-cultural differences in confidence. In D. J. Hacker, J. Dunlosky, & A. C. Graesser (Eds.), *Handbook of metacognition in education* (pp. 221-239). Routledge.

Manlove, S., Lazonder, A. W., & de Jong, T. (2007). Software scaffolds to promote regulation during scientific inquiry learning. *Metacognition & Learning, 2*, 141-155. https://doi.org/10.1007/s11409-007-9012-y

McKinley, M. P., O'Loughlin, V. D., & Pennefather-O'Brien, E. E. (2017). *Human anatomy* (5th ed.). McGraw Hill Education.

Miller, T. M., & Geraci, L. (2011). Training metacognition in the classroom: The influence of incentives and feedback on exam predictions. *Metacognition & Learning, 6*, 303-314. https://doi.org/10.1007/s11409-011-9083-7

Naug, H. L., Colson, N. J., & Donner, D. G. (2011). Promoting metacognition in first year anatomy laboratories using plasticine modeling and drawing activities: A pilot study of the "blank page" technique. *Anatomical Sciences Education, 4*(4), 231-234.

Nietfeld, J. L., Cao, L., & Osborne, J. W. (2006). The effect of distributed monitoring exercises and feedback on performance, monitoring accuracy, and self-efficacy. *Metacognition Learning, 1,* 159-179. https://doi.org/10.1007/s10409-006-9595-6

O'Loughlin, V. D. (2002). Assessing the effects of using interactive learning activities in a large science class. *Journal on Excellence in College Teaching, 13*(1), 29-42.

Ohtani, K., & Hisasaka, T. (2018). Beyond intelligence: a meta-analytic review of the relationship among metacognition, intelligence, and academic performance. *Metacognition & Learning, 13,* 179-212. https://doi.org/10.1007/s11409-018-9183-8

Roediger, H. L., III, & Karpicke, J. D. (2006). Test-enhanced learning: Taking memory tests improves long-term retention. *Psychological Science, 17*(3), 249-255. https://doi.org/10.1111/j.1467-9280.2006.01693.x

Ross, M. E., Green, S. B., Salisbury-Glennon, J. D., & Tollefson, N. (2006). College students' study strategies as a function of testing: An investigation into metacognitive self-regulation. *Innovative Higher Education, 30*(5), 361-375. https://doi.org/10.1007/s10755-005-9004-2

Rovers, S. F. E., Clarebout, G., Savelberg, H. H. C., de Bruin, A. B. H., & van Merrienboer, J. J. G. (2019). Granularity matters: Comparing different ways of measuring self-regulated learning. *Metacognition & Learning, 14*(1), 1-19. https://doi.org/10.1007/s11409-019-09188-6

Rye, P. D., Wallace, J., & Bidgood, P. (1993). Instructions in learning skills: An integrated approach. *Medical Education, 27*(6), 470-473.

Sawdon, M., & Finn, G. (2014). The "unskilled and unaware" effect is linear in a real-world setting. *Journal of Anatomy, 224,* 279-285. https://doi.org/10.1111/joa.12072

Schraw, G. (1998). Promoting general metacognitive awareness. *Instructional Science, 26*(1), 113-125. https://doi.org/10.1023/A:1003044231033

Schraw, G. (2007). The use of computer-based environments for understanding and improving self-regulation. *Metacognition & Learning, 2,* 169-176. https://doi.org/10.1007/s11409-007-9015-8

Schraw, G., Crippen, K. J., & Hartley, K. (2006). Promoting self-regulation in science education: Metacognition as part of a broader perspective on learning. *Research in Science Education, 36,* 111-139. https://doi.org/10.1007/s11165-005-3917-8

Schutte, A. F. (2016). Who is repeating anatomy? Trends in an undergraduate anatomy course. *Anatomical Sciences Education, 9,* 171-178. https://doi.org/10.1002/ase.1553

Terrell, M. (2006). Anatomy of learning: Instructional design principles for the anatomical sciences. *The Anatomical Record (Part B), 289B,* 252-260. https://doi.org/10.1002/ar.b.20116

Thadani, V., & Bouvier-Brown, N. C. (2016). Textbook-bundled metacognitive tools: A study of LearnSmart's efficacy in General Chemistry. *Journal on Excellence in College Teaching, 27*(2), 77-95. https://digitalcommons.lmu.edu/psyc_fac/8/

Tobias, S., & Everson, H. T. (2009). The Importance of knowing what you know: A knowledge monitoring framework for studying metacognition in education. In D. J. Hacker, J. Dunlosky, & A. C. Graesser (Eds.), *Handbook of metacognition in education* (pp. 107-127). Routledge.

Winne, P. H., & Nesbit, J. C. (2009). Supporting self-regulated learning with cognitive tools. In D. J. Hacker, J. Dunlosky, & A. C. Graesser (Eds.), *Handbook of metacognition in education* (pp. 259-277). Routledge.

Zimmerman, B. J., & Martinez-Pons, M. (1990). Student differences in self-regulated learning: Relating grade, sex, and giftedness to self-efficacy and strategy use. *Journal of Educational Psychology, 82*(1), 51. http://dx.doi.org/10.1037/0022-0663.82.1.51

31

LEARNING TO LOOK
Employing Reflexive Photography in Developing Critical Practice

Brent Oliver, PhD, RSW
and Darlene Chalmers, PhD, RSW

DESCRIPTION OF TEACHING/LEARNING CONTEXT

In North America, experiential learning and field practica in postsecondary programs are critical components in preparing students for clinical practice. Regardless of the discipline, students training for clinical practice are required to develop and demonstrate a variety of important skills and knowledge including critical thinking, self-awareness, and reflexivity. Of the many skills required for clinical practice, teaching and learning reflexivity can be challenging for both educators and students alike. Multiple disciplinary perspectives on reflexivity exist, and there is very little conceptual clarity in defining this important construct. Nonetheless, in the context of clinical practice, reflexivity can be summarized as a process of looking outward to the social and political influences that inform professional practice and looking inward to the internal processes that shape our actions as practitioners (D'Cruz et al., 2007). In the context of teaching and learning, reflexivity involves a student's ability to act in the world and to critically reflect on their actions (D'Cruz et al., 2007). In our shared experience as social work educators, we have identified many challenges in supporting students to develop skills in reflexive practice. Unfortunately, we have found very few effective teaching strategies.

With the belief that photographs can facilitate understanding of one's underlying values and assumptions (Taylor, 2002), we engaged reflexive photography in course work with social work students in postsecondary field practica and in their clinical practice settings. Reflexive photography draws upon the principles of Photovoice, a qualitative research method where images are used as a stimulus for reflection and community change (Wang & Burris, 1997). Photovoice offers a unique way to highlight often overlooked perspectives on social issues and community phenomena. As

Friberg, J. C., Visconti, C. F., & Ginsberg, S. M. (Eds.). *Evidence-Based Education in the Classroom: Examples From Clinical Disciplines* (pp. 279-288).

part of the reflexive photography project, students were required to use digital cameras (phone, iPad [Apple], etc.) to document their learning while in clinical practice and to address questions regarding both the content and the context of their photos. Images hold the potential to convey ideas through metaphor (Lofstrom et al., 2015). Accordingly, the reflexive photography project included a brief narrative text summarizing the student's interpretation of the photo. As part of the assignment, students shared their photos in class and discussed their learning with their peers and the instructor. The images reflected both the students' constructions and interpretations of their learning in practicum and communicated their understanding of client work, the practice setting, and the surrounding context (Lofstrom et al., 2015). During these classroom discussions, students were prompted to consider the sociopolitical and cultural structures embedded in their images and how their understanding of the image is informed by previous knowledge (Reavey, 2011).

Over several years, we successfully piloted reflexive photography in clinically based classrooms within three Canadian universities including Mount Royal University, the University of Regina, and York University (for an example of the assignment, see Appendix). As part of a scholarship of teaching and learning (SoTL) inquiry, we conducted a qualitative research project that explored social work students' experiences with reflexive photography within our three distinct and diverse social work practicum courses (diploma, undergraduate, and graduate). Specifically, we were curious about the learning processes social work students experienced as they participated in the reflexive photography project and how this learning contributed to their professional experiences in practicum and in clinical practice. The following case study describes the insight we drew from the study and the ways this informed our teaching.

REVIEW OF LITERATURE

Building upon the work of Schön (1983), reflexivity involves simultaneous processes of reflection in action and critical analysis. To practice effectively, social workers and other clinical practitioners need to be aware of how their own power and privilege influences their encounters with clients and service users.

The important practices that comprise reflexivity are described by Fook (1999) and include the ability to acknowledge the influence of self in determining and changing a situation, the recognition of unconscious assumptions, the capacity to question, and the ability to tolerate uncertainty. Similarly, D'Cruz and colleagues (2007) described reflexivity as involving the central processes of questioning one's assumptions, addressing issues of power and oppression, and including self in the process. Thus, reflexivity in clinical practice requires engaging one's emotions, acknowledging assumptions, and recognizing personal reactions such that these processes offer the potential to create socially situated practice knowledge (Fook, 1999; Pease, 2006).

The capacity for reflexive practice can develop over time as part of transformative learning experiences and training in clinical practice. Mezirow (1990) described this as learning that involves (1) making meaning of experience, (2) using these interpretations to guide decision making, and (3) critically understanding how underlying beliefs influence the process. These learning processes are a necessary part of clinical practice that is committed to equity and social change (Morley, 2008). Traditionally, reflective journals are a key strategy used to assist students to explore, process, and make meaning of their practice experiences. These journal assignments have served as a long-standing and important tool to foster reflective thinking among social work students (Clarke, 2012). Reflective journals are intended, in part, to create a space for the development of critical reflection and reflexivity and have tended to be the main site where students explore these concepts in relation to their practice experiences. Nevertheless, these tools are seldom effective with all students, and many educators have sought creative alternatives to support the development of reflexivity in critical and professional practice.

SoTL in higher education demonstrates that visual and digital content introduced into the curriculum can support student learning in ways that are more relevant, productive, and sustained (Butterwick & Lipson Lawrence, 2009). Increasingly, there is recognition among educators that visual literacy is vital in preparing students to engage in a rapidly changing world (Little, 2015; Little et al., 2010). Subsequently, educators from a variety of disciplines are turning to visual-based methods to engage and support students in clinically based classrooms.

Under this umbrella, there are diverse evidence-informed approaches in the social sciences, many of which utilize photography to assist students to make meaning of transformative learning experiences. For example, Johnson (2010) described how she used participatory photography in a service-learning course within a Salvadoran adult literacy program. She found that this approach was effective in creating meaningful partnerships in the community and in assisting students to reflect on the links between micro and macro practice. In particular, she highlights how photography assisted in critically recovering knowledge within a marginalized community. Furthermore, Hyde (2015) explored a Literacy through Photography methodology, described as a critical pedagogy that integrates writing and photography into classroom instruction. Here, image-making and writing were used to foster creativity and strengthen students' communication and observation skills. This methodology reportedly helped students to cultivate sociological mindfulness. Specifically, the methodology required students to consider how to represent conceptual ideas visually, frame and shoot photographs, and write creative narrative descriptions, thereby emphasizing critical thinking (Hyde, 2015).

ORIGINAL DATA

With an interest in visual methods and their incorporation in teaching reflexive practice in social work education, the authors undertook a study to explore how visual methods might be a useful teaching and learning approach. Our study objective was to understand the processes of student learning specifically related to professional practice using a reflexive photography assignment. A qualitative research design was used to best answer the research question: What learning processes do social work students experience as they participate in a reflexive photography assignment, and how does this learning appear to contribute to their professional experiences in the practicum and in the field?

As part of the reflexive photography project, the use of digital technology (i.e., phone, iPad [Apple]) was required. Students used these devices to record their learning and questions related to the content and context of their clinical practice. In addition, the reflexive photography assignment included a brief narrative, where students were prompted to document social realities at their practicum and reflect on their impact on emerging practice. Additionally, as part of the assignment, students were asked to choose and share two or three photographs with their peers in the practicum seminar and lead a discussion connecting the images to their learning. Students were encouraged to go beyond simply the content of the photographs and explore both the social context and associated meanings connected to them. In this manner, the photographs stimulated unique interpretations, discussion, and analysis that was shared and explored with the instructor and their peers.

Given our intent to explore students' lived experience of process and their co-construction of meaning with a reflexive photography assignment, we chose to employ grounded theory. Grounded theory is an inductive research approach that can be used to explain social phenomena with real-world, research-to-practice application in a diversity of settings (Charmaz, 2014). Data were collected at three Canadian postsecondary sites with students in diploma, undergraduate, and graduate social work programs. A total of 17 students participated in the study. The mean age of research participants was 28 years old. Data collection, conducted by trained peer research assistants at each site, occurred through face-to-face interviews guided by the use of a semi-structured interview guide. The interview questions aimed to elicit understanding of the experience of using photography and

Figure 31-1. Categories of learning emerging from reflexive photography experiences.

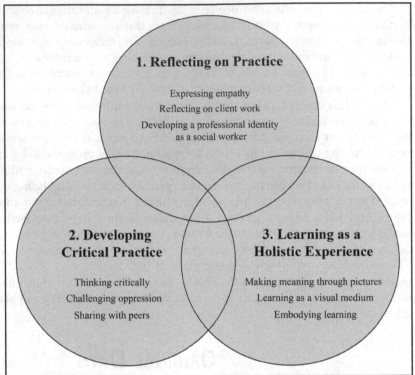

1. **Reflecting on Practice**

Expressing empathy
Reflecting on client work
Developing a professional identity
as a social worker

2. **Developing Critical Practice**

Thinking critically
Challenging oppression
Sharing with peers

3. **Learning as a Holistic Experience**

Making meaning through pictures
Learning as a visual medium
Embodying learning

how such an experience contributed to personal and professional insight. Our data analysis followed grounded theory systematic steps (simultaneous data collection and analysis), including constant comparative analysis (Charmaz, 2014; Strauss & Corbin, 1998) with combined data from across all three collection sites. Our data analysis process also involved team review and discussions of the data and ongoing check-ins with our peer researchers. Data saturation (Charmaz, 2014) resulted in the emergence of three categories and nine subcategories that explained how students' experiences with a reflexive photography assignment shaped understanding of their practice.

Three interrelated categories surfaced from our data collection (Figure 31-1). They included (1) reflecting on practice, (2) developing critical practice, and (3) learning as a holistic experience. Nine subcategories added breadth and depth to the dimensions of each category. Overall, the use of reflexive photography can be understood as both experiential and holistic, touching on the physical, emotional, intellectual, and spiritual domains.

The first category—reflecting on practice—revealed that the assignment permitted intrapersonal exploration. The examination of personal biases and judgments and the hesitancy to embark on a career not yet known was shared by the students through the use of their photographs. During seminar discussions, students were able to externalize these experiences through discussion of the picture. In turn, what emerged was access to peer support and focused conversations with their instructor.

The subcategories—expressing empathy, reflecting on client work, and developing a professional identity—describe the students' increased awareness of others (clients and coworkers). Students also shared greater understanding of the importance of relationships in social work practice. The connection of theory to practice in situ and the requisite skills needed as a professional became apparent as did the discovery of self as a professional in context.

The second category—developing critical practice—describes how the students were able to shift their consciousness outward and reflect on the political and social challenges that confront direct practice. This experience is described in three subcategories: thinking critically, challenging oppression, and sharing with peers. Critical thinking, informed by theory, is a foundational component of social work practice. The reflexive photography assignment provided multiple opportunities to deepen students' thinking. In particular, this included reflecting on and making direct connections to experiences of oppression. Challenging their own deeply held beliefs emerged, and the importance of sharing with peers in a safe environment permitted some risk-taking within the classroom discussion.

The third category—learning as a holistic experience—details how the process of becoming a professional social worker involves all dimensions of one's being. In this category, students shared how their learning involved aspects of themselves that they had not considered previously. Three subcategories further describe how they were able to make meaning through pictures, use a visual medium to learn, and how learning was an embodied experience. Of significance is that students described that the photographs provided immediate opportunities for reflection in the moment (virtually within minutes of taking and viewing the photo). They found that they were able to challenge themselves in their creativity. As such, the assignment was, in part, a paradigm shift for many students in that it permitted a different approach to learning. According to the students, they were able to share and discuss their thinking with their peers and instructor in ways that more easily reflected who they were becoming.

APPLICATION OF LITERATURE/DATA

Findings from this study contributed to our increased understanding of students' perspectives on reflexive photography and its potential as a transformative learning strategy. As coresearchers each of us have been involved in applying this knowledge to improve both student learning and teaching practice. As we analyzed the data from student participants, we were struck by the way in which reflexive photography facilitated an embodied conversation about critical social work concepts and practice experiences. The assignment provided students the opportunity to create and share a photograph as a metaphor for some of the more difficult or challenging learning they experienced in practicum. In articulating transformative learning theory, Mezirow (2009) defined a disorienting dilemma as a significant aspect of the process by which adult learners reflect on and interpret the meaning of their learning experiences. According to Mezirow (2009), this dilemma sets the stage for meaningful learning, which we discovered was also an integral part of the reflexive photography projects in our study. Students often chose to document experiences that they were stuck on, conflicted about, or actively questioned. The photograph served as a creative, informal, and dynamic tool for engaging others in conversation about difficult and often common learning experiences in the field. This shared conversation frequently led to further insight and resolution from a variety of perspectives, where before, there had been only questions and confusion. As such, several students described the experience as validating and supportive, and something they did not get from written reflective assignments. In the interviews with students in our study, many expressed difficulties with reflective journals and described how they were regurgitating material covered in class or just writing what they felt their professor wanted to hear. Consequently, the photos seemed better able to capture the complexity of these experiences than written formats.

One significant outcome from our SoTL project has been a commitment to considering student's perspectives and insights on reflexive photography and applying this in our work with subsequent learners. We actively used insights from student participants in shaping our approach moving forward. Finding student feedback from the study to be validating, we first applied our learning within our practicum-based courses. Second, we expanded upon this approach and adapted reflexive photography for use in other social work courses.

With respect to field practicum, we applied our learning in several ways. Having confirmed that the assignment held value for our students, we continued to use it in class to support their development as practitioners. At Mount Royal University, results from the study were shared with other instructors in the Social Work Diploma program leading to a team discussion regarding reflexivity and effective teaching strategies. This informed program-wide curriculum development, and reflexive photography was added as an assignment to all social work practicum courses. As a team, we now view reflexive photography as an important teaching strategy that is scaffolded into our curriculum such that students move along a continuum from reflection into reflexivity over the course of their social work education. Consequently, the use of reflexive photography has increased consistency within our program and has expanded from one section of 15 practicum students to being used in 15 sections a year.

Learner feedback from this study suggests to us that reflexive photography is a natural means by which to discuss and engage with critical social theory. The photographs were often used by students to communicate their perspective on difficult topics their clients (and themselves) were facing in practicum including stigma, oppression, social exclusion, racism, sexism, and homophobia. This was instructive, as we have often struggled to engage students with these concepts and to facilitate meaningful conversations in the classroom. Established theories in this area of discourse often seem to weigh discussion down and detach it from human experience. Reflexive photography provides another tool or entryway into a discussion of critical concepts that are grounded in both the students' experience and the experience of their clients. In this way, photographs and metaphors provide an opportunity to integrate theory and practice and do so inductively. Rather than starting with theory or concepts and shaping them to fit a student's experience, reflexive photography allows a process that uses photographs to make meaning of practice in a student's words that allows for broader links to established concepts, theories, and a professional framing.

Based on this new understanding, we explored how reflexive photography could be incorporated into additional courses (beyond just practicum). To illustrate, in the social work program at Mount Royal University, key learnings from students related to awareness of critical and structural issues were applied to the curriculum within additional courses, including community development and Indigenous helping practices. We now use reflexive photography to challenge students to think critically about their approach to community practice and Indigenous experiences, and to better understand the role that structural factors play in shaping the lives of their clients.

Rather than as a form of assessment, reflexive photography is being used here as an in-class discussion tool to surface students pre-existing knowledge as a base upon which to further develop a professional lens. For example, in our course on community social work practice, students are asked to create a photograph about an issue they have experienced in the community and post it to an online learning portfolio. In class, they share their photo in a small learning circle and discuss with their peers. Their learning from this discussion is then shared in a full class debrief with the instructor. We used a similar process in a course on social work and Indigenous world views where reflexive photography was effective as a low-risk exercise (no marks attached) to discuss students' perspectives on issues impacting Indigenous communities. Within the safer confines of a small discussion group, students were able to use reflexive photography to engage in dialogue about issues they are often uncomfortable discussing in a large classroom setting. Additionally, the photographs lend well to web-based formats, which provide for creativity and sharing in a broader way as well as instructor review.

At the University of Regina, reflexive photography is used widely throughout the undergraduate field curriculum. However, further consideration was given to its incorporation as a learning tool and assignment for students in other courses, including those focused on critical thinking, practice methods, and research. Insights from these adaptations indicate that reflexive photography can be a useful tool to explore students' preconceived notions of community as well as dispel their discomfort with working cross-culturally.

APPLICATION TO CROSS-DISCIPLINARY CONTEXTS

Scholarship demonstrates the effectiveness of using photography within clinical practice programs. Several studies emanate from within postsecondary education programs where photography has been used in teacher training to assist learners to examine their current attitudes and behaviors toward teaching adults (Taylor, 2003) and their self-awareness and multicultural consciousness (Allen & Labbo, 2001). Additionally, research using photo elicitation methods involved students taking photographs in the field and reflecting on the meaning of participating in college-based outdoor education programs (Loeffler, 2004). While these studies were not conducted under the banner of reflexive photography, many used similar methods to support students in reflecting on their learning. To date, only one study has specifically explored the use of reflexive photography in a clinical practice program. In this research, Amerson and Livingston (2014) used reflexive photography to evaluate the learning processes related to cultural competence during an international service-learning project with nursing students. They concluded that reflexive photography was a more robust method of self-reflection, especially for visual learners. Beyond this scholarship, there is very little research focused on the learning processes associated with reflexive photography.

Nevertheless, we believe our research on reflexive photography has implications for clinical practice programs beyond social work. Reflexive photography would be useful in any professional discipline where critical reflection and transformative learning are valued outcomes. Working cross-culturally and understanding the broader context of their client's experiences in the world is imperative for emerging professionals. Clinical practice programs are important sites for professional socialization, requiring students to engage in reflection—both professional and personal—on how this informs professional values, attitudes, and skills. We found that reflexive photography assisted students to better engage in a dialogue about race, age, class, ability, gender, and sexual diversity, and what this means in clinical practice.

For instance, many students reported that reflexive photography provided them with a powerful experiential means by which they could gain a different perspective on social issues facing their clients. With minimal prompting, these students used the photo as a way to articulate the connections and intersections of discrimination and engage in dialogue about the impact this had on the communities they were working within. The task of creating and communicating about their photos provided an intuitive and inductive process with which to engage with issues that are often only handled conceptually or theoretically in the classroom setting. This provided an enhanced opportunity to position their social location, acknowledge their privilege, and reflect on the role of power in clinical practice. Subsequently, application in other programs, such as nursing, education, clinical psychology, and international development, would likely be efficacious.

ADDITIONAL RESOURCES

- One of the few SoTL studies on reflexive photography in the clinical disciplines:
  - Amerson, R., & Livingston, W. G. (2014). Reflexive photography: An alternative method for documenting the learning process of cultural competence. *Journal Transcultural Learning, 25*(2), 202-210.
- A further resource on the importance of reflection in social work field education:
  - Clarke, N. (2012). Beyond the reflective practitioner. In J. Drolet, N. Clark, & H. Allen (Eds.), *Shifting sites of practice: Field education in Canada*. Pearson Canada.
- Suggestions and strategies on developing visual literacy within curriculum:
  - Little, D. (2015). Teaching visual literacy across the curriculum: Suggestions and strategies. *New Directions for Teaching and Learning, 2015*(141), 87-90.
- A discussion of the use of images and photographs as research data:
  - Lofstrom, E., Nevgi, A., Wegner, E., & Karm, M. (2015). Images in research on teaching and learning in higher education, *Theory and Method in Higher Education Research, 1*, 191-212.

- This chapter discusses the project with further details on methods and findings:
  - ○ Oliver, B., Chalmers, D., & Goitom, M. (2019). Reflexivity in the field: Applying lessons learned from a collaborative scholarship of teaching and learning study exploring the use of reflexive photography in field education. In J. Friberg & K. McKinney (Eds.), *Applying the scholarship of teaching and learning beyond the individual classroom.* Indiana University Press.

- A seminal source on Photovoice:
  - ○ Wang, C., & Burris, M. (1997). Photovoice: Concept, methodology, and use for participatory needs assessment. *Health Education Behavior, 24*(3), 369-387.

REFERENCES

Allen, J, & Labbo, L. D. (2001). Giving it a second thought: Making culturally engaged teaching culturally engaging. *Language Arts, 79*(1), 40-52.

Amerson, R., & Livingston, W. G. (2014). Reflexive photography: An alternative method for documenting the learning process of cultural competence. *Journal Transcultural Learning, 25*(2), 202-210.

Butterwick, S., & Lipson Lawrence, R. (2009). Creating alternative realities: Arts-based approaches to transformative learning. In J. Mezirow, E. W. Taylor (Eds.), *Transformative learning in practice: Insights from community, workplace and higher education* (pp. 35-45). Jossey-Bass Inc.

Charmaz, K. (2014). *Constructing grounded theory.* SAGE Publications.

Clarke, N. (2012). Beyond the reflective practitioner. In J. Drolet, N. Clark, & H. Allen (Eds.), *Shifting sites of practice: Field education in Canada.* Pearson Canada.

D'Cruz, H., Gillingham, P., & Melendez, S. (2007). Reflexivity, its meanings and relevance for social work: A critical review of the literature. *British Journal of Social Work, 37*, 73-90.

Fook, J. (1999). Critical reflectivity in education and practice. In J. Fook & B. Pease (Eds.), *Transforming social work practice: Postmodern critical perspectives* (pp. 195-208). Allen and Unwin.

Hyde, K. (2015). Sociology through photography. *New Directions for Teaching and Learning, 2015*(141), 31-42.

Johnson, M. A. (2010). Teaching macro practice through service learning using participatory photography. *Journal of Community Practice, 18*, 297-314.

Little, D. (2015). Teaching visual literacy across the curriculum: Suggestions and strategies. *New Directions for Teaching and Learning, 2015*(141), 87-90.

Little, D., Felten, P., & Berry, C. (2010). Liberal education in a visual world. *Liberal Education, 96*(2), 44-49.

Loeffler, T. A. (2004). A photo elicitation study of the meanings of outdoor adventure experiences. *Journal of Leisure Research, 26*(4), 536-556.

Lofstrom, E., Nevgi, A., Wegner, E., & Karm, M. (2015). Images in research on teaching and learning in higher education. *Theory and Method in Higher Education Research, 1*, 191-212.

Morley, C. (2008). Teaching critical practice: Resisting structural domination through critical reflection. *Social Work Education, 27*(4), 407-421.

Mezirow, J. (1990). *Fostering critical reflection in adulthood: A guide to transformative and emancipatory learning.* Jossey-Bass Inc.

Mezirow, J. (2009). Transformative learning theory. In J. Mezirow & E. W. Taylor (Eds.), *Transformative learning in practice: Insights from community, workplace and higher education* (pp. 18-33). Jossey-Bass Inc.

Pease, B. (2006). Encouraging critical reflections on privilege in social work and the human services. *Practice Reflexions, 1*(1), 15-26.

Reavey, P. (2011). The return to experience: Psychology and the visual. In P. Reavey (Ed.), *Visual methods in psychology: Using and interpreting images in qualitative research.* Psychology Press.

Schön, D. A. (1983). *The reflective practitioner: How professionals think in action.* Basic Books.

Strauss, A., & Corbin, J. (1998). *Basics of qualitative research: Techniques and procedures for developing grounded theory.* SAGE Publications.

Taylor, E. W. (2002). Using still photography in making meaning of adult educators "teaching belief". *Studies in the Education of Adults, 34*(2), 123-139.

Taylor, E. W. (2003). The relationship between the prior school lives of adult educators and their beliefs about teaching adults. *International Journal of Lifelong Learning Education, 22*(1), 59-77.

Wang, C., & Burris, M. (1997). Photovoice: Concept, methodology, and use for participatory needs assessment. *Health Education Behavior, 24*(3), 369-387.

APPENDIX: REFLEXIVE PHOTOGRAPHY ASSIGNMENT

To facilitate learning and engagement in some of the seminars, we will use reflexive photography. Reflexive photography is a novel way of expressing your perspective and perceptions of your practicum experience, social issues, and the profession of social work. It is a method used to share the meaning of your learning by using a tangible representation of your practicum experience. Photographs can serve as a visual representation of the "humanness" of experience that may not be easily captured in text alone. This assignment creates a space for you to explore, interact, and analyze your practicum environment in a creative way. Photographs permit the opportunity for you to express feelings, to express emotion, and to share the action or physicality of your practicum learning.

In this course, reflexive photography will allow you, as part of your practicum experience, to record, reflect, and communicate your concerns about social issues in your family, community, and society in general. It will also allow you to consider how these topics will influence your future career in social work.

Your task is to take multiple photographs of events, places, or objects that reflect social work issues of interest or importance to you and that are of relevance to your practicum setting. If you do not have access to a camera, please speak with the instructor to make alternate arrangements. Students will present their photographic reflections in one of the seminars during the term. You will select *two* photographs for further discussion with your seminar colleagues at your assigned seminar. You will present your photos in seminar according to the criteria outlined below.

Selecting photographs that embody one's views and experiences is actually more difficult than it may seem. Your assignment is to take a suite of photographs of something related to your practicum placement and/or the practice of social work. There are to be no pictures of people! Pictures copied from the web will not be accepted. Respect for privacy is fundamental and must be your priority. The challenge is not just to see an act and capture it on film, but to see the representation of the act in place. Each photograph and associated reflective piece should capture a "real-life" story or issue, *your* view of it, and its relevance or connection to your placement and/or social work practice.

Evaluation of this assignment includes quality of your photograph, presentation of your reflections on the photograph and your practicum experience, facilitation and leadership of seminar group discussion, and adherence to the assignment instructions.

Photographs

Your photographs will be shared with your peers in your assigned seminar via a brief PowerPoint (Microsoft) presentation. You will create a presentation that consists of three slides: a title slide with your name, followed by your two photo slides. Please name each of your photos by giving them a short caption and include this in your PowerPoint slides beneath the appropriate photo.

Reflective Presentation and Group Discussion

In your assigned seminar, the two photos you selected will be shared with the group via PowerPoint slides, and you will provide a 20- to 25-minute presentation and discussion that gives an overview of the meaning of the photographs, the general themes in your photos, how they relate to your placement and/or the practice of social work, and your personal reflection. It is expected that your presentation will include a critical reflection and analysis of the placement experience and will be followed by a discussion of these issues. You are expected to lead and facilitate this discussion and to come prepared to initiate and stimulate conversation as needed.

To reflect on your photographs, you can use the following questions as guides:

- What do you see there? What is really happening? Why does this challenge/strength/issue exist?
- How does this relate to my/our lives, my practicum placement, and/or the profession of social work?
- What can I/we do about it? What change do you propose?

You took the photos for a reason—it stirred something in you that made you think of the topic. The images and the description should elicit a similar feeling in those who view them.

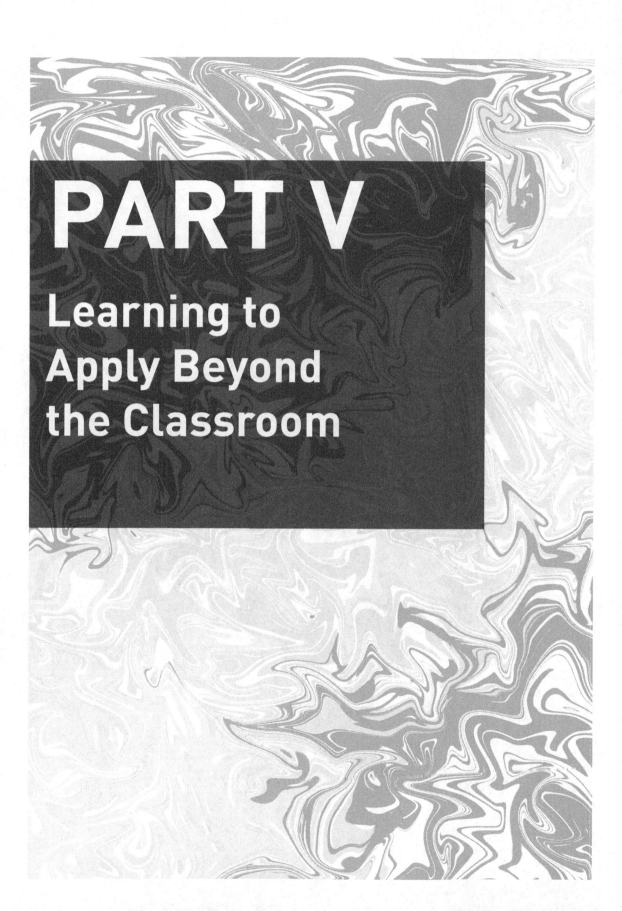

PART V

Learning to Apply Beyond the Classroom

32

ENGAGING STAKEHOLDERS TO IMPROVE PEDAGOGY IN ALLIED HEALTH PLACEMENT PREPARATION

Elizabeth Bourne, PhD, BAppSc(SpPath), CPSP;
Gillian Nisbet, PhD, MMEd, DipNutr, BSc(Hons);
Margaret Nicholson, MEd, BSc, Dip Nut Diet, Dip Ed (Health), AdvAPD;
and Irene Mok, MRC, BA

DESCRIPTION OF TEACHING/LEARNING CONTEXT

A critical role of health professional academics is to prepare and support students undertaking the work integrated learning (WIL) component of their degree program. WIL is an "umbrella term used for a range of approaches and strategies that integrate theory with the practice of work within a purposefully designed curriculum" (Patrick et al., 2008, p. 9). WIL placements enable students to apply theory learned in the classroom to real-world practice in a range of settings, including health (private and public), disability, aged care, education, social welfare, and the corporate sector. In allied health, students are typically guided by clinicians within the workplace, who take on the role of placement educator as part of their normal duties. In Australia, placements are a mandatory component of accredited health degree programs in order to ensure graduates are work-ready, semi-autonomous health professionals. Students are assessed against professional competencies, as determined by the individual allied health disciplines.

Transitioning to placement can be quite a culture shock for many students who until now have predominantly experienced classroom-based teaching methods. Placement is quite different because it requires students to be professional at all times, to proactively engage in their learning, and to critically evaluate their performance through a continual process of assessment and feedback (Stagnitti et al., 2013). Applying and extending the theoretical knowledge and skills gained through classroom learning to the placement context can also be challenging (Bearman et al., 2013). For

Friberg, J. C., Visconti, C. F., & Ginsberg, S. M. (Eds.), *Evidence-Based Education in the Classroom: Examples From Clinical Disciplines* (pp. 291-300).

some students, this is the first encounter with real patients or clients and their families. Combined, these factors can create added anxieties for students in what is already recognized as a stressful time (Hamshire et al., 2012; Keating et al., 2009; Walsh et al., 2010), resulting in a negative impact on student learning. Access to high quality, relevant, and authentic placement preparation is therefore essential to maximize student learning (Molloy & Keating, 2011).

This case study focuses on pedagogy related to the preparation of undergraduate and graduate entry masters allied health student briefing material for use prior to and during the WIL placement component of a student's degree program. Three of our authors are fortunate to work within a centralized portfolio for workplace-based education and research in health: Faculty of Health Sciences, Work Integrated Learning. This is an interprofessional team of academics and professional staff that allows us to capitalize on cross-disciplinary expertise to build specialist capability in WIL, while working closely with our discipline colleagues and external placement providers to ensure clear integration between campus-based and workplace learning. However, as our team has grown, we have noticed a gradual "siloing" toward our individual disciplines of how we operate. In particular, learning outcomes for our preparation for placement briefings have varied, despite students requiring essentially similar preparation across the allied health professions. In addition, our teaching and learning practices have varied from traditional didactic style to interactive workshops and online learning. This project aimed to address this dissonance by transforming the way briefings are delivered in line with current evidence, with content meeting student learning needs. We had the following three specific aims:

1. To improve the quality and consistency of student preparation for placement

2. To facilitate timely student access to relevant educational resources prior to/during placement

3. To reduce duplication in academic staff time spent on tasks related to student preparation for placements

REVIEW OF LITERATURE

We drew on self-determination theory (SDT; Ryan & Deci, 2000) as a framework for the design and development of the student briefing material. SDT helps us understand the motivational processes associated with student learning and performance (see Ten Cate et al., 2011 for a comprehensive appraisal of its relevance to medical education). A key principle of SDT is that people are intrinsically motivated to learn and develop. However, this requires three basic psychological needs: (1) the need for autonomy, (2) the need for competence, and (3) the need for relatedness. Sergis and colleagues (2018) have nicely summarized these terms from Ryan and Deci's earlier work (2000): *Autonomy* refers to "the need to be engaged in tasks in an autonomous manner within a context that is relevant to them" (p. 369); *Competence* refers to "the need for students to feel capable to successfully engage in the learning process" (p. 369); *Relatedness* refers to "the need to be engaged in tasks that allow collaboration and communication with each other" (p. 370). We deliberately included student-centered learning and teaching practices that fostered these three elements as outlined in the following list:

1. Repackaging how we delivered our briefings to incorporate elements of a flipped classroom approach. A flipped classroom has students engage in content prior to attending class, often through online technology. Face-to-face class time is then used to actively engage the learners in meaningful discussion, critical thinking, and problem solving (DeLozier & Rhodes, 2017; Jensen et al., 2015; Taylor et al., 2017). A recent meta-analysis suggests greater academic achievement with a flipped classroom approach compared with the traditional lecture (Chen et al., 2018). Interestingly, cumulative analysis and meta-regressions showed progressively better outcomes by year (Chen et al., 2018), suggesting that academics may be becoming more experienced with this learning and teaching approach. Our team felt this approach would enable us to better facilitate student engagement and skill development compared to our more traditional classroom methods.

2. Ensuring the content of the briefings reflected topic areas considered challenging for students in their transition from the classroom to workplace settings. We were particularly keen to do this in a way that reflected the student voice (Cook-Sather, 2006), but also drew on the experiences of placement educators in the workplace and WIL academics to ensure the relevance of teaching content.

3. Engaging educational/learning design expertise to ensure we were maximizing learning potential through the use of contemporary technologies. As Harris and Walling (2013) proclaim, it is the expertise of the learning designer that melds the science and art of teaching with current and emerging educational technology.

This chapter provides an easy-to-follow, systematic approach to achieve curriculum improvements in student preparation for transition into practice settings. Using underpinning theories of student learning and contemporary teaching methods, such as the flipped classroom, will be of interest to readers wanting to enhance the authenticity and relevance of their student preparation practices in clinical disciplines. Through our example, readers may adopt our approach to WIL preparation within their own setting, or they may use it to more broadly consider the opportunities to enhance their own use of contemporary learning methods or stakeholder consultations in curriculum redesign.

ORIGINAL DATA

Our development of new student briefing learning materials was guided by a resource review and stakeholder consultations across seven allied health disciplines: diagnostic radiography, exercise physiology, nutrition and dietetics, occupational therapy, physiotherapy, rehabilitation counseling, and speech-language pathology. Our iterative needs analysis process is outlined in Figure 32-1.

Review of Existing Resources

We started with a detailed review of the existing student briefing resources across the seven disciplines. By grouping student briefing resources into distinct topic areas, we determined the quantity and quality of resources already available in these topic areas and assessed their suitability for a flipped classroom learning and teaching approach. The review identified eight topic areas that could be redesigned to enhance student preparation: feedback, managing self, professionalism, student-placement educator relationships, using different learning strategies, learning in different contexts, peer learning, and teamwork during placements.

Stakeholder Consultations

We were interested in the views of three key stakeholder groups: academics who deliver the briefings and support students during their placements, external placement educators, and the students who participate in briefings preparation before their placement.

Academics

We surveyed our academic colleagues about their experiences in delivering student briefings. We asked which topics required the most time both in delivery as well as student support and sought our colleagues' perspectives on which areas would benefit the most from redesign. We then conducted a follow-up focus group with academics, which enabled a more detailed exploration of the learning needs within topics. Academics confirmed that feedback, managing self, professionalism, student-placement educator relationships, and using different learning strategies were most suited to educational redesign.

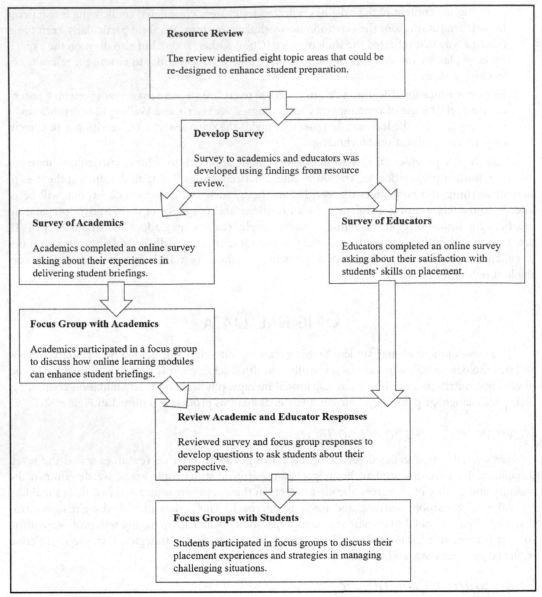

Figure 32-1. Iterative needs analysis process.

Placement Educators

We surveyed workplace clinicians (who were external placement educators of students from our university) on their level of satisfaction with student ability in eight aspects of placement learning, as well as their perception of time involved in supporting students in these aspects. Table 32-1 shows the ranking of topic areas reported to be most time consuming and the corresponding levels of satisfaction with students' ability.

Placement educators rated student-placement educator relationships, using different strategies to maximize learning, and learning in different contexts to be the three most time-consuming areas to support during placement. The project team then compared the findings from the academic and placement educator responses and prioritized areas for further investigation.

TABLE 32-1

Summary of Placement Educator Survey (*n* = 332)

TOPIC	EDUCATOR SATISFACTION (VERY SATISFIED OR SATISFIED)	RANK ORDER FOR SUPPORT NEEDS (WHERE 1 = MOST TIME CONSUMING)	EXAMPLE AREAS OF CONCERN
Feedback	82%	1	• Need for greater self-reflection on skills • Inability to take on constructive feedback
Using different learning strategies	68%	2	• Lack of proactive strategies to improve skills
Learning in different contexts	74%	3	• Adapting to different placement and workplace situations
Managing self	71%	4	• Maintaining self-care • Identifying mental health concerns
Managing student-placement educator relationships	86%	5	• Clarifying student and educator's roles
Professionalism	90%	6	• Understanding of different workplace expectations • Communication etiquette
Teamwork	80%	7	• Assertiveness in communicating ideas
Peer learning	70%	8	• No specific concerns raised

Students

We conducted three student focus groups using a video conferencing platform (Zoom [Zoom Video Communications, Inc]) to further explore three topic areas: feedback, professionalism, and maximizing learning on placement (Zoom, 2021). Student comments gave us a deeper insight into their experiences, both positive and negative, and provided rich examples as well as useful management strategies from a student perspective. The stories about challenging situations with senior colleagues were particularly informative in developing our learning outcomes.

APPLICATION OF LITERATURE/DATA

Our needs analysis and understanding of current educational practices led the team to focus on curriculum improvements in the following areas.

Feedback

Learner feedback is a critical component of educational practice regardless of learning topic, mode, or pedagogy (Carless & Boud, 2018). Many in teaching roles may have experienced students requesting more frequent or varied feedback, and this is no different in the placement context. Similar to other professions (Calleja et al., 2016), our placement educators highlighted poor student responsiveness to feedback, either immediate or over the placement duration, as their paramount area of concern. After we heard from students from a range of disciplines, it became clear to us that what was missing was the development of students' "feedback literacy" (Carless & Boud, 2018, p. 1316). In particular, we needed to help students understand why feedback is so important, what their role and actions should be in the process, and how to participate productively. The following sections discuss these areas in more detail.

Importance of Feedback

We discovered we needed to help more of our students see feedback as an opportunity, to understand that no one is perfect (and particularly not students) but that feedback is being provided to promote learning and growth. We could see that our students did not understand this and, for the most part, interpreted feedback to be judgment rather than formative (Burgess & Mellis, 2015). Other areas that needed reinforcement included understanding that feedback came from diverse sources and forms (e.g., peers, patients or clients, other team members including other professions, broader stakeholders) and was not limited to their direct placement educator.

Understanding Their Role and Actions

We realized students were not often taking on an active learner role in the feedback process and did not understand their role was more than simply to receive feedback comments—in fact, it was a two-way process. Academic and educator comments suggested there was a difference in understanding, where feedback was not seen as being for learning (Henderson et al., 2018) rather than on learning. Each of our stakeholder groups highlighted the importance of using regular self-reflection, asking questions, and using peer supports as sounding boards for how to improve.

How to Participate in Feedback

Both placement educators and academics raised concerns about student skills in this area, for example, student reactions during feedback. Student comments highlighted the benefits of having an open mind and being ready to engage and clarify as part of a feedback conversation, rather than taking on a defensive stance when receiving feedback. Using peers for calibration in relation to self-evaluations and reassessing their own responses to feedback were also raised as useful approaches.

Consequently, after much deliberation, we focused on the following learning outcomes for our feedback learning module, ensuring they were consistent with Bloom's taxonomy level 3 to 4 (Krathwohl, 2002):

- Describe the purposes of feedback
- Discuss why feedback is important during placements
- Identify ways feedback can occur
- Analyze constructive responses to feedback

Professionalism: Dignity

This area of focus was not initially obvious to us from our surveys and focus groups. However, our reading about professionalism revealed this is an area of emerging concern both within research literature for all health professions (Monrouxe & Rees, 2017) as well as current media reports about medical student incidents, including "dignity violations" (Monrouxe & Rees, 2017, p. 137) in hospitals where we also place allied health students. In reviewing our stakeholder contributions, we found examples of our students describing their experiences of their own dignity being violated. These were often mentioned when their clinical contribution to the team was minimized, or even ridiculed, in front of other professionals or patients/clients. While we knew that patient/client dignity was likely to be covered in a range of academic subjects, we felt that student and staff dignity needed to be more explicitly explored prior to placement to protect the safety of our students as well as others they may interact with.

Consequently, for our professionalism dignity learning module, we focused on these specific learning outcomes:

- Explain dignity in the context of health care delivery
- Examine a range of dignity violations
- Analyze the impact of dignity violations on health care professionals, their students, and their patients
- Critique student responses to dignity violations

Maximizing Learning on Placement

Facilitating students to actively participate in their learning has been recommended for inclusion in allied health WIL preparation curriculums (Nagarajan & McAllister, 2015). From our surveys and focus groups, we confirmed the critical importance of spending time reflecting on placement performance and experiences, getting actively involved, and taking initiative as strategies to maximize learning on placement. Placement educator comments suggested they highly valued students who sought to maximize their learning during their placement, regardless of whether the student had a personal interest in the area of practice. Educators were also looking for students to have good self-awareness and to take responsibility for their learning. We recognized that these practices may already be present or develop easily in some students but were more challenging for other students. Regardless, literature confirmed they were also important work readiness skills (Caballero et al., 2011) that students needed as graduate clinicians. We also saw alignment with the competence aspect within our framework of SDT, so we decided they were important to address in our student placement preparation.

Consequently, for our maximizing the learning module, we focused on the following learning outcomes:

- Explain the importance of working within personal competency limits and when to seek support
- Demonstrate active self-reflection skills based on learning experiences
- Implement changes to practice, based on feedback and self-reflection

Educational Design of Online Learning Modules

We worked with educational designers to transform our learning from literature, the resource review, and stakeholder consultations into online learning modules. We wanted to ensure constructive alignment (Biggs, 2014) between learning outcomes, learning activities, and assessment in the modules and utilized storyboarding (Sandars, 2009) to systematically scaffold the content and scenario narratives to meet our chosen learning outcomes. We then commenced preparation of scripts for the video/audio elements as well as the development of other online learning resources, for example, quizzes. We used Smart Sparrow, an online platform, to integrate learning elements into online learning modules (Smart Sparrow, 2018). Smart Sparrow enabled the delivery of interactive digital learning experiences that could be adapted to prompt critical reflection on key areas for individual learners at times and locations that suited them. It was hoped that this flexible design would also enable academics to tailor the learning modules to meet teaching needs for students in early year to near graduate level. Furthermore, some resources could be used in face-to-face tutorials if desired, for example, using the videos with pauses for discussion as needed.

APPLICATION TO CROSS-DISCIPLINARY CONTEXTS

The methodology utilized to develop the student briefings for our project could be applied in a variety of settings to allow academics or educators to create resources that meet the needs of their individual discipline, student level, or workplace site. We recommend performing a detailed needs analysis (online questionnaires, focus groups) and engaging with multiple stakeholders (students, educators, academics) to determine the most relevant topic areas and the specific resource content. We also recommend using an educational designer to guide teams through a storyboard-style process to brainstorm suitable activities to meet identified learning goals. Our experience is that flipped classroom resources can be designed to maintain elements of peer learning and promote student autonomy, relatedness, and competence (Ryan & Deci, 2000). We offer our experiences in developing the online learning component by suggesting consideration of the following design principles:

- Orientation/thought trigger: Engaging scenarios help students activate their own prior knowledge, in keeping with adult learning principles, using formats such as written paragraph, video, or podcast.
- Background (new) information: Brief presentation in a variety of modes (e.g., slide show, podcasts, video).
- Interactive activities: Facilitating student learning through active participation (e.g., reflection on content/principles using relevant case examples, discussion boards, online polls with facility to compare answers to peers).
- Further prompts/information: Providing authentic examples relatable to students (e.g., visual and/or audio [e.g., video or podcast] of students in similar scenarios or being interviewed).
- Feedback/assessment elements: Requiring students to complete sections that enable consolidation of learning. Options include a new scenario to analyze or reflect on, or asking students to generate scenarios or strategies relevant to the presented situations. Online system design features enable automated generic answers to questions along with explanations rather than having to individually mark each student's response. For example, the right answer could be presented following response to multiple-choice questions, with a teaching explanation.
- Extension and referral: Further readings and links to resources suitable for students (e.g., counseling, learning support services).
- Toolbox: Opportunity for students to save any contributions, and add for later reference and/or auditing, as well as direct preparation for planned discussions within the flipped classroom context.

Finally, to ensure longevity and range of application, we recommend that resources developed cover broader fundamental principles, which are unlikely to change quickly and can be readily adapted for different professions. For example, we have chosen topics that are fundamental to many professions and deliberately designed prompt questions within modules to be broad and/or open-ended rather than discipline specific. However, we have also planned contingencies for future modifications, where involved team members will have continued access to all preparation materials (e.g., video scripts) to facilitate minor edits or new topic development if required in the future.

This project has provided an achievable means by which we can transition our students to the workplace setting. The development of targeted dynamic resources will enhance student engagement in learning by presenting information in an engaging and timely manner while also offering efficiencies for academic teachers. Overall, we believe the flipped classroom approach will facilitate better preparation of students to effectively and efficiently assimilate them into busy workplace contexts.

ADDITIONAL RESOURCES

- Delany, C., & Molloy, E. (2018). *Learning and teaching in clinical contexts: A practical guide.* Elsevier.
- Using video in teaching and learning:
  ○ https://le.unimelb.edu.au/supporting-teaching-learning-assessment/video-for-learning-resources
- Feedback for Learning: Closing the Assessment Loop:
  ○ www.feedbackforlearning.org

REFERENCES

Bearman, M., Molloy, E., Ajjawi, R., & Keating, J. (2013). "Is there a Plan B?": Clinical educators supporting underperforming students in practice settings. *Teaching in Higher Education, 18*(5), 531-544. https://doi.org/10.1080/1356251 7.2012.752732

Biggs, J. (2014). Constructive alignment in university teaching. *HERDSA Review of Higher Education, 1*(1), 5-22.

Burgess, A., & Mellis, C. (2015). Feedback and assessment for clinical placements: Achieving the right balance. *Advances in Medical Education and Practice, 6,* 373-381. https://doi.org/10.2147/AMEP.S77890

Caballero, C. L., Walker, A., & Fuller-Tyszkiewicz, M. (2011). The Work Readiness Scale (WRS): Developing a measure to assess work readiness in college graduates. *Journal of Teaching and Learning for Graduate Employability, 2*(2), 41-54.

Calleja, P., Harvey, T., Fox, A., & Carmichael, M. (2016). Feedback and clinical practice improvement: A tool to assist workplace supervisors and students. *Nurse Education in Practice, 17,* 167-173. https://doi.org/10.1016/j.nepr.2015.11.009

Carless, D., & Boud, D. (2018). The development of student feedback literacy: Enabling uptake of feedback. *Assessment & Evaluation in Higher Education, 43*(8), 1315-1325. https://doi.org/10.1080/02602938.2018.1463354

Chen, K. S., Monrouxe, L., Lu, Y. H., Jenq, C. C., Chang, Y. J., Chang, Y. C., & Chai, P. Y. C. (2018). Academic outcomes of flipped classroom learning: A meta-analysis. *Medical Education, 52*(9), 910-924.

Cook-Sather, A. (2006). Sound, presence, and power: "Student voice" in educational research and reform. *Curriculum Inquiry, 36*(4), 359-390. https://doi.org/10.1111/j.1467-873X.2006.00363.x

DeLozier, S. J., & Rhodes, M. G. (2017). Flipped classrooms: A review of key ideas and recommendations for practice. *Educational Psychology Review, 29*(1), 141-151.

Hamshire, C., Willgoss, T. G., & Wibberley, C. (2012). 'The placement was probably the tipping point'—The narratives of recently discontinued students. *Nurse Education in Practice, 12*(4), 182-186.

Harris, P., & Walling, D. R. (2013). The learning designer: Merging art and science with educational technology. *TechTrends, 57*(5), 35-41. http://dx.doi.org/10.1007/s11528-013-0689-2

Henderson, M., Boud, D., Molloy, E., Dawson P., Phillips, M., Ryan, T., & Mahoney, P. (2018). Feedback for learning: Closing the assessment loop—Final report. Canberra: Australian Government Department of Education and Training. http://newmediaresearch.educ.monash.edu.au/feedback/wp-content/uploads/ID16-5366_Henderson_Report_2018.pdf

Jensen, J. L., Kummer, T. A., & Godoy, P. D. D. M. (2015). Improvements from a flipped classroom may simply be the fruits of active learning. *CBE—Life Sciences Education, 14*(1), Article 5.

Keating, J., Dalton, M., & Davidson, M. (2009). Assessment in clinical education. In C. Delany & E. Molloy (Eds.), *Clinical education in the health professions* (pp. 147-172). Churchill Livingstone/Elsevier.

Krathwohl, D. R. (2002). A revision of Bloom's taxonomy: An overview. *Theory Into Practice, 41*(4), 212-218. https://doi.org/10.1207/s15430421tip4104_2

Molloy, E., & Keating, J. (2011). Targeted preparation for clinical practice. In S. Billett & A. Henderson (Eds.), *Developing learning professionals: Integrating experiences in university and practice settings* (pp. 59-82). Springer Netherlands.

Monrouxe, L. V., & Rees, C. E. (2017). *Healthcare professionalism: Improving practice through reflections on workplace dilemmas.* John Wiley & Sons, Inc.

Nagarajan, S., & McAllister, L. (2015). Integration of practice experiences into the allied health curriculum: Curriculum and pedagogic considerations before, during and after work-integrated learning experiences. *Asia-Pacific Journal of Cooperative Education, 16*(4), 279-290. http://search.proquest.com/docview/2231207352/

Patrick, C. J., Peach, D., Pocknee, C., Webb, F., Fletcher, M., & Pretto, G. (2008). The WIL (Work Integrated Learning) report: A national scoping study. *Queensland University of Technology.* http://hdl.voced.edu.au/10707/228658

Ryan, R., & Deci, E. (2000). Self-determination theory and the facilitation of intrinsic motivation, social development, and well-being. *The American Psychologist, 55*(1), 68-78. https://doi.org/10.1037/0003-066X.55.1.68

Sandars, J. (2009). Twelve tips for using podcasts in medical education. *Medical Teacher, 31*(5), 387-389.

Sergis, S., Sampson, D. G., & Pelliccione, L. (2018). Investigating the impact of flipped classroom on students' learning experiences: A self-determination theory approach. *Computers in Human Behavior, 78,* 368-378.

Smart Sparrow. (2018). www.smartsparrow.com

Stagnitti, K., Schoo, A., & Welch, D. (2013). *Clinical fieldwork placement in health professions.* (2nd ed.). Oxford University Press.

Taylor, A. T., Olofson, E. L., & Novak, W. R. (2017). Enhancing student retention of prerequisite knowledge through pre-class activities and in-class reinforcement. *Biochemistry and Molecular Biology Education, 45*(2), 97-104.

Ten Cate, O. T. J., Kusurkar, R. A., & Williams, G. C. (2011). How self-determination theory can assist our understanding of the teaching and learning processes in medical education. AMEE guide No. 59. *Medical Teacher, 33*(12), 961-973.

Walsh, J. M., Feeney, C., Hussey, J., & Donnellan, C. (2010). Sources of stress and psychological morbidity among undergraduate physiotherapy students. *Physiotherapy, 96*(3), 206-212.

Zoom. (2021). www.zoom.us

ORAL ASSESSMENTS FOR CADAVERIC ANATOMY IN PHYSICAL THERAPY EDUCATION

Melissa A. Carroll, PhD, MS

DESCRIPTION OF TEACHING/LEARNING CONTEXT

Ensuring that all students are progressing to competence can be difficult for anatomical educators. As a science focused on human body structure and function, students often approach the content with rote memorization techniques. True success and integration of anatomical science, however, requires learners to understand the logical arrangement, layout, and relationship of body structures. A variety of assessment methods were used in both cadaver lab and also in the didactic classroom for a graduate-level physical therapy course. The intention of implementing formative assessments was to increase the student interaction with the material outside of a designated class lecture, quiz, or exam. Over the last 5 years, the assessments have been modified, but the intention was to assist student use of anatomic terminology, comprehension, and application within a clinical or research setting. The ultimate goal was to increase the exposure and comfort with the material and use in an applied fashion with the interaction of colleagues and direct feedback from peers.

Doctor of Physical Therapy (DPT) students are required to learn human anatomy—a foundational science for physical therapy practice. Several DPT programs have human anatomy courses, where anatomy education is supplemented by cadaver dissection. The cadaver laboratory introduces students to three-dimensional body structures beyond the small animal dissection or comparative anatomy courses that the students had in prior training. Several situational factors exist and need to be considered prior to implementing effective formative assessments, including the American Physical Therapy Association national standards, external stakeholders, institutional beliefs, and the local program mission and vision. Specific situational factors that affect anatomy courses, both positively and negatively, include access to cadaveric materials, the instructor-to-student ratio, the

Friberg, J. C., Visconti, C. F., & Ginsberg, S. M. (Eds.). *Evidence-Based Education in the Classroom: Examples From Clinical Disciplines* (pp. 301-311).

course sequence, the course structure, the integration within the curriculum and parallel course-work, the prior knowledge and training of the students, composition of the student cohort, availability and qualifications of instructors, and the approach to teaching and learning. Each of these factors also create a unique learning environment within the microcosm of the cadaver lab instruction. Furthermore, cadaveric anatomy courses force a behavioral change through the addition of multiple sensory inputs and cognitive challenges.

It is a common theme among medical professionals, who have prior cadaver dissection experience, that the smell of the embalming fluids rapidly brings back memories of their training and time within the cadaver laboratory. The olfactory perception distinctly creates a learning environment that is unparalleled to several other arenas. Students also use their hands and kinesthetic feedback in a true exploratory fashion to discover different textures and investigate the layered arrangement of tissue, muscles, nerves, vessels, and cartilage—some even have the possibility of feeling a patient's pathology prior to learning about the cognitive aspects of pathoanatomic theory. Visually, students are also exposed to monochromatic and contrasting depth of tones, shapes, and direction of structural tissues, organs, and systems. Sounds are not only delivered through the instructor's voice, but also by peer–peer communications and through the movement of fluids, dissection instruments, and the HVAC system in the room, adding a background of white noise to the laboratory environment. The only sense that is not exploited in the cadaver lab is taste; therefore, cadaveric anatomy provides a multifactorial environment for stimulating learning and instruction.

In physical therapy education programs, anatomy educators have an ability to transform students' learning through innovative teaching approaches. One shared goal of anatomy educators should be to foster the transition from surface (rote memorization) to deep learning (application, analysis, and synthesis) within a clinically relevant context (Choudhury & Freemont, 2017; Samarasekera et al., 2015). A few assessments used in my courses have been both structured and unstructured oral assessments (viva voces), discipline-specific review of published literature, and in-class immediate feedback assessment techniques. Each assessment was developed from ideas within the published literature to provide a means for assessing and measuring anatomical knowledge in physical therapy students. Evidence to teach physical therapy students anatomy was (and still is) sparse, so several references were from medical education and had to be modified to fit within my classroom.

This chapter describes the implementation of formative assessments, specifically oral assessments, used in a human cadaveric anatomy course and explores the use of targeted teaching and learning strategies for anatomy in physical therapy education. By no means is this chapter designed to describe the best methods; however, it highlights some ideas of assessment techniques that have worked, have failed, have been modified, and have received positive feedback from student learners. Therefore, this chapter addresses the success (and failures) of the assessment-based approaches I have used to achieve the cognitive, psychomotor, and affective goals of cadaveric education. Data are presented from the published evidence and from a variety of student-generated sources that include course evaluations, requested feedback, and reflection activities.

REVIEW OF LITERATURE

One challenge in teaching cadaveric anatomy is the design and implementation of effective student learning objectives and assessments (Choudhury & Freemont, 2017; Kang et al., 2012; Samarasekera et al., 2015; Winkelmann, 2007). Additionally, there is conflicting evidence regarding the utility of cadaver-based anatomical education (McLauchlan et al., 2004). Some believe cadaver dissection is just a time-honored tradition and can be replaced by technology, whereas others are convinced that cadaver dissection is uniquely superior to any other teaching modality for anatomical education.

The cadaveric laboratory component is designed to supplement the theoretical content discussed within the didactic portion of the anatomy course. However, it is a challenge to understand how to measure knowledge acquisition in order to provide students with motivation to dissect, to keep a clean dissection, and to discuss the dissection tasks. A few of my goals were to efficiently use laboratory time, to increase relevant conversation (fodder of anatomical or clinical relevance), and to encourage the students to use each other as experts rather than wait for me, the sole instructor, to work the room. While completing my Teaching Goals Inventory (Angelo & Cross, 1993), I recognized that teaching specific anatomical concepts was less important than helping students develop higher order thinking and metacognitive skills. It was my belief that implementation of oral assessments held the student accountable to prepare for the lab, to create useful dissections, and to share with their cohort through near-peer teaching and reciprocal peer teaching (RPT) assignments.

It has been difficult for educators and researchers to explicitly demonstrate facilitation of deep learning in the cadaver lab. The push for evidence-based medical education has, in some ways, overshadowed the autonomy that each anatomical educator has had to make the best decision for their classroom (Bergman et al., 2013). Cognitive load theory has also helped to explain the promotion of deep and surface learning through classroom management and teaching (Jong, 2010). Defining intrinsic, extrinsic, and extraneous cognitive load within the anatomy curriculum can be helpful to determine the depth of the content delivered, assessed, and learned by students. Intrinsic cognitive load is defined as the amount of interconnectivity between the content or topics discussed for a specific educational program (Jong, 2010). Anatomical education has a high intrinsic cognitive load—each part of the body depends on its interaction with another to truly understand the whole. Faculty instruction and course design can mediate some of the cognitive load through connecting student learning to prior knowledge—constructivist learning theory (Bergman et al., 2013).

Implementing and mirroring a constructivist approach to teaching and learning is preferred over rote memorization (Choudhury & Freemont, 2017; Pandey & Zimitat, 2007). Constructivist learning and study techniques are the most appropriate for long-term comprehension, understanding, application, and analysis within anatomical science. Deep learning parallels the constructivist theory of education, whereas the instructor surveys the prior and current knowledge of each student and attends to direct the class past discrepancies or learning bottlenecks and alternative mental models. This approach can be aided by structured or planned formative assessments or integrated or improvised formative assessments (Nicol & Macfarlane-Dick, 2006). Each has a goal of providing both student and teacher with a sample of progress, enhancing metacognition for the student and fodder for the instructor to ponder and modify the class or individual approach to the student if necessary.

Several assessment methods have been used and found to be successful in the cadaver laboratory, yet the published evidence is inconsistent regarding support toward assessment modalities (Brenner et al., 2015; Choudhury & Freemont, 2017; Meyer et al., 2016). One consistent thought is the need for multiple assessment strategies for different learning objectives (Choudhury & Freemont, 2017; Samarasekera et al., 2015). Metacognition influences student learning and study time (Medina et al., 2017) and using the best pedagogical and andragogical assessments for cadaveric based anatomy can enhance metacognitive skills. Assessments range from standardized case-based practical examinations, bell ringer (i.e., steeplechase, flaggers, tagged, objective structured clinical examinations) station identifications, multiple-choice questions, single-best-answer questions, essay-based questions, and computerized identification (Brenner et al., 2015; Choudhury & Freemont, 2017). Although there is much debate regarding the best approach to teaching, learning, and assessment in cadaver-based anatomy education, there is consensus on the use of multiple modalities and assessment techniques.

Formative assessments are different from active learning activities (Nicol & Macfarlane-Dick, 2006; Samarasekera et al., 2015). Each formative assessment is low stakes and contributes to the student's progress with the course material. They can be combined with the idea of active learning, metacognition, and reflection processes to allow the students and instructors to gauge the processes of learning and progress with the course material (Medina et al., 2017). It is important for the students to have a pulse on their learning procedures so that they can adjust and seek help from colleagues, faculty, or teaching assistants. The evidence supports that implementation of formative assessments can promote student metacognition, self-regulation, and redirection regarding student learning (Medina et al., 2017; Nicol & Macfarlane-Dick, 2006). These activities are critical for bottleneck topics, which can handicap some students from progressing through the course and obtaining the necessary competence for clinical practice.

The idea of oral assessments, specifically in physical therapy education emerged, for me, from an article by Fabrizio (2013) where he posited that the traditional spotter exams were limited in scope to the assessment of student anatomical knowledge. Oral assessments can increase clinical integration and metacognition by allowing learners an opportunity to think out loud and receive directed feedback (Brenner et al., 2015; Medina et al., 2017; Samarasekera et al., 2015). As a formative assessment, using oral assessments in the cadaver lab provides students with a guided opportunity to prioritize, "chunk," and organize information while challenging the students to demonstrate a higher level of Bloom's taxonomy (i.e., application, analysis, and synthesis).

As with most assessments, there are several advantages and disadvantages of using oral assessments. The assessment itself has good face validity, allows flexibility in the delivery, and challenges the students to verbally express competence (Ganji, 2017; Samarasekera et al., 2015). In contrast, there are questions regarding the reliability of oral assessments because student performance may be influenced by anxiety, contrast errors and assessor bias, inconsistent scoring, and difficulty standardizing the questions (Ganji, 2017). For these reasons, the oral assessment was used as a low-stakes formative assessment with a pass or fail component to enhance efficiency, motivation, and instruction in the cadaver lab.

Kang and colleagues (2012) determined that there was a way to promote student interest and motivation in the cadaver lab through the use of structured questions and tasks to encourage the use of the donor dissection rather than the resources in the textbook or the internet. They found that students reflected positively on the experience, but 75% did not incorporate the study method after the prompting (Kang et al., 2012). Studies have identified that students' choice of study techniques can determine, or influence, the final academic achievement scores; however, this evidence is varied or weak at best. Anecdotally, the theory makes sense—stating that student reliance on rote memorization will not allow deeper connections with the material, and therefore, pose a threat to long-term storage and use of the concepts. Implementing formative assessments, specifically oral assessments, in my cadaveric anatomy course provided students with a measured target and reference point to gauge their metacognitive progress within the course.

APPLICATION OF LITERATURE/DATA

The human anatomy course provides an inherent group collaboration through a shared goal of completing dissection tasks throughout the semester. At the beginning of the semester, students were randomly assigned to dissection groups made up of five or six students. The formative assessments were designed to provide opportunities to apply the learned anatomic knowledge or skills within controlled assessments and encourage the students to work together with trust and collaboration. This enhanced the nontechnical skills of working within a health care team, management of conflict and different personalities, taking ownership and leadership, quick and efficient conversations regarding the task at hand, isolation of the main topic points, and reduction of the minutia. Students were held accountable to each other, to the assignment, and to the instructor through semi-structured rubrics. One of the assessments included peer-peer collaboration and near-peer grading; another used group work analysis of published literature; and lastly, a low stakes quiz format was used with an immediate feedback assessment technique, providing a formative component to the summative assessment. Some formative assessments were used primarily for the classroom setting, and the oral assessment was specifically adapted for the cadaver lab.

In an attempt to increase the anatomic comprehension and use of medical terminology, the use of oral assessments was appealing. The published evidence did not explicitly identify grading rubrics or time limitation for each assessment (Brenner et al., 2015; Fabrizio, 2013), so creating the goal and structure of the assessment needed to be prioritized. Planning the original oral assessment in 2014 took group dynamics into consideration—no team member could speak more than once during the assessment unless each person on the team already had an opportunity, as spokesperson, to answer a question on behalf of the team (see Appendix A). There were direct recall questions (i.e., definitions of anatomic terms), student identification of the dissected structures on the donor-cadaver, in addition to descriptions of the structure's origin, insertion, course, and distribution. Additionally, the group had to apply the theoretical concepts from the didactic portion of the course to describe it in the cadaver lab. There have been advantages to the implementation of oral assessments; student feedback has been overwhelmingly positive, with the typical constructive criticism:

- "I think the oral assessments should be revised a bit. First off, I could never hear [the proctor] very well when [they] were asking the questions while everyone else was talking in the lab, plus it was just distracting having everyone else talking during it. I would suggest that [the instructor] just write the questions, print them, and have [the proctor] hand them out. That way we don't have them ahead of time and then [the proctor] can just ask for our answer for each question on the sheet when [they] come over to each table."

- "Oral assessments have become less valuable. I put less effort into and have gotten less out of them over time as they have become to [sic] repetitive. I like and respect the idea of working with our [team] mates to learn how to work with future colleagues however different types of assessments would be beneficial to 'spicy things up' [sic]."

After 3 years, in 2017, I modified the oral assessments. Rather than structured questions asked by a proctor, the students received an assessment topic that was distributed via a lottery system. The topics aligned with the course objectives and the assessment instructions provide several prompt questions identified at different levels of Bloom's taxonomy (see Appendix B). Assessment day contains a student preparatory phase, where the students have 15 minutes to prepare a logical and cohesive 10-minute maximum presentation for their peers on a topic that they were provided. This modification from the original oral assessments was due to several factors, primarily because the students commented in person, on reflections, or on course evaluations that they would like the opportunity to hear every group's major (higher order) questions on the oral assessments in preparation for the summative exams. Meanwhile, as an instructor, it was hard to grade my original assessment design. The challenge in grading came with time and providing effective feedback. It was a requirement for each student to participate in the oral assessment conversation and be assessed by an unbiased clinical partner or associated faculty member. This required scheduling and training of the assessor to ensure appropriate grading, and a duplicate effort by the instructor to listen to an audio recording of the assessments to determine group participation. A summary of modifications is provided in Table 33-1.

With the updated oral assessment format, grading and scheduling became easier. Student listeners (audience members) were required to grade each presentation (peer to peer) and each student group member was required to self-reflect on team dynamics, participation, and overall performance. Additionally, the course instructor also asked open-ended questions after each presentation to prompt the presenting group to think on the spot and the audience to identify or recognize any inaccuracies of the presentation or to prompt deeper connections (if the presentation had missed key concepts). For successful implementation, this requires the administering faculty members to be able to think quickly and prepare questions based on the presentation that the students created.

Self-reflection rubrics were provided for each student to complete at the end of the assessment day. Students were prompted to reflect specifically on the preparatory phase, including the proposed presentation plan in comparing it to the actual presentation delivered to the class. The rubric provided space for students to reflect on the organization, content, presentation, and participation—the same criteria used in the audience grading and a more structured grading rubric used by the

TABLE 33-1

Comparison Between Structured and Semi-Structured Oral Assessments

	2014	2017

Questions	• Structured exam question bank
	  ◦ Variability between assessment groups
	  ◦ May not have accurately assessed objectives
		• Limited/structured topics
		  ◦ Variability in presentation between groups
		  ◦ Topics specifically related to course/lecture objectives

Taxonomy	• Questions specifically structured based on Bloom's taxonomy—no prompts or follow-up questions from assessor	• Integrated synthesis of Bloom's taxonomy—requires skilled assessor
Grading	• Unbiased proctor/assessor with rubric—requires training of assessor	• Assessment rubrics provided to audience of peers, presentation partners, and instructor—no training necessary

instructor. Often students reflected on the growth and progress made between each oral assessment while also indicating areas for improvement. Sample comments are provided in Table 33-2, demonstrating metacognitive monitoring and evaluating skills (Medina et al., 2017).

In my opinion, the oral assessments work because they incorporate an ideal of RPT, which enhances the novice-to-novice instruction that may loosen, avoid, or break the bottlenecks and barriers for some students. In my courses, I use these oral assessments after a learning module is complete, and the students have to review, summarize, and synthesize the content without knowing which topic they may be assigned within the lab. This differs from traditional RPTs that give students weeks to prepare to teach the class, supported by faculty scrutiny of the lesson plan or ensuring that the student teachers are providing the necessary course objectives. This also reduces the negative impact of students perceiving their colleagues with less confidence than the instructor or being upset that specific content was not addressed by a "professional" because each student presents on the same day with the same opportunity for preparation (e.g., outside of self-learning and studying prior to the assessment) and each student presents as a team of five or six students. Course evaluation comments positively discussed the use of oral assessments:

- "Keeping up with the oral assessments and quizzes helped challenge our thoughts and reinforce everything we learned in smaller sections, to better prepare us for bigger exams and the future."
- "The oral assessments I [thought] were great because they challenged us to think and work as a group. Another reason I like them is because it helped me realize I know a lot more about a subject than I thought."
- "I think the oral assessments really helped me to gain skills in communication with my [team] mates, especially when trying to explain what I thought something was but then also trying to listen to others as what they described something as [sic]."
- "I think the oral assessments were a great way to practice synthesizing information from class with identification in lab to try and answer a question we were not expecting."
- "The oral assessments were a big factor in learning what content I really mastered and what content I still had to study more effectively."

TABLE 33-2

Sample Self-Reflection Comments
Demonstrating Student Metacognition

	SELF-REFLECTION
Organization	• "Next time we could organize the flow of the talk to be even better." • "Of the three oral assessments we have completed so far, I feel that this one was the most organized…. We stayed together and brainstormed as a team really effectively." • "Our group did well with time to make sure we got our main points down with enough time to divide the information amongst ourselves."
Content	• "Compared to other groups I felt like we were lacking, but in terms of our topic and question, I felt as though we covered all of the material necessary." • "Everyone was able to collaborate and add information…so we could present multiple points on each and answer the question to its entirety." • "During the [preparation] phase of the oral assessment, we immediately knew what we were going to talk about and how we were going to set it up. Our whole [team] felt very confident with the material."
Presentation	• "We greatly improved in this oral assessment in presenting." • "We did not rush through this one like we did with others." • "We need to work on identification of things on the donor (cadaver)."
Participation	• "I feel that we could definitely improve in trusting one another when it comes to discussion of content, as some voices were heard and trusted more than others." • "We lack cohesiveness at times because no one wants to admit they are wrong." • "Personally, I felt I did a better job calming my nerves to not only speak clearly but also was able to adequately present the information I had." • "We were confident with this material, and I think it showed in our presentation. We also seemed to slow down and take our time both when preparing and during the actual presentation, which was helpful for everybody involved."
Additional Comments	• "This was our smoothest oral assessment so far, and I think we are growing as a team. We were a little nervous going into the assessment, but after we wrote down all of our thoughts, we all felt pretty confident on our performance." • "I am really proud of our [team]. Our last oral assessment did not go as well as we wanted, and we came back and executed this one really well." • "The questioning was very fair, and I really feel that I got a lot out of this oral presentation. At the end of the day, it feels great knowing our presentation went well, but what feels even better is learning about various structures from fellow classmates I hadn't seen before, or knew the location of."

APPLICATION TO CROSS-DISCIPLINARY CONTEXTS

Anatomy is a foundational science for several health care professionals—teaching and learning anatomy in discipline-specific coursework should address the anatomical need and clinical reasoning for each profession. Anatomy education should be context-specific and should consider how the clinical professional thinks, applies, and reasons through patient care. It is imperative that anatomical educators reflect on how to teach anatomy to achieve competence in clinical practice. Other clinically based disciplines should consider what is foundational anatomy knowledge and determine what would demonstrate anatomical competence within the clinical field.

Content discussed within this chapter is easily modifiable and can be implemented in all clinically related learning environments. Primarily, the instructor determines the direction of assessment, and therefore, a clinical partner would be well suited to join in the administration, proctoring, or creation of the subject areas. Junior faculty may benefit the most from assistance or collaboration with a clinical partner due to inexperience with teaching or with the needs of the health care field.

ADDITIONAL RESOURCES

- This resource is a great overview of all assessment techniques used within anatomy education:
  - Brenner, E., Chirculescu, A. R. M., Reblet, C., & Smith, C. (2015). Assessment in anatomy. *European Journal of Anatomy, 19*(1), 105-124.
- This article compares the pros and cons of oral assessments in a critical review:
  - Ganji, K. K. (2017). Evaluation of reliability in structured viva voce as a formative assessment of dental students. *Journal of Dental Education, 81*(5), 590-596.
- This textbook provides a compilation of perspectives, approaches, and advice for anatomy education:
  - Chan, L. K., & Pawlina, W. (Eds.). (2015). *Teaching anatomy: A practical guide.* Springer International Publishing.

Suggested Readings

- Bentley, B. S., & Hill, R. V. (2009). Objective and subjective assessment of reciprocal peer teaching in medical gross anatomy laboratory. *Anatomical Sciences Education, 2*(4), 143-149.
- Gest, T. R., & Francois, W. (2015). Developing multiple-choice questions for anatomy examinations. In L. K. Chan & W. Pawlina (Eds.), *Teaching anatomy: A practical guide* (pp. 291-297). Springer International Publishing.
- McNulty, J. A., Ensminger, D. C., Hoyt, A. E., Chandrasekhar, A. J., Gruener, G., & Espiritu, B. (2012). Study strategies are associated with performance in basic science courses in the medical curriculum. *Journal of Education and Learning, 1*(1), 1-12.
- Samalia, L., & Stringer, M. D. (2012). A dissecting competition for medical students. *Anatomical Sciences Education, 5*(2), 109-113.
- Urtel, M. G., Bahamonde, R. E., Mikesky, A. E., Udry, E. M., & Vessely, J. S. (2006). On-line quizzing and its effect on student engagement and academic performance. *Journal of Scholarship of Teaching and Learning, 6*(2), 84-92.
- Youdas, J. W., Hoffarth, B. L., Kohlwey, S. R., Kramer, C. M., & Petro, J. L. (2008). Peer teaching among physical therapy students during human gross anatomy: Perceptions of peer teachers and students. *Anatomical Sciences Education, 1*(5), 199-206.
- Youdas, J. W., Krause, D. A., & Hellyer, N. J. (2015). Teaching anatomy to students in a physical therapy education program. In L. K. Chan & W. Pawlina, *Teaching anatomy: A practical guide* (pp. 373-380). Springer International Publishing.

REFERENCES

Angelo, T. A., & Cross, K. P. (1993). The teaching goals inventory. In T. A. Angelo & K. P. Cross (Eds.), *Classroom assessment techniques: A handbook for college teachers* (pp. 13-23). Jossey-Bass Inc.

Bergman, E. M., Sieben, J. M., Smailbegovic, I., Bruin, A. B., Scherpbier, A. J., & van der Vleuten, C. P. (2013). Constructive, collaborative, contextual, and self-directed learning in surface anatomy education. *Anatomical Sciences Education, 6*(2), 114-124.

Brenner, E., Chirculescu, A. R. M., Reblet, C., & Smith, C. (2015). Assessment in anatomy. *European Journal of Anatomy, 19*(1), 105-124.

Choudhury, B., & Freemont, A. (2017). Assessment of anatomical knowledge: Approaches taken by higher education institutions. *Clinical Anatomy, 30,* 290-299.

Fabrizio, P. A. (2013). Oral anatomy laboratory examinations in a physical therapy program. *Anatomical Sciences Education, 6*(4), 271-276.

Ganji, K. K. (2017). Evaluation of reliability in structured viva voce as a formative assessment of dental students. *Journal of Dental Education, 81*(5), 590-596.

Jong, T. D. (2010). Cognitive load theory, educational research, and instructional design: Some food for thought. *Instructional Science, 38,* 105 134.

Kang, S. H., Shin, J.-S., & Hwang, Y.-I. (2012). The use of specially designed tasks to enhance student interest in the cadaver dissection laboratory. *Anatomical Sciences Education, 5*(2), 76-82.

McLauchlan, J. C., Bligh, J., Bradley, P., & Searle, J. (2004). Teaching anatomy without cadavers. *Medical Education, 38*(4), 418-424.

Medina, M. S., Castleberry, A. N., & Persky, A. M. (2017). Strategies for improving learning metacognition in health professional education. *American Journal of Pharmaceutical Education, 81*(4), 1-14.

Meyer, A. J., Innes, S. I., Stomski, N. J., & Armson, A. J. (2016). Student performance on practical gross anatomy examinations is not affected by assessment modality. *Anatomical Sciences Education, 9*(2), 111-120.

Nicol, D. J., & Macfarlane-Dick, D. (2006). Formative assessment and self-regulated learning: A model and seven principles of good feedback practice. *Studies in Higher Education, 31*(2), 199-218.

Pandey, P., & Zimitat, C. (2007). Medical students' learning of anatomy: Memorisation, understanding and visualisation. *Medical Education, 41,* 7-14.

Samarasekera, D. D., Gopalakrishnakone, P., & Gwee, M. C. (2015). Assessing anatomy as a basic medical science. In L. K. Chan & W. Pawlina (Eds.), *Teaching anatomy: A practical guide* (pp. 279-289). Springer International Publishing.

Winkelmann, A. (2007). Anatomical dissection as a teaching method in medical school: A review of the evidence. *Medical Education, 41*(1), 15-22.

APPENDIX A: ORAL ASSESSMENT INSTRUCTIONS 2014

DeSales University—Doctor of Physical Therapy Program

Oral Examination

Goal: Formative assessment; students are responsible for meeting the following two objectives:
1. Discuss the basic anatomical concepts and relationships within the unit
2. Demonstrate concept integration and problem-solving skills

Instructions: At the dissection table, the dissection group is responsible for identifying structures and answering questions posed by the instructors and/or proctors. Questions will vary from simple identification to integration of concepts across courses.

Grading: Pass or fail; all students at the table share the same grade, unless there is an obvious inequity in responses. Once a question is asked, students will have a maximum of 1 minute to discuss their response and then choose a representative to answer the question for the team. This representative should NOT be the same person every time.

Examiner Script Prior to Exam Administration: Your dissection table has been chosen to participate in today's oral examination. This is one of four oral examinations that you will receive during the semester. This is a group assessment; every member of your dissection group will receive the same grade. Each member of your team should contribute to the discussion prior to conveying your group answer. Every member of the team will also be responsible for being the group spokesperson for at least one question. If a group member is not contributing, it is possible for the examiners to make the determination to grade each member individually. Therefore, it is important that you demonstrate your ability to work together to come to one answer.

APPENDIX B: ORAL ASSESSMENT INSTRUCTIONS 2017

DeSales University—Doctor of Physical Therapy Program

Human Anatomy Series: Oral Examinations

Goal: Formative assessment; (1) discuss the basic anatomical concepts and relationships of the unit and (2) assess complex integration and problem-solving skills. Successful completion of this assessment will address DPT Program Learning Outcome #4, specific Psychomotor Course Objectives #1 through #5, and specific Affective Course Objectives #3.

Instructions: At the dissection table, the group is responsible for preparing a 10-minute presentation based on a topic provided by the instructor, which identifies relevant anatomical structures, defines anatomical terminology, and describes muscle attachments, actions, and innervation. Topics will vary from table to table but will be centrally related to the region discussed in class.

Each group will have 15 minutes of preparation time to work and submit a presentation plan— *The use of supplemental resources (e.g., lecture notes, atlases, O/I handout, the internet) is strictly prohibited.*

Grading: Pass (≥ 8/10) or fail (< 8/10); all students at the table share the same grade, unless there is an obvious inequity. It is important that students demonstrate an ability to work together as a team, meaning that each student shares the responsibility of creating a cogent presentation that adequately addresses the topic provided. Each member of the dissection team should provide contributions to the group presentation. This presentation is considered as an instructional opportunity between the dissection tables (as student-teachers) to the other classmates (as student-learners).

Make sure to point out relevant structures on your dissection demonstration.

Recommended Concepts to Discuss: The following suggestions are not exhaustive. The following have been organized by Bloom's taxonomy purely as suggestions for the presentation. Although these suggestions can provide an organized structure for the presentation order, students do NOT have to follow each suggestion as listed.

Knowledge and comprehension:
- Define the relevant anatomical terminology.
- Identify the main musculoskeletal structures involved.
- Explain the relevant articulating structures (joints and osteology).
- Discuss the origin, insertion, innervation, and primary action of the musculoskeletal structures.
- Identify the neurovasculature and discuss the origin, termination, and course of each structure.

Application, analysis, and synthesis:
- Demonstrate the normal movements of the relevant musculoskeletal structures.
- Indicate the structures involved in creating the combined movements (if applicable).
- Differentiate between agonist and antagonist movements (and the structures involved).
- Propose the effective loss seen from an injury to relevant neurovasculature.

34

OBJECTIVE STRUCTURED CLINICAL EXAMINATIONS FOR DEVELOPMENT OF PROFESSIONAL COMPETENCY

Nancy E. Krusen, PhD, OTR/L
and M. Nicole Martino, MS, OTR/L

DESCRIPTION OF TEACHING/LEARNING CONTEXT

Health and social service professions have a demand for learners to master a broad variety of clinical competencies within a short amount of time. Increasingly, complex health care environments require that students arrive at their clinical education placements with a strong set of skills. We developed a set of Objective Structured Clinical Examinations (OSCEs) to supplement existing assessment in an entry-level clinical doctoral program in occupational therapy (Krusen & Rollins, 2019). OSCEs are a series of brief stations in which learners show how to complete tasks representative of professional competencies (Miller, 1990). Our intent was to prepare learners to transition from didactic coursework to fieldwork with minimal difficulty. Across professions, clinical education may be referred to as *fieldwork, practice placement, internship, practica, residency, or affiliation*. We use the term *fieldwork* in this chapter. We also use the terms *student* and *learner* interchangeably.

This chapter describes implementation of OSCEs as evidence-based education. Following brief skills checkouts across multiple courses, we conducted a cumulative OSCE to establish its feasibility to assess readiness for fieldwork. We also report analysis of data from the first OSCE, including lessons learned from our case-based experience.

Friberg, J. C., Visconti, C. F., & Ginsberg, S. M. (Eds.). *Evidence-Based*
Education in the Classroom: Examples From Clinical Disciplines (pp. 313-318).

REVIEW OF LITERATURE

Harden and colleagues (1975) introduced OSCEs to evaluate clinical competency of medical students. They suggested that OSCEs provided more control over variables, allowing for a more objective assessment. This type of examination provided an opportunity to assess specific skills, as well as to assess the abilities of learners to problem solve. Due to its structured nature, OSCEs can be replicated for future examinations. Numerous studies have investigated OSCEs as a supplemental approach for evaluation of clinical skills of learners; however, the vast majority of the work in this area has focused on medical students.

Little research was available regarding the use of OSCEs within the profession of occupational therapy. Edwards and Martin (1989) were the first to design OSCEs for occupational therapy students, using it as a formative and summative tool to assess student performance. It was introduced to first-year occupational therapy students to test their skills with physical assessments of patients (Edwards & Martin, 1989), followed by assessment in the second year after a pediatrics course and an introductory clinical practice course. Edwards and Martin (1989) suggested OSCEs to increase objectivity. OSCEs allowed them to use the same rating checklist, as each student was tested on the same information, increasing reliability. OSCEs were also time efficient, requiring only 2 hours for 20 students rather than 15 hours for a traditional practical examination.

OSCEs are widely used across multiple professions, including dentistry, pharmacy, medicine, midwifery, and nursing. Several qualitative studies (Al Nazzawi, 2017; Awaisu et al., 2010; Khan et al., 2016; Raheel & Naeem, 2013) evaluated student perceptions related to OSCEs, reporting student perception of the OSCE as fair and acceptable while also describing it as mentally difficult and challenging. Researchers also reported student perceptions of learning included stress, time, and a positive learning environment as important factors (Al Nazzawi, 2017; Hemingway et al., 2014; Pierre et al., 2004; Raheel & Naeem, 2013). The most common recommendation across a variety of stakeholders included more flexibility in time limits and more opportunity for preparation for specific competencies (Al Nazzawi, 2017; Awaisu et al., 2010; Jay, 2007; Khan et al., 2016; Raheel & Naeem, 2013). A study by Nasir and colleagues (2014) suggested student perception of OSCEs was a vital indicator for successful implementation because it provided constructive feedback regarding practicality, validity, and reliability.

APPLICATION OF LITERATURE/DATA

After reviewing the literature and attending a conference session with nitty-gritty details about how to implement an OSCE, faculty decided to include the assessment on a trial basis. We scheduled an OSCE as a culminating activity for a competencies course at the end of 2 years of didactic work, just prior to the start of full-time clinical experiences. Faculty believed OSCEs fit within transformative learning theory, the foundation of the curriculum design for the program. Mezirow (1981) posed transformative learning theory as a process through which learners confront challenges as a prompt for reflection and growth.

A team of 12 faculty and community practitioners brainstormed a broad variety of potential OSCE scenarios, using a Decoding the Disciplines approach to identify circumstances in which students or novice practitioners often get stuck (Middendorf & Shopkow, 2018). Scenarios crossed a variety of age ranges, practice settings, diagnoses, and events. A small faculty team narrowed potential scenarios from 30 to 24, matching OSCE items to categories within a profession-specific fieldwork performance evaluation document. Each OSCE scenario focused on a narrow competency, accompanied by a practitioner-generated checklist of specific skills. The team identified some skills as *mandatory* to pass and some as *nice to have*, by consensus. The team used a blueprint or grid to map OSCE characteristics with administrative requirements, such as a computer or equipment (Table 34-1).

TABLE 34-1

Sample of Organizational Blueprint

STATION	AREA OF PRACTICE	SETTING	CLIENT AGE	SCENARIO DESCRIPTION (PERFORMANCE SKILL #)	BLOOM'S DOMAIN	ADMIN
E	Professional	Any	Adult	Accept negative feedback from supervisor (#38 responds constructively to feedback)	Affective, organization	Rater
K	Communication	School	Child	Record directions for occupational therapy assistant intervention with child (#32 clearly and effectively communicates verbally and nonverbally)	Cognitive, applying	Recorder/ computer

The pilot OSCE included 20 stations, 17 scenarios, and 3 rest stations interspersed equally throughout the rotation. We used 11 faculty/community practitioners to serve as raters or simulated patients during the OSCE. The team designed individual schedules for each of the 40 learners, including required learning accommodations. Twenty learners began OSCE simultaneously at different stations. Each scenario allowed 5 minutes for task completion followed by 1 minute for travel to the next station. Some OSCE stations were connected in sets. Learners completed one task at the first station, followed by a related task at the next station. Some OSCE stations had simulated patients, and some stations were unattended with learners responding to video, digital, or paper data.

OSCE stations included a mix of cognitive, affective, and psychomotor skills, all involving application to daily practice. A few examples included:

- Identify the level of evidence (according to a given standard) for each of the three article abstracts
- Based on the abstracts in the previous station, recommend an intervention approach for a family, with your rationale
- Engage in a clear, explicit conversation identifying boundaries with a patient who has fallen in love with you
- Complete a cognitive assessment based on a patient interaction
- Record an audio transfer-of-service message to an occupational therapy assistant

The OSCE team collected data as part of regular course evaluation as a scholarship of teaching and learning study for course improvement. Data included individual checklist scores for each station. Students also received an overall rating or Global Rating Scale at each attended station (Queen's University Belfast, 2012). We also collected data about learners' perceptions of OSCEs via ratings of each station and a Qualtrics survey with Likert-type items and open-ended items.

Quantitative analysis examined the relationship of each station to the parent category. Qualitative analysis revealed four dimensions of learning: temporal, real world, being open to the process, and bottlenecks (Krusen & Martino, 2020).

Temporal concerns included feeling a press for time during rotations, balanced by an opportunity to move on. While thinking on the spot was daunting, there was no time to obsess about the scenario just completed; each new task brought a fresh start. Learners perceived the variety of issues to be reflective of the real world, with a demand to improvise for the unexpected. Scenarios required thinking, feeling, and doing to meet expectations across many contexts.

Most, but not all, students were open to the process of learning. As with any general population, some people experienced greater distress than eustress. Learners described anxiety about the unexpected, individual scenarios, and not knowing what to study ahead of time. Heightened emotions led to difficulty paying attention, making connections to information learned during the previous 2 years, and applying practical solutions to everyday dilemmas. Students described having blind spots and a difficult time reading and attending to the content.

Faculty used data from the OSCE to modify their respective course assignments. This supported clearer connections between student learning objectives and assignments. For example, many learners reported difficulty reading article abstracts (Station A) and rating the level of evidence according to the gold-standard Oxford scale. Oxford scale level of evidence standards were included and available with scenario materials. Reported difficulties included reading "so much material" and recall of the foundational information. For this example of program evaluation, the faculty responsible for teaching evidence-based practice courses modified assignments to include reading in a compressed time frame, reading to identify levels of evidence, and reading to make treatment recommendations. Faculty clarified with students the value of repeating a task to support their development from novice to expert. Though all learners passed the pilot OSCE, we were prepared to run a make-up session for remediation. The team tentatively scheduled raters and new scenarios in reserve.

APPLICATION TO CROSS-DISCIPLINARY CONTEXTS

We implemented OSCEs for discipline-specific and general competencies. Discipline-specific scenarios required learners to demonstrate specialized knowledge and skills for the profession of occupational therapy. General competencies, universal to health and social service professions, included written and oral communication, evidence-based inquiry, critical thinking, health/information literacy, and ethical reasoning. OSCEs could also target interprofessional skills, such as teamwork, cultural agility, safety, and professional growth. While we connected OSCEs to Bloom's taxonomy, we believe other perspectives on assessment to be valuable and merit further inquiry (Anderson & Krathwohl, 2001). Fink's (2013) taxonomy of significant learning could be helpful to make explicit additional aims for the OSCE (e.g., integrating, caring, learning how to learn). Assessing noncognitive variables (e.g., creativity, persistence, motivation, ability to overcome adversity) might frame success in a different way (Sedlacek, 2017).

OSCEs may be applied to assessment within a module, course, or program. Some health professions programs currently use OSCEs as a cumulative assessment of student competency that is mandatory for graduation. While our team originally intended OSCEs to be summative, learners used the experience as formative. Learners identified strengths, describing pride in their performance. They also identified areas for growth, generating goals for improvement before moving on to clinical placements. OSCEs have a place as both types of assessment. Summative assessment may serve as building blocks for larger scale programmatic purposes. OSCE competencies may connect student learning objectives to course goals to program evaluation, creating a trail of breadcrumbs to meet accreditation standards. Formative assessment supports confidence, realistic self-appraisal, and goal setting, all valuable for professional development.

We learned some lessons in the case of using OSCEs. We are happy to share what we believe are universal lessons across clinical professions. Educators need to be prepared to adapt, to model the flexibility learners may develop for implementation in daily practice. Life is filled with improvisation. We created contingency plans for scenarios and distressed participants. We had backup video and paper cases, we eliminated scoring for a station when technology failed, and we scheduled bio-breaks. We provided all participants with a mechanism to reach the OSCE stage manager in case of emergency. We reduced the number of OSCE stations to 12 for the next cohort for choreographic relief to room and rater scheduling.

It was important to involve community practitioners with insight into the way things happen on a daily basis. The process of decoding the discipline (Middendorf & Shopkow, 2017) is relevant across professions. Practitioners helped identify places in fieldwork where learners get stuck along the path from novice to expert, referred to as *bottlenecks*. Learners also identified bottlenecks from their OSCE experience. Each stakeholder group offered perspectives different from faculty that were equally valuable in learning.

While we believe OSCEs to be an effective approach in assessing competence prior to fieldwork, we also see the need for future scholarship of teaching and learning study to examine education using Kirkpatrick-based outcome levels (Milota et al., 2019). Examining change in learner behavior within other contexts, change in delivery of services or care, and/or direct benefit to clients as a result of OSCEs would close the loop in establishing powerful evidence-based education.

ADDITIONAL RESOURCES

Several resources provided useful information in implementing OSCEs:

- Queen's University Belfast has an extensive website for OSCE examiner training. The site includes background information, formats, setting standards, global scores, and common dilemmas:
  - https://www.med.qub.ac.uk/osce/background_Scores.html
- The Decoding the Disciplines website lays out a step-by-step process to help students move from novice to expert ways of thinking and practicing. The process of decoding is logical and practical:
  - http://decodingthedisciplines.org/
- The following article by Harden and colleagues (1975) is the original work proposing OSCEs to assess clinical competence. They proposed control of complexity; assessment of knowledge, skill, and attitudes; feedback for students; and program evaluation:
  - Harden, R. M., Stevenson, M., Downie, W. W., & Wilson, G. M. (1975). Assessment of clinical competence using objective structured examination. *British Medical Journal, 1*(5955), 447-451. https://doi.org/10.1136/bmj.1.5955.447
- The Medical Council of Canada has a website for OSCE candidate orientation. The site contains history, definitions, what to expect, and tips for success:
  - https://mcc.ca/examinations/osce-orientation/

REFERENCES

Al Nazzawi, A. A. (2017). Dental students' perception of the objective structured clinical examination (OSCE): The Taibah University experience, Almadinah Almunawwarah, KSA. *Journal of Taibah University Medical Sciences, 13*(1), 64-69. https://doi.org/10.1016/j.jtumed.2017.09.002

Anderson, L. W., & Krathwohl, D. R. (2001). *A taxonomy for teaching, learning, and assessing: A revision of Bloom's taxonomy of educational objectives*. Longman.

Awaisu, A., Abd Rahman, N., Nik Mohamed, M., Bux Rahman Bux, S., & Mohamed Nazar, N. (2010). Malaysian pharmacy students' assessment of an objective structured clinical examination (OSCE). *American Journal of Pharmaceutical Education, 74*(2), 34. https://doi.org/10.5688/aj740234

Edwards, M., & Martin, A. (1989). Objective structured clinical examination as a method of occupational therapy student evaluation. *Canadian Journal of Occupational Therapy, 6*(3), 128-131. https://doi.org/10.1177/000841748905600306

Fink, L. (2013). *Creating significant learning experiences: An integrated approach to designing college courses* (Revised and updated ed.). Jossey-Bass Inc.

Harden, R., Stevenson, M., Downie, W., & Wilson, G. (1975). Assessment of clinical competence using objective structured examination. *British Medical Journal, 1*(5955), 447-451. https://doi.org/10.1136/bmj.1.5955.447

Hemingway, S., Stephenson, J., Roberts, B., & McCann, T. (2014). Mental health and learning disability nursing students' perceptions of the usefulness of the objective structured clinical examination to assess their competence in medicine administration. *International Journal of Mental Health Nursing, 23*(4), 364-373. https://doi.org/10.1111/inm.12051

Jay, A. (2007). Students' perceptions of the OSCE: A valid assessment tool? *British Journal of Midwifery, 15*(1), 32-37. https://doi.org/10.1016/j.jtumed.2017.09.002

Khan, A., Ayub, M., & Shah, Z. (2016). An audit of the medical students' perceptions regarding objective structured clinical examination. *Education Research International, 2016,* 1-4. https://doi.org/10.1155/2016/4806398

Krusen, N., & Martino, M. N. (2020). Occupational therapy students' perceptions of an OSCE: A qualitative descriptive analysis. *Journal of Occupational Therapy Education, 4*(1).

Krusen, N. E., & Rollins, D. (2019). Design of an OSCE to assess clinical competence of occupational therapy students. *Journal of Occupational Therapy Education, 3*(1). https://encompass.eku.edu/jote/vol3/iss1/11

Mezirow, J. (1981). A critical theory of adult learning and education. *Adult Education Quarterly, 32,* 3-24. https://doi.org/10.1177/074171368103200101

Middendorf, J., & Shopkow, L. (2018). *Overcoming student learning bottlenecks.* Stylus.

Miller, G. E. (1990). The assessment of clinical skills/competence/performance. *Academic Medicine, 65*(9), 63-37.

Milota, M. M., van Thiel, G. J. M. W., & van Delden, J. J. M. (2019). Narrative medicine as a medical education tool: A systematic review. *Medical Teacher, 41*(7), 802-810. https://doi.org/10.1080/0142159X.2019.1584274

Nasir, A. A., Yusuf, A. S., Abdur-Rahman, L. O., Babalola, O. M., Adeyeye, A. A., Popoola, A. A., & Adeniran, J. O. (2014). Medical students' perception of objective structured clinical examination: A feedback for process improvement. *Journal of Surgical Education, 71*(5), 701-706. http://dx.doi.org/10.1016/j.jsurg.2014.02.010

Pierre, R., Wierenga, A., Barton, M., Branday, J., & Christie, C. (2004). Student evaluation of an OSCE in paediatrics at the University of the West Indies, Jamaica. *BMC Medical Education, 4,* 22-28. https://doi.org/10.1186/1472-6920-4-22

Queen's University Belfast. (2012). OSCE examiner training and development. https://www.med.qub.ac.uk/osce/background_Scores.html

Raheel, H., & Naeem, N. (2013). Assessing the objective structured clinical examination: Saudi family medicine undergraduate medical students' perceptions of the tool. *Journal of the Pakistan Medical Association, 63*(10), 1281-1284.

Sedlacek, W. (2017). *Measuring noncognitive variables: Improving admissions, success, and retention for underrepresented students.* Stylus.

35

Developing Culturally Responsive Practitioners Through an International Education Experience

Colleen F. Visconti, PhD, CCC-SLP
and K. Chisomo Selemani, MA, CCC-SLP

Description of Teaching/Learning Context

We live in an increasingly global society. The U.S. Census Bureau projects that by 2044, more than half the population will consist of individuals from what are currently recognized as under-represented or minority groups (Colby & Ortman, 2014). As such, it is imperative to train future and current health care professionals with an understanding of culturally responsive practices. In academic programs, international education can be an excellent mechanism by which to engage in multicultural and international considerations. However, when doing so, it is important to operate within best practices in both the specific health care field and international education. Furthermore, where service learning is considered, best practices in community engagement must also be implemented.

The Speech-Language Pathology (SLP) program at Baldwin Wallace University has intentionally incorporated a service-oriented study abroad program within the graduate program. In this program, first-year SLP graduate students travel with faculty to Zambia, Africa, a country with cultures and systems that are perceived to be very different from the United States. Opportunities to engage with community partners in Zambia are available year-round. The students and faculty involved with the SLP 2B in Zambia program have the opportunity to travel to meet those individuals and to see one of the fastest developing African nations. This experience provides the graduate SLP students with a unique opportunity to develop necessary skills for clinical practice. The SLP 2B in Zambia program ensures that speech-language pathology students go beyond the classroom and have a real-world experience, which challenges them in ways a traditional classroom could not.

Friberg, J. C., Visconti, C. F., & Ginsberg, S. M. (Eds.). *Evidence-Based Education in the Classroom: Examples From Clinical Disciplines* (pp. 319-326).

Utilizing a bidirectional approach, students and faculty work together with professionals in Zambia, with all groups sharing their expertise in order to begin to work with individuals with communication disabilities and their families.

During the travel component of the program, the students participate in various service and educational exchange activities, such as collaboration with health care professionals and educators within various community partnerships, parent/patient education, dynamic assessment, and criterion-referenced screenings, among other activities. The sites include educational settings, clinic-centered health care facilities, and community-based health care sites. In addition to the time spent with community partners during service and educational exchange activities, faculty and students host an invited guest—community partners from a variety of different industries (e.g., fashion, business, hospitality, health care)— almost every night. At the end of the night, the students and faculty engage in a time of guided reflection. While much of the focus of this program has been the academic, service, and educational exchange components, there is also a strong focus on cultural exchange. Some of the student's cultural experiences come through the service and educational exchange days. The rest of the cultural experiences come in the form of other opportunities, such as the dinnertime sessions, trips to local markets, galleries, boutiques, and a longer 2-day trip to Livingstone, Zambia. In Livingstone, the students visit Victoria Falls, go on a game drive (i.e., safari), and visit other places of interest. Thus, students are given the opportunity to explore two of Zambia's major cities.

The program has elements of all three fields: communication sciences and disorders (CSD), international education, and community engagement. As such, the faculty have worked to engage in best practices within these different but converging fields. The SLP 2B in Zambia program is a part of the developing Baldwin Wallace University in Zambia initiative, which was honored by two of the highest regarded institutions for international education in 2018. The Baldwin Wallace University in Zambia program was the recipient of the Institute of International Education's 2018 Andrew Heiskell Award, Honorable Mention for Innovation in International Education, and 2018 NAFSA: Association of International Educators' Senator Paul Simon Spotlight Award.

REVIEW OF LITERATURE

According to a recent study conducted by the Institute of International Education, going to places that students consider to be "different" from what is familiar yields increased skills in problem solving and other transferable or "soft" skills (Stipek et al., 2018). These skills—problem solving, tolerance with ambiguity, empathy, among others—are the intangible but necessary qualities of successful health care providers.

Best practices in community engagement encourages reciprocity in relationships, regular contact and collaboration, reflection, and humility (Principles of Ethical and Effective Service, n.d.). At the inception of the SLP 2B in Zambia program, three CSD faculty members conducted two exploratory trips (May 2015 and May 2016), which had dedicated time for asking questions regarding expectations for exchange activities from community partners in Zambia. In May 2018, an advisory board that consisted of community partners from various industries was formally instituted. This advisory board structure acts as a formal channel by which the university can receive feedback from the community. The information gathered from the advisory board has been used to change existing elements of the program, and it has ensured that successful pieces of the program continue. The relationships with community partners and development of an advisory board are fundamental and generalizable components of this program. These interactions have informed the structure of the SLP 2B in Zambia service-oriented study abroad program.

TABLE 35-1

Overview of General Logistics of the Speech-Language Pathology 2B in Zambia Program

YEAR	COURSE CREDIT	PREDEPARTURE MEETINGS	# OF FACULTY	# OF STUDENTS	# OF DAYS ON TRIP	# OF SERVICE DAYS
2017	0	45 minutes/week for 11 weeks	4*	18	15	6
2018	1	50 minutes/week for 15 weeks	4	21	13	5
2019	1	50 minutes/week for 15 weeks	3	19	15	8

Note: *Two CSD faculty and one computer science faculty member who had all been on an exploratory trip, and one administrator with a background in education who had not been on an exploratory trip.

ORIGINAL DATA

The student preparation and the trip itself has changed over the past 3 years (Table 35-1). Initially, students were required to attend 11 predeparture meetings with no class credit associated with predeparture or the study abroad experience. Based on student, faculty, and community partner feedback, predeparture and in-country activities were assigned course credit through the officially developed elective course, CSD 563—SLP 2B in Zambia, implemented prior to the 2018 program. Student feedback after the 2017 program suggested that this course should have a greater focus on cultural aspects, in addition to the previously incorporated discussions of community engagement and reflective practices. The course now covers the following topics over the 15-week spring semester: reflective practices, cultural aspects (general classifications of culture, identity and culture, and elements of Zambian culture), group dynamics, the impact of cultural aspects on interpersonal communication, community engagement, the development of culturally appropriate materials for screening and treatment, and trip logistics.

In an effort to investigate the impact of the SLP 2B in Zambia study abroad program on student outcomes related to cultural competence, qualitative research was conducted. This research reviewed students' perceptions of their experiences through written reflections.

Students completed three written reflections: two during the predeparture course and one within 4 weeks of returning from the trip. In addition, students also completed an anonymous survey upon their return regarding the trip, which was sent out by the Office of Explorations and Study Abroad.

In order to determine if the SLP 2B in Zambia program is effectively developing culturally responsive practitioners, a qualitative research study was conducted. Subsequently, institutional review board approval was obtained, and the authors analyzed the final reflective essays for each cohort of students that has participated in this program (i.e., 2017 to 2019). The American Speech-Language-Hearing Association (n.d., para. 1) states that "cultural competence involves understanding and appropriately responding to the unique combination of cultural variables and the full range of dimensions of diversity that the professional and client/patient/family bring to interactions." Standard 3.1.1B of the Council on Academic Accreditation in Audiology and Speech-Language

TABLE 35-2

Cultural Responsiveness for Each Cohort by Student Learning Outcome

COHORT	SLO #1: SELF m (SD)	SLO #2: INDIVIDUALS SERVED m (SD)	SLO #3: INDIVIDUAL AND FAMILY m (SD)	SLO #4: INDIVIDUAL AND RELATED SERVICES m (SD)
2017	2.44 (0.511)	1.67 (0.970)	1.22 (0.732)	1.61 (0.608)
2018	2.57 (0.507)	2.38 (0.509)	2.19 (0.814)	2.00 (0.775)
2019	3.00 (0.000)	2.63 (0.496)	2.53 (0.513)	2.74 (0.562

M = mean; SD = standard deviation; SLO = student learning outcome.

Pathology (CAA) identifies four components of cultural competency within the field (CAA, 2020). Faculty in the CSD program utilized the CAA standards to develop four learning outcome statements (see Appendix A). The final reflective essay for each student was evaluated to determine the impact of the service-oriented study abroad experience on meeting the cultural responsiveness learning outcomes (see Appendix B).

Cultural responsiveness performance for each cohort is shown in Table 35-2. The sophistication of each cohort's performance has improved as changes have been made to the service-oriented study abroad program. Analysis of variance by cohort showed significant differences ($p = .000$) for all variables. Therefore, as the program added a specific course that more intentionally taught students about culture in preparation for their time abroad, the students performed better. Then, based on results from a focus group with community partners in Zambia who recommended that the number of service days be increased, revisions were again made to the program. This led to improvements in the learning outcomes, as exhibited by reflections that contained content that demonstrated the student's ability to not only compare and differentiate, but to also integrate or synthesize the cultural experience with regards to self, the individual served, the individual and family, and the individual and related services.

APPLICATION OF LITERATURE/DATA

Students participating in the SLP 2B in Zambia program complete pre- and post-surveys distributed by the study abroad office, along with several written reflections before, during, and after the study abroad experience. In addition, focus group data were collected in Zambia with the advisory board that consisted of community partners and stakeholders who work in various industries but are based in Zambia, primarily in Lusaka. The advisory board members provided the program with the Zambian perspective regarding the bidirectional relationship. The information obtained has informed the development of the overall Baldwin Wallace University in Zambia initiatives, including exploratory trips and current undergraduate and graduate study abroad programs.

Based on the post-survey data, student reflections, and feedback from our community partners in Zambia, the program will continue to use the predeparture course and the increased number of service days as one of the pedagogical approaches to assisting students in becoming culturally responsive practitioners. In addition, all students, whether they choose to travel to Zambia or not, will be required to enroll in the course in order to provide all students with specific knowledge about reflective practices, cultural aspects (general classifications of culture, identity and culture, and elements of Zambian culture), group dynamics, the impact of cultural aspects on interpersonal communication, community engagement, and the development of culturally appropriate materials for screening and treatment.

APPLICATION TO CROSS-DISCIPLINARY CONTEXTS

The framework used in the SLP 2B in Zambia program can be easily replicated in other courses. As part of the greater Baldwin Wallace University in Zambia initiative, other programs on campus have either implemented or considered implementing this approach. Two faculty from the departments of film studies and theater at Baldwin Wallace University modeled their Words in Action Project 2019 after the SLP 2B in Zambia course, and led their inaugural program in Spring 2019. Per student evaluations and informal feedback from community partners, this program was quite successful. Additionally, other faculty from other departments in the College of Education and Health Sciences have completed an exploratory trip and are considering developing programs with a similar framework. These considerations are of vital importance for those seeking to participate in international education and service-oriented activities abroad. In fact, the notion of cultural competence in global interactions is fairly well understood. As stated by Hyter and colleagues (2017) "global competencies have been discussed in the literature of various disciplines, including business, education, health care, global studies, and nursing" (p. 11). The presence of these discussions suggests the need for resources in international education across disciplines. This framework acts as an evidence-based resource that considers best practices in community or civic engagement and international education.

Often, it is not just the actions or the events related to an educational experience that make it successful, it is the mindset, attitudes, or affective considerations underlying that educational experience. This is exceptionally imperative when considering international education and service learning. In this case, students from Baldwin Wallace University are engaging in activities in Zambia. This is an example of people from a minority world country engaging in activities with people from a majority world country. One must bear in mind that countries like the United States exist as part of the minority of the world, and countries like Zambia exist as part of the majority of the world. In such interactions, a high degree of care and consideration must occur. Therefore, it is important for students and faculty to examine their existing theoretical and epistemological frameworks as it pertains to parts of the world that are perceived to be quite different. The process of reflection, verbal or written, is quite useful in examination of one's existing epistemologies, or ways of knowing. The SLP 2B in Zambia course requires students and faculty to engage in regular reflective exercises where participants are posed questions such as, "How can we enter a community with an asset-based mindset?"; "In what ways is this community similar?"; or "Let's challenge our existing perception of wealth to think beyond socioeconomic status, in what other ways can a community be wealthy?" Taking time to reflect before, during, and after travel is imperative and easily generalizable to any field. Furthermore, reflective practice encourages the possibility of high-quality international interactions regardless of discipline.

ADDITIONAL RESOURCES

- Body, R., & McAllistair, L. (2009). *Ethics in speech language pathology.* Wiley-Blackwell.
- Carastathis, A. (2016). *Intersectionality: Origins, contestations, horizons.* University of Nebraska Press.
- Comhlámh. (2015). Irish code of good practice for volunteer sending agencies. https://comhlamh.org/code-of-good-practice/

- Crenshaw, K. (2005). Mapping the margins: Intersectionality, identity politics, and violence against women of color. In R. K. Bergen, J. L. Edleson, & C. M. Renzetti (Eds.), *Violence against women: Classic paper* (pp. 282-313). Pearson Education.
- Geller, E., & Foley, G. (2009). Broadening the "ports of entry" for speech-language pathologists: A relational and reflective model for clinical supervision. *American Journal of Speech-Language Pathology, 18*, 22-41.
- Hyter, Y. D., & Sales-Provance, M. B. (2019). *Culturally responsive practices in speech, language and hearing sciences.* Plural Publishing.
- Pickering, M., & McAllister, L. (2000). A conceptual framework for linking and guiding domestic cross-cultural and international practice in speech-language pathology. *Advances in Speech Language Pathology, 2*(2), 93-106.

REFERENCES

American Speech-Language-Hearing Association. (n.d.). Cultural competency. (Practice Portal). https://www.asha.org/PRPSpecificTopic.aspx?folderid=8589935230&section=Overview

Colby, S. L., & Ortman, J. M. (2014). Projections of the size and composition of the U.S. population: 2014 to 2060, current population reports, P25-1143, U.S. Census Bureau, Washington, DC. https://www.census.gov/content/dam/Census/library/publications/2015/demo/p25-1143.pdf

Council on Academic Accreditation in Audiology and Speech-Language Pathology. (2020). *Standards for accreditation of graduate education programs in audiology and speech-language pathology (2017).* https://caa.asha.org/wp-content/uploads/Accreditation-Standards-for-Graduate-Programs.pdf

Hyter, Y. D., Roman, T. R., Staley, B., & McPherson, B. (2017). Competencies for effective global engagement: A proposal for communication sciences and disorders. *Perspectives of ASHA Special Interest Group, SIG 17, 2*(1), 9-19.

Principles of Ethical and Effective Service. (n.d.). Stanford Haas Center for Public Service. https://haas.stanford.edu/about/our-approach/principles-ethical-and-effective-service

Stipek, A., Loveland, E., Morris, C., Calvert, L., Johannes, W., & Childs, S. (2018). Study abroad matters: Linking higher education to the contemporary workplace through international experience. *Global Education Research Reports.* https://www.iie.org/en/Research-and-Insights/Publications/Study-Abroad-Matters

APPENDIX A: CULTURAL RESPONSIVENESS LEARNING OUTCOME STATEMENTS

1. The speech-language pathology graduate students will articulate the impact of their own set of cultural and linguistic variables (e.g., age, ethnicity, linguistic background, national origin, race, religion, gender, sexual orientation) on the delivery of effective services for individuals with disabling communication impairments.

2. The speech-language pathology graduate students will compare and contrast the impact of the cultural and linguistic variables (e.g., age, ethnicity, linguistic background, national origin, race, religion, gender, sexual orientation) of the individuals with disabling communication impairments on the delivery of effective services.

3. The speech-language pathology graduate students will investigate the interaction of cultural and linguistic variables between the caregivers and the individuals with disabling communication impairments in order to maximize service delivery.

4. The speech-language pathology graduate students will examine the characteristics (e.g., age, demographics, cultural and linguistic diversity, educational history and status, medical history and status, cognitive status, physical and sensory abilities) of the individuals with disabling communication impairment and articulate how these characteristics impact the clinical services provided.

Appendix B: Rating Overall Quality of Cultural Responsiveness for Each Learning Outcome

VALUE	IDENTIFIER	DESCRIPTION
0	No evidence	The reflection provides no evidence regarding the learning outcome.
1	Identify or recognize	The reflection lists, identifies, and recognizes the cultural aspect of the learning outcome but does not move beyond that.
2	Compare or differentiate	The reflection includes information that compares, contrasts, or makes statements that differentiate between the cultural aspects of the learning outcome.
3	Integrate or synthesize	The reflection includes information that shows a depth of understanding of the cultural aspect through the discussion of similarities, differences, or application of information in making informed decisions.

FINANCIAL DISCLOSURES

Dr. Hilary Applequist has no financial proprietary interest in the materials presented herein.

Dr. Cassandra Barragan has no financial proprietary interest in the materials presented herein.

Dr. Dana Battaglia has no financial or proprietary interest in the materials presented herein.

Dr. Ann R. Beck has no financial or proprietary interest in the materials presented herein.

Dr. Carole Bennett has no financial or proprietary interest in the materials presented herein.

Dr. Sarah Bolander has no financial or proprietary interest in the materials presented herein.

Dr. Chelsey M. Bahlmann Bollinger has no financial or proprietary interest in the materials presented herein.

Dr. Elizabeth Bourne received partial funding from a University of Sydney DVC Strategic Education small grant that was awarded in December 2018.

Dr. Tim Brackenbury has received financial support through the M. Neil Browne Professorship at Bowling Green State University.

Dr. Judi Brooks has no financial or proprietary interest in the materials presented herein.

Dr. Melissa A. Carroll has no financial or proprietary interest in the materials presented herein.

Dr. Susan L. Caulfield has no financial or proprietary interest in the materials presented herein.

Dr. Darlene Chalmers has no financial or proprietary interest in the materials presented herein.

Dr. Andrea Coppola has no financial or proprietary interest in the materials presented herein.

Dr. Julie L. Cox is an employee at Western Illinois University where the course was taught using the description provided in the chapter.

Dr. Mary Culshaw has no financial or proprietary interest in the materials presented herein.

Dr. Kathy Doody has no financial or proprietary interest in the materials presented herein.

Amy Egli has no financial or proprietary interest in the materials presented herein.

Krystina Eymann has no financial proprietary interest in the materials presented herein.

Dr. Karen A. Fallon has no financial or proprietary interest in the materials presented herein.

Diane Fenske has no financial or proprietary interest in the materials presented herein.

Dr. Jennifer C. Friberg is employed in a position at Illinois State University that focuses on the scholarship of teaching and learning. She receives royalties from Plural Publishing and Indiana University Press for other texts focused on evidence-informed teaching and learning.

Dr. Katrina Fulcher-Rood has no financial or proprietary interest in the materials presented herein.

Dr. April Garrity has no financial or proprietary interest in the materials presented herein.

Dr. Sarah M. Ginsberg has no financial or proprietary interest in the materials presented herein.

Dr. Jennine M. Harvey-Northrop is employed by Illinois State University. She would like to acknowledge funding for this work via two teaching and learning innovation grants from the Center for Teaching and Learning at Illinois State University.

Amber Herrick has no financial or proprietary interest in the materials presented herein.

Dr. Leslie A. Hoffman has no financial or proprietary interest in the materials presented herein.

Dr. Polly R. Husmann has no financial or proprietary interest in the materials presented herein.

Dr. Keiko Ishikawa has no financial or proprietary interest in the materials presented herein.

Dr. Casey Keck has no financial or proprietary interest in the materials presented herein.

Dr. Louise C. Keegan has no financial or proprietary interest in the materials presented herein.

Dr. Marla Kniewel has no financial proprietary interest in the materials presented herein.

Dr. Nancy E. Krusen has no financial proprietary interest in the materials presented herein.

Dr. Eric Kyle has no financial proprietary interest in the materials presented herein.

Dr. Carey Leckie has no financial or proprietary interest in the materials presented herein.

Dr. Mary-Jon Ludy's work in this chapter was supported by an Ohio Department of Higher Education grant from 2016 to 2018.

M. Nicole Martino has no financial or proprietary interest in the materials presented herein.

Dr. Lydia McBurrows has no financial or proprietary interest in the materials presented herein.

Dr. Jean McCaffery has no financial or proprietary interest in the materials presented herein.

Lauren H. Mead has no financial or proprietary interest in the materials presented herein.

Dr. Andi Beth Mincer has no financial or proprietary interest in the materials presented herein.

Irene Mok received partial funding from a University of Sydney DVC Strategic Education small grant that was awarded in December 2018.

Dr. Joy Myers has no financial or proprietary interest in the materials presented herein.

Margaret Nicholson received partial funding from a University of Sydney DVC Strategic Education small grant that was awarded in December 2018.

Dr. Gillian Nisbet received partial funding from a University of Sydney DVC Strategic Education small grant that was awarded in December 2018.

Dr. Brent Oliver has no financial or proprietary interest in the materials presented herein.

Dr. Christina Y. Pelatti receives a salary from Towson University where the research was conducted.

Dr. D. Mark Ragg has no financial or proprietary interest in the materials presented herein.

Amanda Reddington has no financial or proprietary interest in the materials presented herein.

Haleigh M. Ruebush has no financial or proprietary interest in the materials presented herein.

Dr. Ken Saldanha has no financial or proprietary interest in the materials presented herein.

Dr. Eric J. Sanders has no financial or proprietary interest in the materials presented herein.

Dr. Allison Sauerwein has no financial or proprietary interest in the materials presented herein.

Dr. Amanda G. Sawyer has no financial or proprietary interest in the materials presented herein.

Dr. Jean Sawyer has no financial or proprietary interest in the materials presented herein.

Dr. Audra F. Schaefer has no financial or proprietary interest in the materials presented herein.

Heather Schmuck has no financial or proprietary interest in the materials presented herein.

Dr. Pamela Schuetze has no financial or proprietary interest in the materials presented herein.

Dr. Scott Seeman has no financial or proprietary interest in the material presented herein.

K. Chisomo Selemani has no financial or proprietary interest in the material presented herein.

Dr. Maryam S. Sharifian has no financial or proprietary interest in the materials presented herein.

Dr. Amanda B. Silberer has no financial or proprietary interest in the material presented herein.

Dr. Lisa R. Singleterry has no financial or proprietary interest in the material presented herein.

Heidi Verticchio has no financial or proprietary interest in the material presented herein.

Dr. Lisa A. Vinney's work reported on in Chapter 19 was supported by two teaching and learning innovation grants from Illinois State University.

Dr. Colleen F. Visconti has no financial or proprietary interest in the material presented herein.

Dr. Kaitlyn P. Wilson receives a salary from Towson University where the research was conducted.

Dr. Stephanie P. Wladkowski has no financial or proprietary interest in the material presented herein.

Dr. Andrea Gossett Zakrajsek has no financial or proprietary interest in the material presented herein.

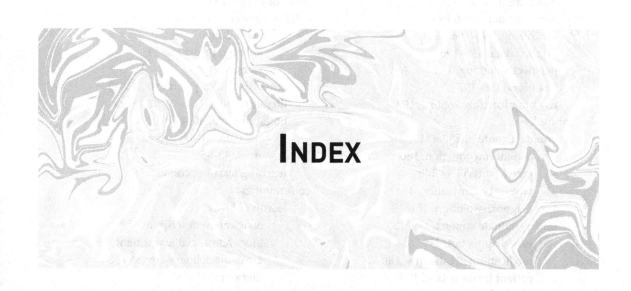

INDEX

Printed in the United States
by Baker & Taylor Publisher Services

Printed in the United States
by Baker & Taylor Publisher Services